Surgical Neuropathology
of Focal Epilepsies:
Textbook and Atlas

This book has been published with the support of the Cleveland Clinic.

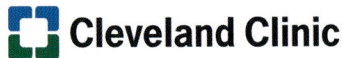

ISBN : 978-2-7420-1399-9

Published by
Éditions John Libbey Eurotext
127, avenue de la République,
92120 Montrouge, France.
Tél. : 01.46.73.06.60
Fax : 01.40.84.09.99
e-mail : contact@jle.com
Site Internet : http://www.jle.com

John Libbey Eurotext
34 Anyard Road, Cobham
Surrey KT11 2LA
United Kingdom

© 2015, John Libbey Eurotext. All rights reserved.

Unauthorized duplication contravenes applicable laws.
It is prohibited to reproduce this work or any part of it without authorisation of the publisher or of the Centre Français d'Exploitation du Droit de Copie (CFC), 20, rue des Grands-Augustins, 75006 Paris.

Surgical Neuropathology of Focal Epilepsies: Textbook and Atlas

Ingmar Blümcke
Harvey B. Sarnat
Roland Coras

■ SURGICAL NEUROPATHOLOGY OF FOCAL
EPILEPSIES: TEXTBOOK AND ATLAS

CONTENTS

Preface | IX

Chapter 1: Introduction
Ingmar Blümcke, Harvey B. Sarnat | 1

Chapter 2: Hippocampal sclerosis (HS)
Ingmar Blümcke | 5

Chapter 3: Malformations of cortical development
Harvey B. Sarnat, Ingmar Blümcke | 18

Chapter 4: Brain tumours associated with early epilepsy onset
Ingmar Blümcke | 54

Chapter 5: Encephalitis
Ingmar Blümcke | 67

Chapter 6: Vascular lesions associated with focal epilepsies
Ingmar Blümcke, Harvey B. Sarnat | 74

Chapter 7: Atlas of neuropathological lesions in epilepsy surgery
Roland Coras, Ingmar Blümcke | 82

Chapter 8: Tables: Clinico-pathological findings in epilepsy surgery | 146

Chapter 9: Recommendations for neuropathological work-up and microscopic evaluation of epilepsy surgery specimens | 151

About the authors

Ingmar Blümcke, Department of Neuropathology, University Hospital Erlangen, Germany.

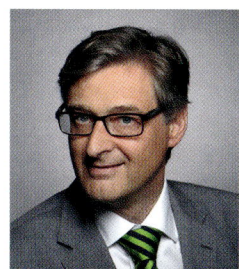

Dr. Blümcke was born on March 4th, 1965 and is full professor and director of the Dept. of Neuropathology at the University Hospital Erlangen in Germany. He graduated from medical school at Kiel University, Germany in 1991. Until 1994, he was a post-doctoral fellow in Marco Celio's lab at the University of Fribourg, Switzerland, working on the cellular distribution of calcium-binding proteins parvalbumin, calbindin & calretinin as well as perineuronal nets in the mammalian central nervous system. Between 1994 and 2001, Dr. Blümcke trained as resident of Neuropathology at the University Hospital in Bonn under the supervision of Prof. Otmar D. Wiestler. Since then, his scientific interest addresses the clinical and molecular neuropathology of human epilepsies. He published more than 200 scientific papers in peer-reviewed journals, with a current h-factor of 53 (> 950 citations in 2014; Thomson Reuters' web of science), served on many editorial boards and co-authored almost 20 book chapters on neuropathology and epilepsy surgery. Dr. Blümcke received the Alfred Hauptman Award of the German Epilepsy Society in 2011, chairs the commission of Diagnostic Methods of the International League Against Epilepsy (2013-2017), as well as the European Epilepsy Brain Bank and German Neuropathology Reference Centre for Epilepsy surgery.

In 2015, he received the IBE and ILAE Ambassador for Epilepsy Award.

Dr. Blümcke organised the 1st International Summer School for Neuropathology and Epilepsy Surgery (INES) in 2013 in Erlangen, Germany. This Summer School took place in Erlangen also in 2014, and became now an annually migrating histopathology and microscopy training course for epilepsy associated human brain specimens. In 2015, the Summer School was invited to Campinas (Brazil). Future Summer Schools will be envisaged in different regions of the world, *i.e.*, USA, China, Germany, Namibia, Japan. Please mail to bluemcke@uk-erlangen.de for any further information. Our Summer School is kindly supported by CEA (ILAE's commission on European affais), ILAE (International League against Epilepsy), IBRO (International Brain Research Organisation), ISN (International Society for Neuropathology), DGfE (German ILAE chapter), and DGNN (German ISN chapter).

Roland Coras, Department of Neuropathology, University Hospital Erlangen, Germany.

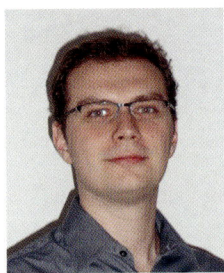

Dr. Coras was born in 1980. He is senior neuropathologist at the Department of Neuropathology in Erlangen with particular training and experience in clinical neuropathology of human focal epilepsies. He studied at the Friedrich-Alexander University Erlangen-Nuremberg School of Medicine from 2000-2007 and developed experimental skills in isolation, proliferation and differentiation of adult neuronal stem cells using human epileptic brain samples the morpho-functional organisation of the mesial temporal lobe as well as co-registration of neurosurgical brain specimens with MRI and intracerebral neurophysiological recordings. Dr. Coras is also in charge of the German Neuropathology Reference Centre for Epilepsy Surgery and European Epilepsy Brain Bank (together with Prof. Blümcke and Dr. Spreafico), and actively works with the Task Force for Neuropathology on ILAE Classification schemes for FCD, HS and tumours with early epilepsy onset.

Dr Coras received the 1st Werner Rosenthal young investigators award of the German Society for Neuropathology and Neuroanatomy (DGNN) in 2010.

Harvey B. Sarnat, Neuropathology and Clinical Neurosciences, University of Calgary, Faculty of Medicine, Alberta Children's Hospital, Research Institute Calgary, Canada.

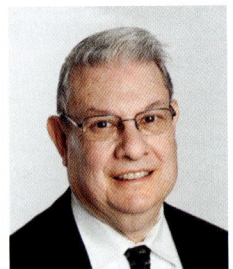

Dr. Sarnat was born in 1941. He is Professor of Paediatrics, Pathology (Neuropathology) and Clinical Neuroscience at the Faculty of Medicine, University of Calgary. He received his Bachelor of Science in Zoology, Master of Science in Neuroanatomy and Doctor of Medicine at the Univ. of Illinois, Chicago, USA. His research focused on Neuroembryology and developmental neuropathology as well as metabolic encephalomyopathies. He has published more than 170 peer-reviewed scientific papers, served on many editorial boards and co-authored almost 100 book chapters on Paediatric Neurology and Neuropathology. An additional research interest of Dr. Sarnat is comparative neuroanatomy and evolutionary theory.

Preface

Ingmar Blümcke

The idea to publish the *Surgical Neuropathology of Focal Epilepsies: Textbook and Atlas* arose from our many discussions at local, national and international meetings, as well as multi-head microscopy sessions around the world, in which the demand for a specialised reference handbook became more evident than ever. At my very first attendance at a national epilepsy symposium hosted in Kiel, Germany, in 1995, neuropathology findings were neither discussed with the audience, nor were any posters presented describing epilepsy-associated brain lesions. This situation has dramatically changed over the past 20 years as interest and requests for a systematic histopathological evaluation of human epilepsy tissue has increased at high speed, in both clinical practice and research. Still, no neuropathology textbook or atlas has been made available in these years, with the exception of Lahl, Villagran and Teixeira's *Neuropathology Atlas of Focal Epilepsies* published by John Libbey (London-Paris-Rome-Sydney) in 2003. However, their compilation of a large series of epilepsy patients operated at the Bielefeld-Bethel centre in Germany has not been updated since Dr. Lahl's retirement.

Meanwhile, the International Summer School for Neuropathology and Epilepsy Surgery (INES) was successfully launched in 2013 and goes into its 3rd year of continuous training for students, residents, lecturer, professors and researchers interested in morpho-functional analysis of human epilepsy brain tissue. An INES booklet is provided for each participant, and represents the backbone for our first edition of this textbook. Herein, all three authors reviewed their professional experience in surgical and post-mortem neuropathological studies to compile a coherent summary of clinico-pathological findings, current classification schemes, useful protocols and research data for major histopathological entities of brain lesions encountered in modern epilepsy surgery programmes, which are hippocampal sclerosis, brain tumours associated with early onset epilepsy, malformations of cortical development, brain inflammation and malformative vascular lesions. In his chapter on malformations of cortical development, Harvey Sarnat further emphasises timing and molecular signalling pathways of human cortical development as foundation to better understand the various histomorphological lesion patterns and their phenotypes. Our atlas is edited by Roland Coras and includes 32 case presentations compiled of macroscopic and microscopic images together with a summary of clinical data and magnetic resonance imaging findings that we think is representative for those brain lesions most commonly observed in epilepsy surgery, and accounting for more than 90% of cases collected at the German Neuropathology Reference Centre for Epilepsy Surgery in Erlangen, Germany. We hope that this textbook will be helpful for your daily practice as neuropathologist, neurologist, neurosurgeon, radiologist, as well as researcher or any other profession with interest in epilepsy to understand and recognise the characteristic cellular signature of a given brain lesion. This first edition does not claim, however, to explain or present any possible variant that may present. It is our professional experience that each patient's brain plasticity can produce variability that we cannot demonstrate *in toto* and we are aware that our readers will present cases at conferences in the near future that we have not yet observed and which will remain difficult to classify according to current classification schemes. Please always keep in mind that this phenotypic variability is a common histopathological feature in many epileptogenic brain lesions!

We hope to meet you some day and share your personal experience with *Neuropathology and Epilepsy Surgery*.

Yours
Ingmar Blümcke
Erlangen July 23rd, 2015

Supported by:

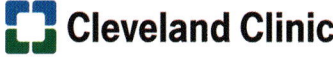
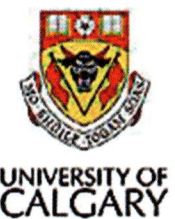
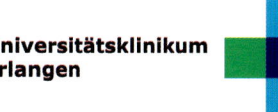

1. Introduction

Ingmar Blümcke, Harvey B. Sarnat

In February 2015, the Executive Board of the World Health Organization (WHO) has acknowledged epilepsy as most common severe neurological disorder[1], affecting more than 50 million people worldwide (Thurman *et al.*, 2011; Moshe *et al.*, 2014). However, epilepsy should not be regarded as a specific disease entity as it includes many different aetiologies, ranging from single genetic point mutations to metabolic dysfunction, as well as developmental, neoplastic or acquired brain lesions. Indeed, the neuropathological spectrum in human epilepsies is broad and it remains another challenging issue to understand how a genetic or acquired brain lesion will generate seizures by recruiting and synchronizing epileptogenic networks. The International League against Epilepsy (ILAE) continuously improves, therefore, concepts for the classification of seizure disorders (Fisher *et al.*, 2005; Berg *et al.*, 2010) and practical clinical definitions of epilepsy (Fisher *et al.*, 2014). These most recent classification systems still reflect the long-standing and often controversial dialogue about the impact of aetiology, dating back to the early work of Sir John Russel Reynolds (1861), John Hughlings Jackson (1870), William Gowers (1881), Henry Gastaut (1953) or William Lennox (1960) (for review, see Shorvon, 2011). In all of these classification schemes, circumscribed brain lesions were recognised and classified as symptomatic epilepsy (synonyms: organic or structural) with a highly precipitating risk to develop spontaneous seizures.

Our survey of 5,603 surgical epilepsy brain tissue specimens collected at the German Neuropathology Reference Centre for Epilepsy Surgery indeed demonstrates a broad spectrum of structural brain lesions resected from patients with drug-resistant localised epilepsies (*Table I*), and the list includes similar categories of epilepsy-associated brain lesions already described by Walter Dandy early in 1932 (Dandy, 1932). The neuropathology data bank also reveals a long duration of epilepsy with a mean of 15.8 years from epilepsy onset to surgery! These figures are important to recognise, considering the many side effects of chronic anti-epileptic drug (AED) treatment (Kwan *et al.*, 2010), the impact of seizures and disease load on cognitive impairment (Helmstaedter and Elger, 2009), as well as the observation that early surgery is predictive for successful long-term seizure control (Simasathien *et al.*, 2013). To improve therapeutic options and outcome in these difficult-to-treat focal epilepsies, knowledge of underlying aetiologies and their detection by epilepsy-specific morpho-functional biomarkers may help to clarify the risk and benefit of early surgery in the near future.

With advancement in imaging technologies, structural brain lesions are increasingly recognised in patients suffering from chronic focal or generalised seizures (Colombo *et al.*, 2009; Huppertz *et al.*, 2009; Wagner *et al.*, 2011; Berkovic and Jackson, 2014; Bernasconi and Bernasconi, 2014; Coan *et al.*, 2014; Coras *et al.*, 2014), and epilepsy surgery has been established as reliable treatment strategy (Wiebe *et al.*, 2001), when pharmaco-treatment has failed two adequate trials of tolerated, appropriately chosen and used AED schedules (whether as monotherapies or in combination) to achieve sustained seizure control (Kwan *et al.*, 2010). However, the epileptogenic brain region may extend beyond an MRI visible lesion and needs careful electrophysiological evaluation to also clarify, whether a suspected structural brain lesion is localised inside the seizure focus, and whether the considered surgical resection field will compromise any functionality, in particular when located in the dominant hemisphere or close to eloquent areas. These important and challenging questions can often be answered by advanced diagnostic procedures only, including invasive or stereo-EEG recordings (Bartolomei *et al.*, 2008; Kahane and Bartolomei, 2010; Gonzalez-Martinez *et al.*, 2013).

---

1. For further information, see <http://apps.who.int/gb/ebwha/pdf_files/EB136/B136_R8-en.pdf>; <http://www.who.int/en/>; https://www.youtube.com/watch?v=SshVn6MUGxA>

In our cohort of patients suffering from intractable focal seizures and submitted to epilepsy surgery, characteristic histological patterns were recognised in 93.5% (*Table I*). These included hippocampal sclerosis (HS, syn: Ammon's horn sclerosis), brain tumours with early epilepsy onset (gangliogliomas, dysembryoplastic neuroepithelial tumours), malformations of cortical development (focal cortical dysplasia, nodular heterotopia, hemimegalencephaly, polymicrogyria, cortical tubers), malformative vascular lesions (cavernomas, arterio-venous malformations, Sturge-Weber syndrome), glial scars (bleeding, ischemic or traumatic brain injuries) or inflammatory lesions (Rasmussen or limbic encephalitis). The ranking of most frequent neuropathological categories varied, however, between children and adults (see tables in chapter 9). Whereas 45% of our adult patient's cohort suffered from temporal lobe epilepsies (TLE) with HS, focal cortical dysplasias (FCDs) in the frontal lobe were most common in children. In both cohorts, 5.3-6.9% of submitted tissue samples did not reveal any specific alteration and were reported histopathologically as non-lesional. This does not imply, that histologically "normal" tissue is functionally normal, as many molecular alterations have the propensity to increase susceptibility for seizures (or decrease seizure thresholds), but escape light microscopy detection. With more advanced and refined analysis protocols such alterations may be recognised, *i.e.* acquired channelopathies (Bernard *et al.*, 2004) and altered glial networks (Steinhauser and Boison, 2012). However, histopathologically confirmed non-lesional cases can result also from sampling errors. We recommend, therefore, to apply standardised laboratory protocols for tissue procurement based on the identification of anatomical landmarks (Blümcke and Muhlebner, 2011). Therefore, we have included proposals for standardised laboratory work-up and tissue procurement, which may help to better assess 1) regions of interest within a given specimen (en bloc resections are always recommended) as well as 2) morpho-functional correlations with any other diagnostic information obtained from *i.e.* imaging or EEG.

Table I

Principle histopathological categories of brain lesions associated with drug-resistant focal epilepsies submitted for epilepsy surgery in Germany, Austria and Switzerland

	All cases		Onset age	OP	Duration epilepsy
Hippocampal Sclerosis	2,071	36.8%	11.4	33.6	22.3
Tumours	1,160	20.7%	16.9	27.2	10.4
Malformations	1,067	19.0%	6.0	17.7	11.6
No lesion	363	6.5%	13.1	28.0	14.9
Scars	321	5.7%	10.9	25.4	14.5
Vascular lesions	305	5.4%	23.4	34.5	11.1
Dual pathology	209	3.7%	9.5	26.7	17.2
Encephalitis	95	1.7%	11.3	18.4	7.2
Double pathology	12	0.2%	6.8	11.9	5.3
Total/mean	**5,603**		**12.2**	**27.9**	**15.8**

Data retrieved from the German Neuropathology Reference Centre for Epilepsy Surgery. Age at Onset/OP = age of patients at onset of spontaneous seizure activity (in years) and surgery (in years), respectively; duration of epilepsy before surgical treatment (in years). We kindly thank the following colleagues for their continuous support of the German Neuropathology Reference Centre for Epilepsy Surgery from Aachen: J. Weiß, H. Clusmann; Berlin: Thomas Nickolas Lehmann, Hans-Joachim Meencke; Bielefeld-Bethel: C.G. Bien, A. Ebner, R. Schulz, T. Kalbhenn, H. Pannek, T. Polster; Bonn: A. Becker, J. Schramm, C.E. Elger, C.G. Bien; Düsseldorf: G. Reifenberger; Erlangen: R. Coras, G. Haaker, H. Hamer, K. Rössler, M. Buchfelder, H. Stefan; Freiburg/Kehl-Kork: J. Zentner, T. Freimann, C. Schewe, B. Steinhoff; Greifswald: S. Vogelgesang, U. Runge; Göttingen: W. Brück; Heidelberg: A. von Deimling, D. Capper; Tübingen/Ulm: H. Lerche, Y. Weber; Marburg: F. Rosenow A. Hermsen; Munich: S. Noachter, P. Winkler; Münster: W. Paulus; Radeberg: T. Mayer; Salzburg: E. Trinka, P. Winkler; Vogtareuth: H. Holthausen, T. Pieper, P. Winkler, M. Kudernatsch, Vienna: M. Feucht, A. Mühlebner, T. Czech; Zurich: T. Grunwald, G. Krämer.

In previous decades, neuropathologists have not always been amongst the leading figures to unravel the impact of aetiology in seizure disorders. More recently, this notion changed into a "neuropathology renaissance" (Blümcke and Spreafico, 2012; Blümcke *et al.*, 2014). The opportunity to specify clinico-pathologic subtypes that allows prediction of a patient's risk for favourable or unfavourable seizure control following surgery will make the difference (Miyata *et al.*, 2013), and many epilepsy surgery programs appreciate an advanced neuropathology work-up of resected human brain tissue (Blümcke and Muhlebner, 2011). Prominent examples for such joint efforts promoting the notion that "cause matters" are ILAE's first consensus classification systems for FCDs (Blümcke *et al.*, 2011) and HS (Blümcke *et al.*, 2013).

According to these proposals, neuropathology assessment of surgical epilepsy specimens and reports should apply consensus terminologies following standardised protocols, which you will find also in the appendix of this first textbook on neuropathology in epilepsy surgery. Notwithstanding, such standardised procedures and protocols will be primordial to the implementation of evidence-based medicine, which is still very much lacking in the field of epilepsy surgery. This general principle is applicable to chemotherapy protocols in oncology, to surgical approaches to nucleus pulposis herniation in the vertebral column, to the prevention and treatment of shunt infections, and to the neuropathological examination and reporting of resections of epileptic foci. Standardisation does not impede innovation or creativity; on the contrary, it facilitates creativity by providing a foundation upon which to innovate. One purpose of our textbook thus is to attempt to standardise the latter, with the goal of establishing an essential infrastructure for systematic neuropathological examinations in this specialised brain tissue.

In conclusion, a neuropathology report should refer to 1) anatomical landmarks and their orientation, 2) clarification the histopathological diagnosis according to most recent consensus classification systems and 3) whether resection borders are lesion-free. This could be of particular importance if a lesion is located in or adjacent to eloquent cortex. Such an approach is usually not required in diagnostic neuropathology routine, *i.e.* when assessing diffusely infiltrating malignant brain tumours. Auxiliary clinical information from the epilepsy centre should include representative MR imaging findings and is helpful to correlate with the histopathology report. The neuropathology laboratory should be responsible for standardised tissue processing, which also guarantee sufficient tissue procurement for other (consented) research projects and ensure that selected tissue does contain expected cellular components (either lesional, perilesional or histologically normal). Further histopathological assessment should systematically apply recommended stainings to achieve a specific diagnosis according to international consensus or WHO classification systems.

References

Bartolomei F, Chauvel P, Wendling F. Epileptogenicity of brain structures in human temporal lobe epilepsy: a quantified study from intracerebral EEG. *Brain* 2008; 131: 1818-30.

Berg AT, Berkovic SF, Brodie MJ, *et al.* Revised terminology and concepts for organization of seizures and epilepsies: report of the ILAE Commission on Classification and Terminology, 2005-2009. *Epilepsia* 2010; 51: 676-85.

Berkovic SF, Jackson GD. "Idiopathic" no more! Abnormal interaction of large-scale brain networks in generalized epilepsy. *Brain* 2014; 137: 2400-2.

Bernard C, Anderson A, Becker A, Poolos NP, Beck H, Johnston D. Acquired dendritic channelopathy in temporal lobe epilepsy. *Science* 2004; 305: 532-5.

Bernasconi N, Bernasconi A. Epilepsy: Imaging the epileptic brain-time for new standards. *Nature Rev Neurology* 2014; 10: 133-4.

Blümcke I, Muhlebner A. Neuropathological work-up of focal cortical dysplasias using the new ILAE consensus classification system – practical guideline article invited by the Euro-CNS Research Committee. *Clin Neuropathol* 2011; 30: 164-77.

Blümcke I, Spreafico R. Cause matters: a neuropathological challenge to human epilepsies. *Brain Pathol* 2012; 22: 347-9.

Blümcke I, Russo GL, Najm I, Palmini A. Pathology-based approach to epilepsy surgery. *Acta Neuropathol* 2014; 128: 1-3.

Blümcke I, *et al.* International consensus classification of hippocampal sclerosis in temporal lobe epilepsy: A Task Force report from the ILAE Commission on Diagnostic Methods. *Epilepsia* 2013; 54: 1315-29.

Blümcke I, *et al.* The clinico-pathological spectrum of Focal Cortical Dysplasias: a consensus classification proposed by an ad hoc Task Force of the ILAE Diagnostic Methods Commission. *Epilepsia* 2011; 52: 158-74.

Coan AC, Kubota B, Bergo FP, Campos BM, Cendes F. 3T MRI quantification of hippocampal volume and signal in mesial temporal lobe epilepsy improves detection of hippocampal sclerosis. *AJNR Am J Neuroradiol* 2014; 35: 77-83.

Colombo N, Salamon N, Raybaud C, Ozkara C, Barkovich AJ. Imaging of malformations of cortical development. *Epileptic Disord* 2009; 11: 194-205.

Coras R, Milesi G, Zucca I, *et al.* 7T MRI features in control human hippocampus and hippocampal sclerosis: An ex vivo study with histologic correlations. *Epilepsia* 2014; 55: 2003-16.

Dandy WE. *The Practice of Surgery. The Brain.* Hagerstown: Prior, 1932.

Fisher RS, van Emde Boas W, Blume W, *et al.* Epileptic seizures and epilepsy: definitions proposed by the International League Against Epilepsy (ILAE) and the International Bureau for Epilepsy (IBE). *Epilepsia* 2005; 46: 470-2.

Fisher RS, Acevedo C, Arzimanoglou A, *et al.* ILAE official report: a practical clinical definition of epilepsy. *Epilepsia* 2014; 55: 475-82.

Gonzalez-Martinez J, Bulacio J, Alexopoulos A, Jehi L, Bingaman W, Najm I. Stereoelectroencephalography in the "difficult to localize" refractory focal epilepsy: early experience from a North American epilepsy center. *Epilepsia* 2013; 54: 323-30.

Helmstaedter C, Elger CE. Chronic temporal lobe epilepsy: a neurodevelopmental or progressively dementing disease? *Brain* 2009; 132: 2822-30.

Huppertz HJ, Kroll-Seger J, Kloppel S, Ganz RE, Kassubek J. Intra- and interscanner variability of automated voxel-based volumetry based on a 3D probabilistic atlas of human cerebral structures. *Neuroimage* 2009; 49: 2216-24.

Kahane P, Bartolomei F. Temporal lobe epilepsy and hippocampal sclerosis: lessons from depth EEG recordings. *Epilepsia* 2010; 51 (Suppl 1): 59-62.

Kwan P, Arzimanoglou A, Berg AT, *et al.* Definition of drug resistant epilepsy: consensus proposal by the ad hoc Task Force of the ILAE Commission on Therapeutic Strategies. *Epilepsia* 2010; 51: 1069-77.

Miyata H, Hori T, Vinters HV. Surgical pathology of epilepsy-associated non-neoplastic cerebral lesions: A brief introduction with special reference to hippocampal sclerosis and focal cortical dysplasia. *Neuropathology* 2013; 33: 442-58.

Moshe SL, Perucca E, Ryvlin P, Tomson T. Epilepsy: new advances. *Lancet* 2015; 385: 884-98.

Shorvon SD. The causes of epilepsy: changing concepts of etiology of epilepsy over the past 150 years. *Epilepsia* 2011; 52: 1033-44.

Simasathien T, Vadera S, Najm I, Gupta A, Bingaman W, Jehi L. Improved outcomes with earlier surgery for intractable frontal lobe epilepsy. *Ann Neurol* 2013; 73: 646-54.

Steinhauser C, Boison D. Epilepsy: crucial role for astrocytes. *Glia* 2012; 60: 1191.

Thurman DJ, et al. Standards for epidemiologic studies and surveillance of epilepsy. *Epilepsia* 2011; 52 (Suppl 7): 2-26.

Wagner J, Weber B, Urbach H, Elger CE, Huppertz HJ. Morphometric MRI analysis improves detection of focal cortical dysplasia type II. *Brain* 2011; 134: 2844-54.

Wiebe S, Blume WT, Girvin JP, Eliasziw M. A randomized, controlled trial of surgery for temporal-lobe epilepsy. *N Engl J Med* 2001; 345: 311-8.

2. Hippocampal sclerosis (HS)

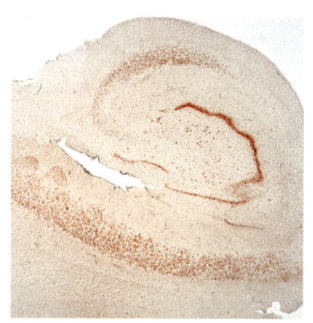

Ingmar Blümcke

Hippocampal sclerosis (HS) is the most common histopathological abnormality observed in adults with drug-resistant temporal lobe epilepsy (TLE) (Cavanagh and Meyer, 1956; Bruton, 1988; Blümcke et al., 2002; de Lanerolle et al., 2003; Blümcke et al., 2012; Cendes et al., 2014). In our series of 5,603 epilepsy patients submitted to surgical resection for various aetiologies and compiled in the Neuropathology Reference Centre for Epilepsy Surgery in Erlangen, Germany, HS was identified in 36.8% of the entire patient cohort (45% when only adults), with an additional 3.7% showing dual pathology, that is, HS in combination with tumours, vascular lesions, cortical malformations (except focal cortical dysplasia [FCD] Type IIIa, see below), or inflammation (Blümcke and Spreafico, 2012). Although the pathogenesis of HS remains to be identified and may be multi-layered, clinical histories follow a characteristic schedule in many patients. Approximately 50% of patients suffer from an "initial precipitating injury" before the age of 4 years (Mathern et al., 1995; Blümcke et al., 2002). In this cohort, complex febrile seizures are the most frequently noted events (Shinnar et al., 2012; Lewis et al., 2014). Birth trauma, head injury or meningitis are other early childhood lesions observed in TLE patients. The mean age at onset of spontaneous complex partial seizures is 11.4 years. Structural, molecular or functional analyses were usually not obtained at this early period. Diagnosis of HS is confirmed after a long period of unsuccessful antiepileptic medication (Kwan et al., 2010), with a mean age at time of surgery of 33.6 years and history of epileptic seizures of 22.3 years. As in most other series reported so far, both genders were equally affected. The prevalence of familial TLE remains uncertain. However, several forms of familial TLE have been described (Cendes et al., 1998; Crompton et al., 2010) and family history of seizures is quite common in patients with TLE (Yasuda et al., 2010).

Surgical resection offers postoperative seizure control at 2 years in 60-80% of patients with drug-resistant TLE (Engel et al., 1993; Arruda et al., 1996; Bien et al., 2001; Wiebe et al., 2001; Wieser et al., 2003; Janszky et al., 2005; von Lehe et al., 2006; Blümcke et al., 2007; Blümcke et al., 2009; Stefan et al., 2009). Long-term follow-up studies present less favourable results (Jeha et al., 2006; Jeha et al., 2007; Jehi et al., 2010; de Tisi et al., 2011; Bulacio et al., 2012; Bien et al., 2013; Jehi et al., 2015), supporting the notion that TLE is a heterogeneous condition in terms of 1) network properties and prognostic features (Stefan and Pauli, 2002; Wieser, 2004; Kahane and Bartolomei, 2010; Thom et al., 2010a; Bonilha et al., 2012); 2) degree and pattern of structural MRI anomalies within the ipsilateral temporal lobe (Bernasconi et al., 2003; Townsend et al., 2004; Sankar et al., 2008; Bernhardt et al., 2014); or 3) lesions outside the temporal lobe (Bernasconi et al., 2004; Bernhardt et al., 2010).

HS is characterized at the histopathological level by segmental pyramidal cell loss in cornu ammonis' sector CA1 (Sommer's sector), CA3 and CA4 (Bratz's sector, hilus or endfolium), whereas CA2 pyramidal and dentate gyrus granule cells are more seizure resistant (Blümcke et al., 2012). Various interneuronal cell populations are also affected, i.e. neuropeptide Y- and somatostatin – immunoreactive interneurones and/or mossy cells in the CA4 sector (Blümcke et al., 2000a; de Lanerolle et al., 2003). Neuronal loss is invariably associated with reactive astrogliosis, which results in stiffening of the tissue and which established the traditional term of "Ammon's horn sclerosis" (Sommer, 1880). Several histopathological classification systems have been proposed in the past based on a qualitative or semi-quantitative analysis of regional cell loss, extent and severity of gliosis, or axonal reorganization (Wyler et al., 1992; Proper et al., 2001; Blümcke et al.,

2007; Thom et al., 2010b; Blümcke et al., 2012; Miyata et al., 2013). Herein, we will refer to the ILAE consensus classification system for HS (Blümcke et al., 2013b), which refers to semi-quantitative assessment of segmental cell loss patterns within hippocampal subfields (Table I, Figure 2). Notwithstanding, the microscopic analysis and classification will require anatomically intact hippocampus specimens preferably obtained at the mid-body level of en bloc resections.

An intriguing question relates to mechanisms of selective neuronal vulnerability between these morphologically similar neuronal/pyramidal cell populations (Blümcke et al., 1996c; Blümcke et al., 1999b; Blümcke et al., 2000a; Blümcke et al., 2001; Aliashkevich et al., 2003) and how neuronal loss can contribute to hypersynchronized (epileptic) network activity. Such pathomechanisms include, besides others, aberrant neuronal circuitries (aberrant mossy fibre sprouting; Figures 1C, 1F) (Sutula et al., 1989), cellular reorganization patterns in epilepsy-resistant inhibitory neurones (Sloviter, 1991; Sloviter et al., 1991; DeFelipe et al., 1993; Blümcke et al., 1999c), and molecular rearrangement/plasticity of ion channel and neurotransmitter receptor expression (Blümcke et al., 1996b; Blümcke et al., 1996a; Blümcke et al., 1999a; Blümcke et al., 2000b; Becker et al., 2003; Bernard et al., 2004). The majority of hippocampal specimens reveal alterations within the dentate gyrus, i.e. granule cell dispersion (Houser, 1990; Blümcke et al., 2009). In addition, variable cell loss can be detected within adjacent cortical regions, including the subiculum, entorhinal cortex, and amygdala (Du et al., 1993; Yilmazer-Hanke et al., 2000). Cortical dyslamination and increased numbers of heterotopic white matter neurones within the ipsilateral temporal lobe may also occur in HS (Marusic et al., 2007; Thom et al., 2009).

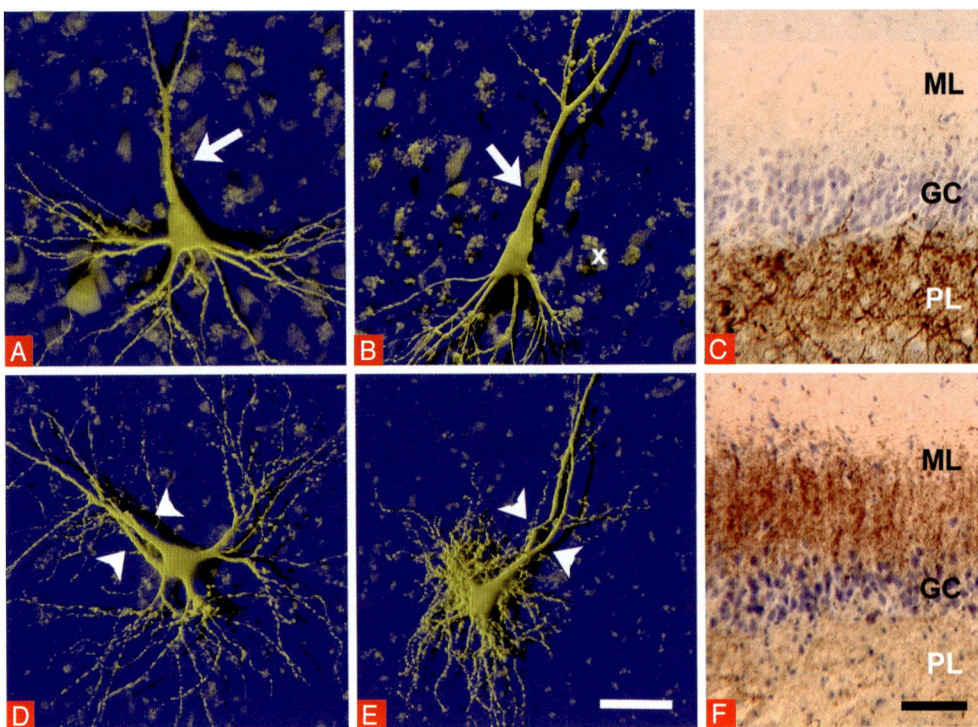

Figure 1

Cellular and axonal reorganisation patterns in hippocampal sclerosis

Confocal laser scanning microscopy and 3D-reconstruction of single neurones of the human hippocampus injected with Lucifer Yellow (Blümcke et al., 1999c). A-B: Typical shape and orientation of pyramidal cells (arrows point to apical dendrites) obtained from post-mortem controls (x labelled autofluorescent lipofuscin granules which were numerous in the elderly human brain). D-E: In HS patients, CA4 pyramidal cells showed increased dendritic arborisation patterns and often more than one apical dendrite (arrowheads). This structural abnormality is likely to occur during early life and may directly compromise neuronal signalling and network activity. C, F: Timm-staining of the dentate gyrus in a non-epileptic control (C) compared to patient with HS (F). Brownish coloured Zink-containing axonal boutons of mossy fibres are located typically in the polymorphic layer (PL). In HS-patients, axonal collaterals of mossy fibres aberrantly invade the molecular layer (ML). GC: granule cell layer. Scale bar in E = 40 µm, in F = 100 µm.

The international consensus classification system of HS (ILAE 2013)

ILAE Category	Patterns of subfield-specific neuronal loss and gliosis			
	HS ILAE Type 1	HS ILAE Type 2[d]	HS ILAE Type 3[e]	No-HS/gliosis only
DG[a]	0 – 2	0 – 1	0 – 2	0 – 1
CA4[b]	2	0 – 1	1 – 2	0 – 1
CA3[b]	0 – 2	0 – 1	0 – 2	0 – 1
CA2[b]	0 – 2	0 – 1	0 – 1	0 – 1
CA1[b]	2	1 – 2	0 – 1	0 – 1
SUB[c]	0 – 1	0 – 1	0 – 1	0 – 1

Table I

HS classification system (modified from Blümcke et al. 2013)

Semi-quantitative scoring system based on microscopic examination of formalin-fixed, paraffin-embedded surgical specimen (4 μm section thickness), haematoxylin and eosin staining and NeuN immunohistochemistry (recommended). The scoring system refers to neuronal loss (NeuN immunoreactivity) and is defined for CA1 to CA4 as following: 0 = no obvious neuronal loss or moderate astrogliosis only; 1 = moderate neuronal loss and gliosis (GFAP); 2 = severe neuronal loss (majority of neurones lost) and fibrillary astrogliosis. a = Scores for the Dentate Gyrus (DG): granule cell layer is normal (score = 0), dispersed (score 1; can be focal) or shows severe granule cell loss (score 2; can be focal). It should be assessed only in regions without curvature of the dentate gyrus. b = by visual inspection, neuronal loss may become detectable at approximately 30-40% cell loss. Quantitative methods will be more reliable for scoring (Blümcke et al., 2007); c = the subiculum shows usually no or only moderate neuronal loss (score = 0-1), distinguishing HS in TLE from neurodegenerative disorders (Montine et al., 2012). d = most prominent cell loss in CA1; may affect also CA3 and CA4, but this would be more subtle and usually detectable only by quantitative assessment. e = prominent cell loss in CA4 and DG; may affect also CA3 and CA1, but this would be more subtle and usually detectable only by quantitative assessment.

• No-HS/gliosis only

Despite electrophysiological evidence for generation of seizures in the mesial temporal lobe, about 20% of surgical TLE cases (*en bloc* resected specimens) do not show significant neuronal loss with reactive gliosis only (Blümcke *et al.*, 2007). Cell density measurements in TLE series obtained from surgery or post-mortem examinations did not show significant differences from age-matched autopsy controls (Bruton, 1988; de Lanerolle *et al.*, 2003; Thom *et al.*, 2005a; Blümcke *et al.*, 2007; Thom *et al.*, 2010b). This grading scale contrasts, therefore, with Wyler's classification system, in which 10% neuronal loss was assigned to HS Wyler grade 1. Reactive gliosis is usually detectable in no-HS specimens. Different patterns of gliosis can be histopathologically distinguished (Sofroniew and Vinters, 2010), acknowledging the continuum of changes ranging from reversible astroglial hypertrophy with preservation of cellular domains (herein referred to as "reactive astrogliosis") to long-lasting rearrangement of tissue structure (herein referred to as "fibrillary astrogliosis"). With growing evidence for glia-mediated modulation or triggering of seizures (Fedele *et al.*, 2005; Steinhauser and Boison, 2012; Aronica *et al.*, 2013; Devinsky *et al.*, 2013), reactive gliosis may play a pivotal role in hippocampal epileptogenicity despite lack of segmental neuronal loss, and may be similar to non-lesional kindling models of rodent epilepsy (Mody, 1993; Mathern *et al.*, 1998). Also see *Figure 2A* and our case presentation in chapter 7.1.

• HS ILAE Type 1 (classical and severe patterns of hippocampal sclerosis)

The largest group of HS specimens presents with a classical or severe pattern of segmental neuronal loss, representing approximately 60-80% of all TLE-HS cases in reported series (Bruton, 1988; Davies *et al.*, 1996; Blümcke *et al.*, 2002; de Lanerolle *et al.*, 2003; Blümcke *et al.*, 2007; Thom *et al.*, 2010b). The CA1 segment is most severely affected (with > 80% cell loss; Blümcke *et al.* 2012). Other segments also show significant neuronal loss, affecting 30-50% of pyramidal neurones in CA2, 30-90% of neurones in CA3, and 40-90% of neurones in CA4 (*Figure 2C, D*). The dentate gyrus is frequently affected by 50-60% granule cell loss. Due to the large variability in granule cell pathology without a clear association with clinical outcome (Blümcke *et al.*, 2009; Stefan *et al.*, 2009), granule cell pathology patterns do not account for the ILAE subtype classification. Microscopic agreement studies from the ILAE Task Force for Neuropathology could not reliably distinguish between so-called classic and severe/total cell loss patterns in HS (Wyler et al., 1992; Blümcke et al., 2007; Thom et al., 2010b), and this terminology will not be used further on. Please see also *Figure 2C* and our case presentation in chapter 7.2.

• "Atypical" HS ILAE Type 2 (predominant CA1-sclerosis)

This subtype presents histopathologically with predominant neuronal loss in CA1, affecting almost 80% of CA1 pyramidal cells. All other sectors show mild cell loss barely visible by qualitative microscopic inspection, *i.e.* in CA2 < 20%, in CA3 < 20% and in CA4 < 25% of principal cells (*Table I*). This pattern is detectable in approximately 5-10% of surgical case series of HS, and similar to that described earlier (de Lanerolle et al., 2003). DG pathology patterns may include granule cell dispersion, but usually lack severe granule cell loss (Blümcke et al., 2007). Compared to HS Type 1, preceding events in HS Type 2 were documented at later age (mean 6 years). Please see also *Figure 2E* and our case presentation in chapter 7.3.

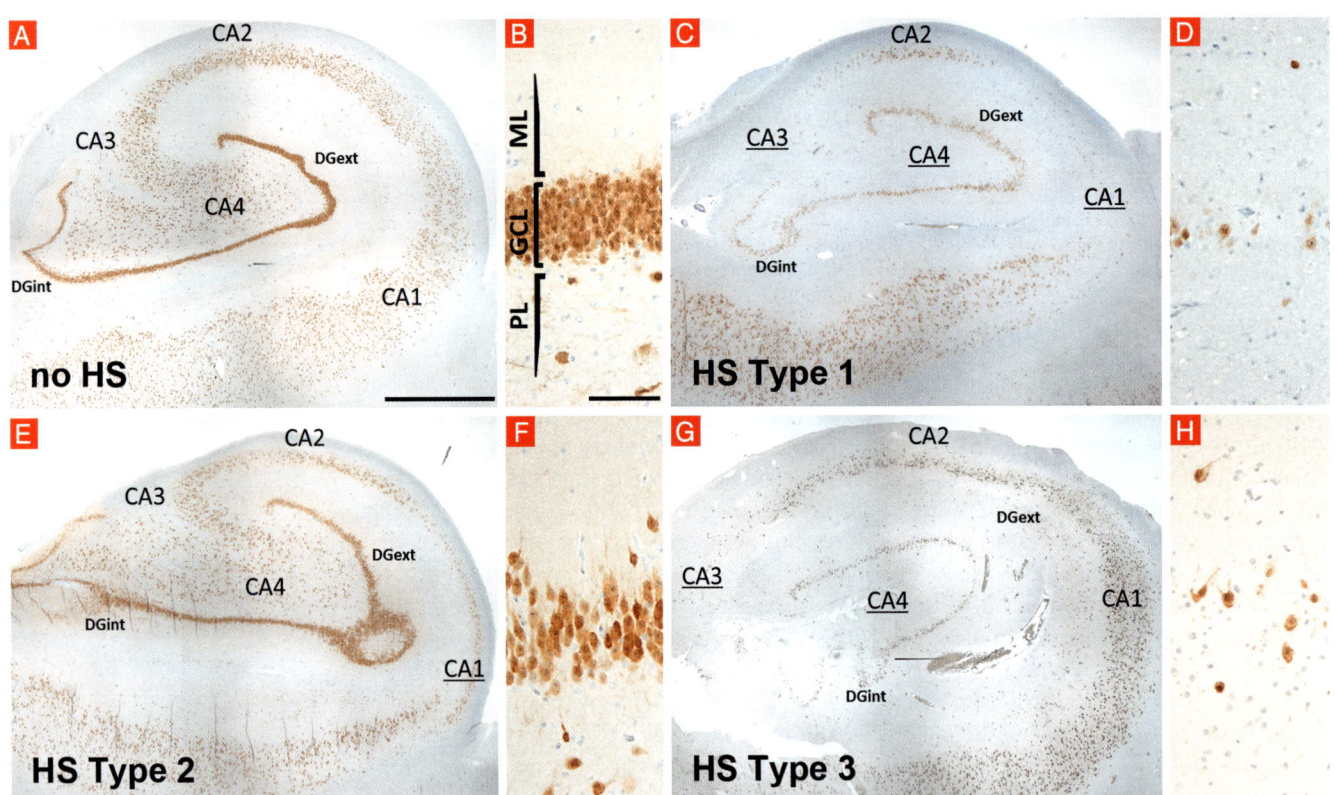

Figure 2

Histopathological HS subtypes (ILAE classification system from 2013)

A: No hippocampal sclerosis, gliosis only (no-HS): Microscopic inspection does not reveal significant cell loss in any hippocampal subregion. **C: Hippocampal sclerosis ILAE Type 1** shows preferential pyramidal cell loss in both CA4 and CA1 sectors. Damage to sectors CA3 and CA2 is more variable, but also encountered in this example. **E: Hippocampal sclerosis ILAE Type 2 (CA1 predominant neuronal loss and gliosis):** This is an atypical HS pattern characterised by neuronal loss primarily involving CA1 compared with other subfields where damage is not detectable by visual inspection. **G: Hippocampal sclerosis ILAE Type 3 (CA4 predominant neuronal loss and gliosis):** This subtype is characterised by severe cell loss in CA4 and variable cell loss patterns in CA3. **B, D, F and H:** higher magnification of the dentate gyrus (corresponding sections shown in A, C, E and G) with regular density of granule cells and layer architecture in no-HS and HS Type 2. In contrast, severe granule cell loss can be observed in HS Type 1 and 3. NeuN immunohistochemistry: all neurones were labelled in brown colour with haematoxylin counterstaining using 4 µm thin paraffin embedded sections (Wolf et al., 1996). DGext/DGint: external/internal limbs of Dentate Gyrus, PL: polymorphic layer; GCL: granule cell layer; ML: molecular layer. Scale bar in A = 2,000 µm (applies also for E and G). Scale bar in C = 1.5 mm. Scale bar in B = 100 µm (applies also for D, F and H).

- **"Atypical" HS ILAE Type 3 (predominant CA4-sclerosis)**

Predominant cell loss can be observed in CA4, (approximately 50% cell loss) and the dentate gyrus (35% cell loss), whereas CA3 (< 30%), CA2 (< 25%) and CA1 (< 20%) are moderately affected (Blümcke *et al.*, 2012). It is another rare HS subtype detectable in approximately 4-7.4% of all TLE surgical cases (Bruton, 1988; Blümcke *et al.*, 2007; Thom *et al.*, 2010b), and probably similar to that described in 1966 by Margerison and Corsellis as end-folium sclerosis (Margerison and Corsellis, 1966). It is likely that HS Type 3 will be more often associated with a dual pathology such as Rasmussen's encephalitis or other large (extra-temporal) lesions (Mathern *et al.*, 1997; Wang *et al.*, 2013). Mean age of first events were described to occur later than HS Type 1 (Blümcke *et al.*, 2007). See also *Figure 2G* and our case presentation in chapter 7.4.

Hippocampal sclerosis associated with focal cortical dysplasia (FCD Type IIIa)

An intriguing issue remains the association between TLE and focal cortical dysplasia. Despite the many published results neither a distinct aetiology nor a clinico-pathological phenotype for TLE with FCD has been identified, which elicits continuous debate (Spreafico and Blümcke, 2010). HS is frequently associated with other pathologies, and electro-clinical as well as imaging abnormalities in TLE-HS patients often extend beyond the hippocampus, suggesting a more widespread substrate for the generation or persistence of seizures (Chassoux *et al.*, 2000; Chabardes *et al.*, 2005; Fauser and Schulze-Bonhage, 2006; Barba *et al.*, 2007; Bartolomei *et al.*, 2010; Bernhardt *et al.*, 2014). The Neuropathology Task Force of the ILAE Diagnostic Methods Commission has classified, therefore, architectural abnormalities in TLE patients with HS as FCD Type IIIa (Blümcke *et al.*, 2011). It has not yet been clarified whether FCD Type IIIa is an acquired pathology with accompanying reorganizational dysplasia resulting from some initial injury that has also produced hippocampal sclerosis, or follows its own maldevelopmental pathomechanism distinct from that resulting in hippocampal sclerosis *per se*. The latter would favour the hypothesis that HS is the consequence of chronic epileptogenicity of the temporal lobe due to the dysplasia. Several aspects argue, however, for a common aetiology between HS and FCD Type IIIa. Patients from both groups have a similar onset age and a similar history of febrile seizures as an initial precipitating injury (Marusic *et al.*, 2007); no other clinical differences have yet been identified between HS and HS/FCD Type IIIa cases (Thom *et al.*, 2009). Accordingly, post-surgical outcome is similar in patients with HS compared to HS with FCD Type IIIa (Tassi *et al.*, 2010). Another well-recognized clinical challenge is that of ipsilateral temporal lobe atrophy with temporal polar grey/white matter blurring, visible on MRI in up to 70% of TLE-HS patients (Choi *et al.*, 1999; Meiners *et al.*, 1999; Mitchell *et al.*, 1999). It was often regarded as a sensitive radiological FCD marker, but the correlation between 7T MRI and histopathology including electron microscopy showed severe and patchy myelin loss in temporal white matter as underlying substrate, rather than cortical/subcortical dysplasia (Garbelli *et al.*, 2012). Whether these temporo-polar histological changes might relate with the electro-clinical temporo-polar type of TLE-HS (Chabardes *et al.*, 2005) remains another interesting issue to be clarified.

Clinico-pathological correlation with postsurgical outcome

The electro-clinical and pathology spectrum of TLE-HS indicate that structural and functional disturbances reach beyond the hippocampus (Wieser, 2004; Thom *et al.*, 2010a; Bonilha *et al.*, 2012). We can clinically define subgroups ranging from focal mesial to more extensive "temporal plus" types (Kahane and Bartolomei, 2010), which could result from a gradually evolving process (Bartolomei *et al.*, 2008). Indeed, neuropathological investigations of extra-hippocampal tissue have detected cell loss in adjacent temporal lobe structures (Wyler *et al.*, 1992; Du *et al.*, 1993;

Mathern et al., 1995; Yilmazer-Hanke et al., 1997; de Lanerolle et al., 2003; Blümcke et al., 2007; Thom et al., 2010b). An intriguing issue will be, therefore, to identify the missing links between clinical and pathology patterns of TLE-HS. A reliable consensus classification system is a step forward to achieve this goal by using a common terminology for any prospective evaluation of clinico-pathological HS types with respect to postsurgical seizure control and amelioration/aggravation of frequent co-morbidities, such as memory impairment and mood disorders.

In the light of published reports, the ILAE classification system may facilitate prediction of postsurgical outcome in TLE patients (Blümcke et al., 2007; Stefan et al., 2009; Thom et al., 2010b; Johnson et al., 2014; Na et al., 2015). According to these retrospective studies, the best outcome was achieved in patients presenting with HS ILAE Type 1 (60-80% seizure freedom 1-2 years after surgery), with current indications that fewer patients with atypical HS patterns (HS ILAE Type 2 and HS ILAE Type 3) became seizure free. The integration of data from retrospective studies is confounded by different surgical approaches and completeness of resection (including hippocampus, amygdala, entorhinal cortex, and anterior temporal lobe), the extent of mesial temporal resection, different lengths of follow up periods, the presence of a second pathology, all of which could influence postsurgical seizure control.

Other indicative clinical features of TLE have been also correlated with HS subtypes. For example, TLE patients with normal appearing hippocampus and HS ILAE Type 3 (CA4 predominant sclerosis) had a later onset and shorter epilepsy duration compared with HS ILAE Types 1 and 2 (Blümcke et al., 2007; Thom et al., 2010b). Regarding initial precipitating injuries (IPIs), defined by significant seizure and non-seizure events before age 4 years (Mathern et al., 1995), overall 40-60% of patients present with an IPI before epilepsy onset, most frequently as prolonged and complex febrile seizures (34%-70%). Other IPIs include encephalitis, anoxia, head trauma, birth trauma or intracerebral bleeding. There is some evidence to support that an IPI, in particular early febrile seizures more often associate with HS ILAE Type 1 than HS Types 2, 3 or no-HS (Van Paesschen et al., 1997; Blümcke et al., 2007). In a prospective study of 199 children with febrile seizures, 11.5% of the infants had evidence for acute hippocampal damage and abnormalities in hippocampal development (Shinnar et al., 2012). However, any retrospective evaluation of early FS in series of adult TLE patients will remain difficult and need confirmation in such an prospective trial (Hesdorffer et al., 2012).

Regarding the extent of hippocampal pathology and resection, only one randomized controlled surgical trial has been conducted so far (Schramm et al., 2011). By comparing 2.5 vs. 3.5 cm resection of the hippocampus and parahippocampus in 207 TLE patients, the authors could detect no differences in outcome with respect to complete seizure control (Engel class I). Clinical experience and neuroimaging studies also support that sclerosis is not always uniform along the anterior-posterior axis (Coras et al., 2014b; Thom, 2012), which may influence surgical planning (Bronen et al., 1994; Bernasconi et al., 2003). Post-mortem based neuropathology studies of HS have confirmed variation in the extent and pattern of neuronal loss along the longitudinal axis, raising the possibility that poor outcome may also relate to residual HS in the hippocampal remnant (Thom et al., 2012). In conclusion, current evidence suggests TLE-HS as a group of closely related syndromes with variable patterns of hippocampal histopathology, rather than a single disease. It awaits further clarification if such patterns result also from seizure progression and epilepsy burden. However, knowledge of different HS subtypes may lead to a refinement in diagnostic and surgical approaches to improve long-term outcome (Thom et al., 2010a; Bonilha et al., 2012).

Dentate gyrus pathology is an indicator for memory impairment

It remains an intriguing observation that dentate granule cell loss significantly associates with deficient memory acquisition and recall in TLE patients (Pauli et al., 2006; Blümcke et al., 2009; Coras et al., 2010; Coras et al., 2014a). Experimental data confirmed dentate gyrus granule cells to play a major role in memory acquisition (Eriksson et al., 1998; Gage, 2000; van Praag et al., 2002; Schmidt-Hieber et al., 2004; Nakashiba et al., 2012), i.e. pattern separation and rapid pattern completion (Nakashiba *et al.*, 2012), whereas hippocampal CA1 neurones are implicated in consolidation of a long-term memory (Remondes and Schuman, 2004), place memory and autobiographical memory retrieval (Bartsch *et al.*, 2006; Bartsch *et al.*, 2010; Bartsch *et al.*, 2011). The population of dentate granule cells is pathologically affected in the majority of HS patients (Blümcke *et al.*, 2002). Lesional patterns in this anatomical distinct compartment range from granule cell dispersion (GCD), which occurs in almost 50% of patients (Blümcke *et al.*, 2009), to severe cell loss in HS Type 1. Neuropathological criteria for granule cell alterations include increased granule cell lamination above 10 layers with smaller perikarya and larger intercellular gaps, as well as heterotopic clusters and bilamination in the molecular layer (Wieser, 2004). Since grading scales for granule cell pathology are not yet internationally standardized, clinico-pathological studies yielded complementary but also controversial results (Sagar and Oxbury, 1987; Houser, 1990; Mathern *et al.*, 1997; Thom *et al.*, 2005b; Blümcke *et al.*, 2009).

Our current understanding of granule cell pathology patterns were fundamentally influenced from developmental neurobiological studies of the dentate gyrus and its propensity to generate neurones throughout life (Altman, 1962; Eriksson *et al.*, 1998; Gage, 2000; van Praag *et al.*, 2002; Siebzehnrubl and Blümcke, 2008; Clelland *et al.*, 2009; Aimone *et al.*, 2011; Cameron and Glover, 2015). Hippocampal progenitor cells reside in the "polymorphic zone" just beneath the inner part of the dentate gyrus; their processes extend into the granule cell layer, passing between granule cells. Assembly of the granule cell layer follows different migratory streams building first its internal limb, from which newly generated granule cells progressively expand into lateral direction, thus forming the external limb (Altman and Bayer, 1990a, b, c). Most intriguingly, the neurogenic capacity of the dentate gyrus is maintained throughout life, including the human brain (Eriksson *et al.*, 1998; Coras *et al.*, 2010; Spalding *et al.*, 2013). The obvious association between HS and GCD led to the hypothesis that newly generated granule cells were aberrantly integrated into the dentate gyrus and compromised the tri-synaptic hippocampal pathway, thereby increasing seizure susceptibility (Parent *et al.*, 1997). Recurrent mossy fibre sprouting (mossy fibres are axonal projections of granule cells, see *Figure 1F*) has long been recognized in animal models of temporal lobe epilepsy (Tauck and Nadler, 1985) as well as in surgical human hippocampal specimens (Sutula *et al.*, 1989). Seizure induced granule cell neurogenesis and/or dispersion could then represent a key pathomechanism in the epileptic hippocampus (Parent *et al.*, 1997). Further studies challenged this assumption showing that irradiation of hippocampal precursor cells did not abolish mossy fibre sprouting after experimental induction of status epilepticus (Parent *et al.*, 1999). However, newly generated granule cells integrate not only anatomically and functionally into the granule cell layer (as destined) or heterotopically into the molecular layer (GCD) but also into CA4 (Parent *et al.*, 2006). The relevance of neurogenesis for aetiology of TLE and its architectural abnormalities within the human hippocampus still remains to be clarified (Scharfman and Gray, 2007).

Patients with TLE present with a broad spectrum of memory impairment, which can be assessed during clinical examination (Wada and Rasmussen, 1960; Hermann *et al.*, 1992; Helmstaedter and Elger, 2009; Wilson *et al.*, 2015). Surgical resection of the epileptic hippocampus as well as advanced neuroimaging studies offer the unique possibility to anatomically study the differential contribution of hippocampal subfields to compromized learning and memory in humans (Sass *et al.*, 1991; Rausch and Babb, 1993; Chelune, 1995; Pauli *et al.*, 2006). As a recent example, memory profiles were obtained from intracarotid amobarbital testing and non-invasive verbal memory assessment in a series of 100 consecutive TLE patients undergoing epilepsy surgery, and correlated with histopathologically quantified cell loss pattern in hippocampal subfields obtained from same patients using the ILAE classification system (Coras *et al.*, 2014a). Interestingly, patients with CA1 predominant cell loss (HS ILAE Type 2) did not show declarative (short-term) memory impairment and their memory performance was indistinguishable from patients without any hippocampal cell loss. In contrast, patients with neuronal loss affecting all hippocampal subfields including CA1, CA4 and dentate gyrus (HS ILAE Type 1), or predominant cell loss in CA4 and partially affecting also CA3 and DG (HS ILAE Type 3) showed significantly reduced declarative memory capacities (Pauli *et al.*, 2006; Blümcke *et al.*, 2009; Coras *et al.*, 2010; Coras *et al.*, 2014a). In conclusion, our studies suggest that normal (short term) learning in the human brain depends on intact regenerative potential of dentate granule rather than CA pyramidal cells.

Molecular neuropathology studies and animal models decipher pathogenic mechanisms of hippocampal sclerosis

In this textbook, we will not review or discuss all molecular, cellular and electro-physiologic abnormalities of "epileptic" neurones and glial cells that have been discovered and described for this disease condition in recent decades (Blümcke et al., 1999a; Sisodiya et al., 2007; Blümcke et al., 2012). It is tempting to speculate, however, that a common molecular trait of up-stream regulatory events exists leading to HS and/or chronic seizure manifestation, and such up-stream regulatory events may involve either epigenetic chromatin modifications (Kobow and Blümcke, 2011, 2012; Kobow et al., 2013a; Kobow et al., 2013b) or the adenosine deficiency hypothesis of epileptogenesis (Boison et al., 2011). Both mechanisms are able to severely modify down-stream gene expression cascades in affected brain regions and are closely related to each other. Animal models remain, therefore, important to study molecular and pathophysiologic mechanisms of epileptogenesis (Coulter et al., 2002). A single injection of pilocarpin (or kainic acid) into the animal's peritoneum or directly into the hippocampus elicits status epilepticus, which is often used experimentally to study pathogenic mechanisms of TLE (Nadler et al., 1978). Other models require subthreshold electrical stimulation of the limbic system following intrahippocampal or amygdala electrode implantation (Mody and Heinemann, 1987). Only few experimental paradigms have tried, however, to specifically reproduce human hippocampal pathology or even establish different HS subtypes. Notwithstanding, very long disease duration in many TLE patients will make this attempt difficult to address in experimental animals. One study aimed at this specific issue postulating that classical hippocampal sclerosis (ILAE Type 1) results from a single excitatory event by producing prolonged hippocampal excitation in awake rats without causing convulsive status epilepticus (Norwood et al., 2010). In their model, spontaneous hippocampal-onset seizures began 16-25 days post-injury, before hippocampal atrophy developed, as demonstrated by sequential magnetic resonance imaging. The model correlates well with the early onset hypothesis of HS Type 1 in TLE patients (Blümcke et al., 2009; Blümcke et al., 2013a) suffering from initial precipitating injuries before 4 years of age. It also supports the concept that TLE with HS is not a single epileptic disease but may evolve from different aetiologies. However, previous studies in HS ILAE Type 1 lead us to the following pathomechanistic model (*Figure 3*). Initial precipitating injuries (IPIs) may result from or induce a maturational delay of mesial temporal lobe structures and their functional organization (Blümcke et al., 2002; Blümcke,

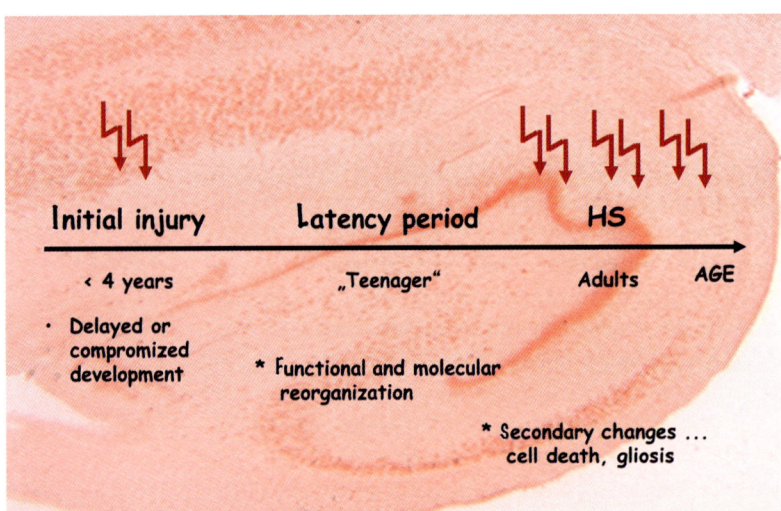

Figure 3

A pathomechanistic model for hippocampal sclerosis (ILAE Type 1)

During the clinical latency period, which usually extends into the "teenager period", a number of structural and molecular reorganisation mechanisms can be assumed. Notwithstanding, such a model is difficult to assess in human surgical tissue specimens obtained from an end-stage of the disease. However, there is ample evidence from animal models of limbic epilepsy indicating a number of activity dependent reorganisational events preceding the onset of spontaneous seizure activity. In particular, neurotransmitter receptor complexes dramatically change their molecular composition in a region-specific manner. Such modulatory changes can functionally reduce seizure threshold levels in the hippocampus (Brooks-Kayal et al., 1998; Shumate et al., 1998; Becker et al., 2003; Bernard et al., 2004).

2009). Whether a genetic/epigenetic component plays a role, *i.e.* affecting neurodevelopmental signalling pathways such as the reelin cascade, cannot be excluded (Kobow *et al.*, 2009). An interesting finding was the persistence of Cajal-Retzius cells in the molecular layer of the dentate gyrus obtained from TLE patients with HS and IPIs (Blümcke *et al.*, 1996c; Blümcke *et al.*, 1999b). We suggested prolonged or abnormal maturatory processes in the affected hippocampus as predisposition/susceptibility factor to generate seizures and subsequent neuronal loss. This hypothesis is supported by the notion that long-term epilepsies "per se" do not inevitably damage the hippocampus as repetitively shown in cohorts of TLE patients with poorly controlled seizures (Thom *et al.*, 2005a).

Following the onset of spontaneous seizure activity within the hippocampal formation and mesial temporal lobe structures during adolescence, secondary changes associated with excitotoxic cellular damage may lead to the full-blown pattern of HS Type 1 (Blümcke *et al.*, 2002). This model does not rule out that segmental neuronal loss can occur already during an earlier period. We do, however, propose that limbic seizure activity on its own cannot induce HS without preceding anatomical and functional alterations in the hippocampus/dentate gyrus network. This assumption is supported by our studies in lesion-associated TLE, in which patients suffer from low-grade tumours, malformations or vascular lesions. In these patients, the hippocampus does not unequivocally reveal neuropathological changes, *i.e.* no-HS, although seizure semiologies and clinical histories can be very similar to HS-associated TLE patients (Blümcke *et al.*, 2002).

Late onset TLE with histopathologically proven HS has been observed after limbic encephalitis (Bien *et al.*, 2007; Kroll-Seger *et al.*, 2009). These patients usually have no latency period which is a different clinical signature from that described above for HS Type 1. It is our assumption and partially also our clinical experience, that hippocampal cell loss patterns reveal significant differences in late onset TLE corresponding to "atypical HS Type 2 or 3 variants" (Wang *et al.*, 2013). Thus, systematic neuropathological evaluation is a helpful tool to characterize distinct pathogenic patterns and to better understand the variability in focal onset, drug-resistant chronic epilepsies.

Definitions and terminology issues

The term HS is used to histopathologically define the pattern of segmental neuronal loss with concomitant astrogliosis in the hippocampal formation (including the dentate gyrus). This scheme applies to patients with TLE. Segmental hippocampal neuronal loss also can be observed in other pathological conditions, including neurodegeneration, aging and ischemia, but patterns of neuronal loss differ significantly (Miyata *et al.*, 2013) and usually involves the subiculum (Nelson *et al.*, 2011; Montine *et al.*, 2012).

HS occurs either isolated or in association with another epileptogenic principal lesion of independent origin (dual pathology), for example tumours, malformations of cortical development, vascular malformations or encephalitis. FCD Type IIIa in the ipsilateral temporal lobe (Blümcke *et al.*, 2011; Blümcke *et al.*, 2013b) should not be considered dual pathology, as its independent nature and pathomechanistic origin await further clarification (Thom *et al.*, 2009). Other examples of difficult-to-classify lesions comprise: FCD ILAE Type IIb occurring within the hippocampal formation, which may present with hippocampal neuronal loss (Thom *et al.*, 2008; Rogerio *et al.*, 2014). This should not be classified as dual pathology. The same applies to epilepsy-associated glio-neuronal tumours overrunning the hippocampus. In all these difficult constellations, we suggest that your histopathology diagnosis refer only to the principal lesion, *i.e.* FCD IIb or ganglioglioma in the hippocampus.

The three ILAE types can be microscopically identified, when an anatomically well preserved surgical specimen is available (*en bloc* resection recommended). The ILAE classification scheme cannot be applied for fragmented specimens without available anatomical landmarks. The histopathology report should than reflect the level of confidence. Possible HS: if cell loss can be identified in CA1 and DG/CA4. Potential HS: if pyramidal cell loss in only one or unclassifiable segment. Histological patterns may vary along the anterior-posterior axis (Thom *et al.*,

2012; Coras *et al.*, 2014b). Although diagnosis should reflect any variability observed, it should usually refer to the mid-body. HS with familial (hereditary) forms of uni- or bilateral HS have been also described (Cendes *et al.*, 1998).

Mesial temporal sclerosis (MTS) is defined as HS plus changes in other structures of the mesial part of the temporal lobe such as amygdala and entorhinal cortex (as evidenced by imaging findings or histopathology).

The term "Ammon's horn sclerosis" (AHS) was coined by Sommer in 1880 (Sommer, 1880) and is often used synonymous to HS.

References

Aimone JB, Deng W, Gage FH. Resolving new memories: a critical look at the dentate gyrus, adult neurogenesis, and pattern separation. *Neuron* 2011; 70: 589-96.

Aliashkevich AF, Yilmazer-Hanke D, Van Roost D, Mundhenk B, Schramm J, Blümcke I. Cellular pathology of amygdala neurons in human temporal lobe epilepsy. *Acta Neuropathol (Berl)* 2003; 106: 99-106.

Altman J. Are new neurons formed in the brains of adult mammals? *Science* 1962; 135: 1127-8.

Altman J, Bayer SA. Migration and distribution of two populations of hippocampal granule cell precursors during the perinatal and postnatal periods. *J Comp Neurol* 1990a; 301: 365-81.

Altman J, Bayer SA. Prolonged sojourn of developing pyramidal cells in the intermediate zone of the hippocampus and their settling in the stratum pyramidale. *J Comp Neurol* 1990b; 301: 343-64.

Altman J, Bayer SA. Mosaic organization of the hippocampal neuroepithelium and the multiple germinal sources of dentate granule cells. *J Comp Neurol* 1990c; 301: 325-42.

Aronica E, Sandau US, Iyer A, Boison D. Glial adenosine kinase – A neuropathological marker of the epileptic brain. *Neurochem Int* 2013; 63: 688-95.

Arruda F, Cendes F, Andermann F, *et al.* Mesial atrophy and outcome after amygdalohippocampectomy or temporal lobe removal. *Ann Neurol* 1996; 40: 446-50.

Barba C, Barbati G, Minotti L, Hoffmann D, Kahane P. Ictal clinical and scalp-EEG findings differentiating temporal lobe epilepsies from temporal "plus" epilepsies. *Brain* 2007; 130: 1957-67.

Bartolomei F, Chauvel P, Wendling F. Epileptogenicity of brain structures in human temporal lobe epilepsy: a quantified study from intracerebral EEG. *Brain* 2008; 131: 1818-30.

Bartolomei F, Cosandier-Rimele D, McGonigal A, *et al.* From mesial temporal lobe to temporoperisylvian seizures: a quantified study of temporal lobe seizure networks. *Epilepsia* 2010; 51: 2147-58.

Bartsch T, Dohring J, Rohr A, Jansen O, Deuschl G. CA1 neurons in the human hippocampus are critical for autobiographical memory, mental time travel, and autonoetic consciousness. *Proc Natl Acad Sci USA* 2011; 108: 17562-7.

Bartsch T, Alfke K, Stingele R, *et al.* Selective affection of hippocampal CA-1 neurons in patients with transient global amnesia without long-term sequelae. *Brain* 2006; 129: 2874-84.

Bartsch T, Schonfeld R, Muller FJ, *et al.* Focal lesions of human hippocampal CA1 neurons in transient global amnesia impair place memory. *Science* 2010; 328: 1412-5.

Becker AJ, Chen J, Zien A, *et al.* Correlated stage- and subfield-associated hippocampal gene expression patterns in experimental and human temporal lobe epilepsy. *Eur J Neurosci* 2003; 18: 2792-802.

Bernard C, Anderson A, Becker A, Poolos NP, Beck H, Johnston D. Acquired dendritic channelopathy in temporal lobe epilepsy. *Science* 2004; 305: 532-5.

Bernasconi N, Bernasconi A, Caramanos Z, Antel SB, Andermann F, Arnold DL Mesial temporal damage in temporal lobe epilepsy: a volumetric MRI study of the hippocampus, amygdala and parahippocampal region. *Brain* 2003; 126: 462-9.

Bernasconi N, Duchesne S, Janke A, Lerch J, Collins DL, Bernasconi A. Whole-brain voxel-based statistical analysis of gray matter and white matter in temporal lobe epilepsy. *Neuroimage* 2004; 23: 717-23.

Bernhardt BC, Bernasconi N, Concha L, Bernasconi A. Cortical thickness analysis in temporal lobe epilepsy: reproducibility and relation to outcome. *Neurology* 2010; 74: 1776-84.

Bernhardt BC, Hong SJ, Bernasconi A, Bernasconi N. Magnetic resonance imaging pattern learning in temporal lobe epilepsy: Classification and prognostics. *Ann Neurol* 2015; 77: 436-46.

Bien CG, Raabe AL, Schramm J, Becker A, Urbach H, Elger CE. Trends in presurgical evaluation and surgical treatment of epilepsy at one centre from 1988-2009. *J Neurol Neurosurg Psychiatry* 2013; 84: 54-61.

Bien CG, Kurthen M, Baron K, *et al.* Long-term seizure outcome and antiepileptic drug treatment in surgically treated temporal lobe epilepsy patients: a controlled study. *Epilepsia* 2001; 42: 1416-21.

Bien CG, Urbach H, Schramm J, *et al.* Limbic encephalitis as a precipitating event in adult-onset temporal lobe epilepsy. *Neurology* 2007; 69: 1236-44.

Blümcke I. Neuropathology of focal epilepsies: a critical review. *Epilepsy Behav* 2009; 15: 34-9.

Blümcke I, Spreafico R. Cause matters: a neuropathological challenge to human epilepsies. *Brain Pathol* 2012; 22: 347-9.

Blümcke I, Thom M, Wiestler OD. Ammon's horn sclerosis: a maldevelopmental disorder associated with temporal lobe epilepsy. *Brain Pathol* 2002; 12: 199-211.

Blümcke I, Cross JH, Spreafico R. The international consensus classification for hippocampal sclerosis: an important step towards accurate prognosis. *Lancet Neurol* 2013a; 12: 844-6.

Blümcke I, Beck H, Lie AA, Wiestler OD. Molecular neuropathology of human mesial temporal lobe epilepsy. *Epilepsy Res* 1999a; 36: 205-23.

Blümcke I, Coras R, Miyata H, Ozkara C. Defining clinico-neuropathological subtypes of mesial temporal lobe epilepsy with hippocampal sclerosis. *Brain Pathol* 2012; 22: 402-11.

Blümcke I, Behle K, Malitschek B, *et al.* Immunohistochemical distribution of metabotropic glutamate receptor subtypes mGluR1b, mGluR2/3, mGluR4a and mGluR5 in human hippocampus. *Brain Res* 1996a; 736: 217-26.

Blümcke I, Suter B, Behle K, *et al.* Loss of hilar mossy cells in Ammon's horn sclerosis. *Epilepsia* 2000a; 41: S174-80.

Blümcke I, Schewe JC, Normann S, *et al.* Increase of nestin-immunoreactive neural precursor cells in the dentate gyrus of pediatric patients with early-onset temporal lobe epilepsy. *Hippocampus* 2001; 11: 311-21.

Blümcke I, Beck H, Scheffler B, *et al.* Altered distribution of the alpha-amino-3-hydroxy-5-methyl-4-isoxazole propionate receptor subunit GluR2(4) and the N-methyl-D-aspartate receptor subunit NMDAR1 in the hippocampus of patients with temporal lobe epilepsy. *Acta Neuropathol* 1996b; 92: 576-87.

Blümcke I, Beck H, Suter B, *et al.* An increase of hippocampal calretinin-immunoreactive neurons correlates with early febrile seizures in temporal lobe epilepsy. *Acta Neuropathol (Berl)* 1999b; 97: 31-9.

Blümcke I, Beck H, Nitsch R, *et al.* Preservation of calretinin-immunoreactive neurons in the hippocampus of epilepsy patients with Ammon's horn sclerosis. *J Neuropathol Exp Neurol* 1996c; 55: 329-41.

Blümcke I, Zuschratter W, Schewe JC, et al. Cellular pathology of hilar neurons in Ammon's horn sclerosis. *J Comp Neurol* 1999c; 414: 437-53.

Blümcke I, Becker A, Klein C, et al. Temporal lobe epilepsy-associated up-regulation of specific metabotropic glutamate receptors: correlated changes in mGluR1 mRNA and protein expression in experimental animals and human patients. *J Neuropathol Exp Neurol* 2000b; 59: 1-10.

Blümcke I, Pauli E, Clusmann H, et al. A new clinico-pathological classification system for mesial temporal sclerosis. *Acta Neuropathol* 2007; 113: 235-44.

Blümcke I, Kistner I, Clusmann H, et al. Towards a clinico-pathological classification of granule cell dispersion in human mesial temporal lobe epilepsies. *Acta Neuropathol* 2009; 117: 535-44.

Blümcke I, et al. International consensus classification of hippocampal sclerosis in temporal lobe epilepsy: a Task Force report from the ILAE Commission on Diagnostic Methods. *Epilepsia* 2013b; 54: 1315-29.

Blümcke I, et al. The clinico-pathological spectrum of focal cortical dysplasias: a consensus classification proposed by an ad hoc Task Force of the ILAE Diagnostic Methods Commission. *Epilepsia* 2011; 52: 158-74.

Boison D, Masino SA, Geiger JD. Homeostatic bioenergetic network regulation – a novel concept to avoid pharmacoresistance in epilepsy. *Expert Opin Drug Discov* 2011; 6: 713-24.

Bonilha L, Martz GU, Glazier SS, Edwards JC. Subtypes of medial temporal lobe epilepsy: influence on temporal lobectomy outcomes? *Epilepsia* 2012; 53: 1-6.

Bronen RA, Anderson AW, Spencer DD. Quantitative MR for epilepsy: a clinical and research tool? *AJNR Am J Neuroradiol* 1994; 15: 1157-60.

Brooks-Kayal AR, Shumate MD, Jin H, Rikhter TY, Coulter DA. Selective changes in single cell GABA(A): receptor subunit expression and function in temporal lobe epilepsy. *Nat Med* 1998; 4: 1166-72.

Bruton CJ. The neuropathology of temporal lobe epilepsy. In: Russel G, Marley E, Williams P, eds. *Maudsley Monographs*, pp. 1-158. London: Oxford University Press, 1988.

Bulacio JC, Jehi L, Wong C, et al. Long-term seizure outcome after resective surgery in patients evaluated with intracranial electrodes. *Epilepsia* 2012; 53: 1722-30.

Cameron HA, Glover LR. Adult neurogenesis: beyond learning and memory. *Ann Rev Psychol* 2015; 66: 53-81.

Cavanagh JB, Meyer A. Aetiological aspects of Ammon's horn sclerosis associated with temporal lobe epilepsy. *Brit Med J* 1956; 2: 1403-7.

Cendes F, Lopes-Cendes I, Andermann E, Andermann F. Familial temporal lobe epilepsy: a clinically heterogeneous syndrome. *Neurology* 1998; 50: 554-7.

Cendes F, Sakamoto AC, Spreafico R, Bingaman W, Becker AJ. Epilepsies associated with hippocampal sclerosis. *Acta Neuropathol* 2014; 128: 21-37.

Chabardes S, Kahane P, Minotti L, et al. The temporopolar cortex plays a pivotal role in temporal lobe seizures. *Brain* 2005; 128: 1818-31.

Chassoux F, Devaux B, Landre E, et al. Stereoelectroencephalography in focal cortical dysplasia: a 3D approach to delineating the dysplastic cortex. *Brain* 2000; 123 (Pt 8): 1733-51.

Chelune GJ. Hippocampal adequacy versus functional reserve: predicting memory functions following temporal lobectomy. *Arch Clin Neuropsychol* 1995; 10: 413-32.

Choi D, Na DG, Byun HS, et al. White-matter change in mesial temporal sclerosis: correlation of MRI with PET, pathology, and clinical features. *Epilepsia* 1999; 40: 1634-41.

Clelland CD, Choi M, Romberg C, et al. A functional role for adult hippocampal neurogenesis in spatial pattern separation. *Science* 2009; 325: 210-3.

Coras R, Pauli E, Li J, Schwarz M, et al. Differential influence of hippocampal subfields on memory formation: insights from patients with temporal lobe epilepsy. *Brain* 2014a; 137: 1945-57.

Coras R, Siebzehnrubl FA, Pauli E, et al. Low proliferation and differentiation capacities of adult hippocampal stem cells correlate with memory dysfunction in humans. *Brain* 2010; 133: 3359-72.

Coras R, Milesi G, Zucca I, et al. 7T MRI features in control human hippocampus and hippocampal sclerosis: An ex vivo study with histologic correlations. *Epilepsia* 2014b; 55: 2003-16.

Coulter DA, McIntyre DC, Löscher W. Animal models of limbic epilepsies: what can they tell us? *Brain Pathol* 2002; 12: 240-56.

Crompton DE, Scheffer IE, Taylor I, et al. Familial mesial temporal lobe epilepsy: a benign epilepsy syndrome showing complex inheritance. *Brain* 2010; 133: 3221-31.

Davies KG, Hermann BP, Dohan FC, Foley KT, Bush AJ, Wyler AR. Relationship of hippocampal sclerosis to duration and age of onset of epilepsy, and childhood febrile seizures in temporal lobectomy patients. *Epilepsy Res* 1996; 24: 119-26.

de Lanerolle NC, Kim JH, Williamson A, et al. A retrospective analysis of hippocampal pathology in human temporal lobe epilepsy: evidence for distinctive patient subcategories. *Epilepsia* 2003; 44: 677-87.

de Tisi J, Bell GS, Peacock JL, et al. The long-term outcome of adult epilepsy surgery, patterns of seizure remission, and relapse: a cohort study. *Lancet* 2011; 378: 1388-95.

DeFelipe J, Garcia Sola R, Marco P, del Rio MR, Pulido P, Ramon y Cajal S. Selective changes in the microorganization of the human epileptogenic neocortex revealed by parvalbumin immunoreactivity. *Cereb-Cortex* 1993; 3: 39-48.

Devinsky O, Vezzani A, Najjar S, De Lanerolle NC, Rogawski MA. Glia and epilepsy: excitability and inflammation. *Trends Neurosci* 2013; 36: 174-84.

Du F, Whetsell WJ, Abou Khalil B, Blumenkopf B, Lothman EW, Schwarcz R. Preferential neuronal loss in layer III of the entorhinal cortex in patients with temporal lobe epilepsy. *Epilepsy Res* 1993; 16: 223-33.

Engel JJ, Van Ness P, Rasmussen TB, Ojemann LM. Outcome with respect to epileptic seizures. In: Engel JJ, ed. *Surgical Treatment of the Epilepsies*, pp. 609-621. New York: Raven, 1993.

Eriksson PS, Perfilieva E, Bjork-Eriksson T, et al. Neurogenesis in the adult human hippocampus. *Nat Med* 1998; 4: 1313-7.

Fauser S, Schulze-Bonhage A. Epileptogenicity of cortical dysplasia in temporal lobe dual pathology: an electrophysiological study with invasive recordings. *Brain* 2006; 129: 82-95.

Fedele DE, Gouder N, Guttinger M, et al. Astrogliosis in epilepsy leads to overexpression of adenosine kinase, resulting in seizure aggravation. *Brain* 2005; 128: 2383-95.

Gage FH. Mammalian neural stem cells. *Science* 2000; 287: 1433-8.

Garbelli R, Milesi G, Medici V, et al. Blurring in patients with temporal lobe epilepsy: clinical, high-field imaging and ultrastructural study. *Brain* 2012; 135: 2337-49.

Helmstaedter C, Elger CE. Chronic temporal lobe epilepsy: a neurodevelopmental or progressively dementing disease? *Brain* 2009; 132: 2822-30.

Hermann BP, Wyler AR, Bush AJ, Tabatabai FR. Differential effects of left and right anterior temporal lobectomy on verbal learning and memory performance. *Epilepsia* 1992; 33: 289-97.

Hesdorffer DC, Shinnar S, Lewis DV, et al. Design and phenomenology of the FEBSTAT study. *Epilepsia* 2012; 53: 1471-80.

Houser CR. Granule cell dispersion in the dentate gyrus of humans with temporal lobe epilepsy. *Brain Res* 1990; 535: 195-204.

Janszky J, Janszky I, Schulz R, Hoppe M, Behne F, Pannek HW, Ebner A. Temporal lobe epilepsy with hippocampal sclerosis: predictors for long-term surgical outcome. *Brain* 2005; 128: 395-404.

Jeha LE, Najm I, Bingaman W, Dinner D, Widdess-Walsh P, Luders H. Surgical outcome and prognostic factors of frontal lobe epilepsy surgery. *Brain* 2007; 130: 574-84.

Jeha LE, Najm IM, Bingaman WE, et al. Predictors of outcome after temporal lobectomy for the treatment of intractable epilepsy. *Neurology* 2006; 66: 1938-40.

Jehi L, Yardi R, Chagin K, et al. Development and validation of nomograms to provide individualised predictions of seizure outcomes after epilepsy surgery: a retrospective analysis. *Lancet Neurol* 2015; 14: 283-90.

Jehi LE, Silveira DC, Bingaman W, Najm I. Temporal lobe epilepsy surgery failures: predictors of seizure recurrence, yield of reevaluation, and outcome following reoperation. *J Neurosurg* 2010; 113: 1186-94.

Johnson AM, Sugo E, Barreto D, et al. Clinicopathological associations in temporal lobe epilepsy patients utilising the current ILAE focal cortical dysplasia classification. *Epilepsy Res* 2014; 108: 1345-51.

Kahane P, Bartolomei F. Temporal lobe epilepsy and hippocampal sclerosis: lessons from depth EEG recordings. *Epilepsia* 2010; 51 (Suppl 1): 59-62.

Kobow K, Blümcke I. The methylation hypothesis: do epigenetic chromatin modifications play a role in epileptogenesis? *Epilepsia* 2011; 52 (Suppl 4): 15-9.

Kobow K, Blümcke I. The emerging role of DNA methylation in epileptogenesis. *Epilepsia* 2012; 53: 11-20.

Kobow K, El-Osta A, Blümcke I. The methylation hypothesis of pharmacoresistance in epilepsy. *Epilepsia* 2013a; 54 (Suppl 2): 41-7.

Kobow K, Jeske I, Hildebrandt M, et al. Increased reelin promoter methylation is associated with granule cell dispersion in human temporal lobe epilepsy. *J Neuropathol Exp Neurol* 2009; 68: 356-64.

Kobow K, Kaspi A, Harikrishnan KN, et al. Deep sequencing reveals increased DNA methylation in chronic rat epilepsy. *Acta Neuropathol* 2013b; 126: 741-56.

Kroll-Seger J, Bien CG, Huppertz HJ. Non-paraneoplastic limbic encephalitis associated with antibodies to potassium channels leading to bilateral hippocampal sclerosis in a pre-pubertal girl. *Epileptic Disord* 2009; 11: 54-9.

Kwan P, Arzimanoglou A, Berg AT, et al. Definition of drug resistant epilepsy: consensus proposal by the ad hoc Task Force of the ILAE Commission on Therapeutic Strategies. *Epilepsia* 2010; 51: 1069-77.

Lewis DV, Shinnar S, Hesdorffer DC, et al. Hippocampal sclerosis after febrile status epilepticus: the FEBSTAT study. *Ann Neurol* 2014; 75: 178-85.

Margerison JH, Corsellis JA. Epilepsy and the temporal lobes. A clinical, electroencephalographic and neuropathological study of the brain in epilepsy, with particular reference to the temporal lobes. *Brain* 1966; 89: 499-530.

Marusic P, Tomasek M, Krsek P, et al. Clinical characteristics in patients with hippocampal sclerosis with or without cortical dysplasia. *Epileptic Disord* 2007; 9 (Suppl 1): S75-82.

Mathern GW, Pretorius JK, Babb TL. Influence of the type of initial precipitating injury and at what age it occurs on course and outcome in patients with temporal lobe seizures. *J Neurosurg* 1995; 82: 220-7.

Mathern GW, Kuhlman PA, Mendoza D, Pretorius JK. Human fascia dentata anatomy and hippocampal neuron densities differ depending on the epileptic syndrome and age at first seizure. *J Neuropathol Exp Neurol* 1997; 56: 199-212.

Mathern GW, Pretorius JK, Leite JP, et al. Hippocampal AMPA and NMDA mRNA levels and subunit immunoreactivity in human temporal lobe epilepsy patients and a rodent model of chronic mesial limbic epilepsy. *Epilepsy Res* 1998; 32: 154-71.

Meiners LC, Witkamp TD, de Kort GA, et al. Relevance of temporal lobe white matter changes in hippocampal sclerosis. Magnetic resonance imaging and histology. *Invest Radiol* 1999; 34: 38-45.

Mitchell LA, Jackson GD, Kalnins RM, et al. Anterior temporal abnormality in temporal lobe epilepsy: a quantitative MRI and histopathologic study. *Neurology* 1999; 52: 327-36.

Miyata H, Hori T, Vinters HV. Surgical pathology of epilepsy-associated non-neoplastic cerebral lesions: A brief introduction with special reference to hippocampal sclerosis and focal cortical dysplasia. *Neuropathology* 2013; 33: 442-58.

Mody I. The molecular basis of kindling. *Brain Pathol* 1993; 3: 395-403.

Mody I, Heinemann U. NMDA receptors of dentate gyrus granule cells participate in synaptic transmission following kindling. *Nature* 1987; 326: 701-4.

Montine TJ, Phelps CH, Beach TG, et al. National Institute on Aging-Alzheimer's Association guidelines for the neuropathologic assessment of Alzheimer's disease: a practical approach. *Acta Neuropathol* 2012; 123: 1-11.

Na M, Ge H, Shi C, Shen H, et al. Long-term seizure outcome for international consensus classification of hippocampal sclerosis: A survival analysis. *Seizure* 2015; 25: 141-6.

Nadler JV, Perry BW, Cottman CW. Intraventricular kainic acid preferentially destroys hippocampal pyramidal cells. *Nature* 1978; 271: 676-7.

Nakashiba T, Cushman JD, Pelkey KA, et al. Young dentate granule cells mediate pattern separation, whereas old granule cells facilitate pattern completion. *Cell* 2012; 149: 188-201.

Nelson PT, Head E, Schmitt FA, et al. Alzheimer's disease is not "brain aging": neuropathological, genetic, and epidemiological human studies. *Acta Neuropathol* 2011; 121: 571-87.

Norwood BA, Bumanglag AV, Osculati F, et al. Classic hippocampal sclerosis and hippocampal-onset epilepsy produced by a single "cryptic" episode of focal hippocampal excitation in awake rats. *J Comp Neurol* 2010; 518: 3381-407.

Parent JM, Tada E, Fike JR, Lowenstein DH. Inhibition of dentate granule cell neurogenesis with brain irradiation does not prevent seizure-induced mossy fiber synaptic reorganization in the rat. *J Neurosci* 1999; 19: 4508-19.

Parent JM, Elliott RC, Pleasure SJ, Barbaro NM, Lowenstein DH. Aberrant seizure-induced neurogenesis in experimental temporal lobe epilepsy. *Ann Neurol* 2006; 59: 81-91.

Parent JM, Yu TW, Leibowitz RT, Geschwind DH, Sloviter RS, Lowenstein DH. Dentate granule cell neurogenesis is increased by seizures and contributes to aberrant network reorganization in the adult rat hippocampus. *J Neurosci* 1997; 17: 3727-38.

Pauli E, Hildebrandt M, Romstock J, Stefan H, Blümcke I. Deficient memory acquisition in temporal lobe epilepsy is predicted by hippocampal granule cell loss. *Neurology* 2006; 67: 1383-9.

Proper EA, Jansen GH, van Veelen CW, van Rijen PC, Gispen WH, de Graan PN. A grading system for hippocampal sclerosis based on the degree of hippocampal mossy fiber sprouting. *Acta Neuropathol (Berl)* 2001; 101: 405-9.

Rausch R, Babb TL. Hippocampal neuron loss and memory scores before and after temporal lobe surgery for epilepsy. *Arch Neurol* 1993; 50: 812-7.

Remondes M, Schuman EM. Role for a cortical input to hippocampal area CA1 in the consolidation of a long-term memory. *Nature* 2004; 431: 699-703.

Rogerio F, Morita ME, Coan AC, et al. Hippocampal dysplasia with balloon cells: case report and discussion on classification. *J Neurology* 2014; 261: 2022-4.

Sagar HJ, Oxbury JM. Hippocampal neuron loss in temporal lobe epilepsy: correlation with early childhood convulsions. *Ann Neurol* 1987; 22: 334-40.

Sankar T, Bernasconi N, Kim H, Bernasconi A. Temporal lobe epilepsy: differential pattern of damage in temporopolar cortex and white matter. *Hum Brain Mapp* 2008; 29: 931-44.

Sass KJ, Lencz T, Westerveld M, Novelly RA, Spencer DD, Kim JH. The neural substrate of memory impairment demonstrated by the intracarotid amobarbital procedure. *Arch Neurol* 1991; 48: 48-52.

Scharfman HE, Gray WP. Relevance of seizure-induced neurogenesis in animal models of epilepsy to the etiology of temporal lobe epilepsy. *Epilepsia* 2007; 48 (Suppl 2): 33-41.

Schmidt-Hieber C, Jonas P, Bischofberger J. Enhanced synaptic plasticity in newly generated granule cells of the adult hippocampus. *Nature* 2004; 429: 184-7.

Schramm J, Lehmann TN, Zentner J, et al. Randomized controlled trial of 2.5-cm versus 3.5-cm mesial temporal resection in temporal lobe epilepsy – Part 1: intent-to-treat analysis. *Acta Neurochir (Wien):* 2011; 153: 209-19.

Shinnar S, Bello JA, Chan S, et al. MRI abnormalities following febrile status epilepticus in children: The FEBSTAT study. *Neurology* 2012; 79: 871-7.

Shumate MD, Lin DD, Gibbs JWr, Holloway KL, Coulter DA. GABA(A): receptor function in epileptic human dentate granule cells: comparison to epileptic and control rat. *Epilepsy Res* 1998; 32: 114-28.

Siebzehnrubl F, Blümcke I. Neurogenesis in the human hippocampus and its relevance to temporal lobe epilepsies. *Epilepsia* 2008; 49: 55-65.

Sisodiya S, et al. Genetics of epilepsy: epilepsy research foundation workshop report. *Epileptic Disord* 2007; 9: 194-236.

Sloviter RS. Permanently altered hippocampal structure, excitability, and inhibition after experimental status epilepticus in the rat: the "dormant basket cell" hypothesis and its possible relevance to temporal lobe epilepsy. *Hippocampus* 1991; 1: 41-66.

Sloviter RS, Sollas AL, Barbaro NM, Laxer KD. Calcium-binding protein (calbindin-D28K): and parvalbumin immunocytochemistry in the normal and epileptic human hippocampus. *J Comp Neurol* 1991; 308: 381-96.

Sofroniew MV, Vinters HV. Astrocytes: biology and pathology. *Acta Neuropathol* 2010; 119: 7-35.

Sommer W. Erkrankung des Ammonshorns als aetiologisches Moment der Epilepsie. *Arch Psychiatr* 1880b; 10: 631-75.

Spalding KL, Bergmann O, Alkass K, et al. Dynamics of hippocampal neurogenesis in adult humans. *Cell* 2013; 153: 1219-27.

Spreafico R, Blümcke I. Focal cortical dysplasias: clinical implication of neuropathological classification systems. *Acta Neuropathol* 2010; 120: 359-67.

Stefan H, Pauli E. Progressive cognitive decline in epilepsy: an indication of ongoing plasticity. *Prog Brain Res* 2002; 135: 409-17.

Stefan H, Hildebrandt M, Kerling F, *et al*. Clinical prediction of postoperative seizure control: structural, functional findings and disease histories. *J Neurol Neurosurg Psychiatry* 2009; 80: 196-200.

Steinhauser C, Boison D. Epilepsy: crucial role for astrocytes. *Glia* 2012; 60: 1191.

Sutula TP, Cascino G, Cavazos J, Parada I, Ramirez L. Mossy fiber synaptic reorganization in the epileptic human temporal lobe. *Ann Neurol* 1989; 26: 321-30.

Tassi L, Garbelli R, Colombo N, *et al*. Type I focal cortical dysplasia: surgical outcome is related to histopathology. *Epileptic Disord* 2010; 12: 181-91.

Tauck DL, Nadler JV. Evidence of mossy fiber sprouting in hippocampal formation of kainic acid – treated rats. *J Neurosci* 1985; 5: 1016-22.

Thom M, Zhou J, Martinian L, Sisodiya S. Quantitative post-mortem study of the hippocampus in chronic epilepsy: seizures do not inevitably cause neuronal loss. *Brain* 2005a; 128: 1344-57.

Thom M, Mathern GW, Cross JH, Bertram EH. Mesial temporal lobe epilepsy: How do we improve surgical outcome? *Ann Neurol* 2010a; 68: 424-34.

Thom M, Martinian L, Williams G, Stoeber K, Sisodiya SM. Cell proliferation and granule cell dispersion in human hippocampal sclerosis. *J Neuropathol Exp Neurol* 2005b; 64: 194-201.

Thom M, Martinian L, Caboclo LO, McEvoy AW, Sisodiya SM. Balloon cells associated with granule cell dispersion in the dentate gyrus in hippocampal sclerosis. *Acta Neuropathol* 2008; 115: 697-700.

Thom M, Liagkouras I, Martinian L, Liu J, Catarino CB, Sisodiya S. Variability of sclerosis along the longitudinal hippocampal axis in epilepsy: A post mortem study. *Epilepsy Res* 2012; 102: 45-9.

Thom M, Eriksson S, Martinian L, *et al*. Temporal lobe sclerosis associated with hippocampal sclerosis in temporal lobe epilepsy: neuropathological features. *J Neuropathol Exp Neurol* 2009; 68: 928-38.

Thom M, Liagkouras I, Elliot KJ, *et al*. Reliability of patterns of hippocampal sclerosis as predictors of postsurgical outcome. *Epilepsia* 2010b; 51: 1801-8.

Townsend TN, Bernasconi N, Pike GB, Bernasconi A. Quantitative analysis of temporal lobe white matter T2 relaxation time in temporal lobe epilepsy. *Neuroimage* 2004; 23: 318-24.

Van Paesschen W, Connelly A, King MD, Jackson GD, Duncan JS. The spectrum of hippocampal sclerosis: a quantitative magnetic resonance imaging study. *Ann Neurol* 1997; 41: 41-51.

van Praag H, Schinder AF, Christie BR, Toni N, Palmer TD, Gage FH. Functional neurogenesis in the adult hippocampus. *Nature* 2002; 415: 1030-4.

von Lehe M, Lutz M, Kral T, Schramm J, Elger CE, Clusmann H. Correlation of health-related quality of life after surgery for mesial temporal lobe epilepsy with two seizure outcome scales. *Epilepsy Behav* 2006; 9: 73-82.

Wada J, Rasmussen T. Intracarotid injection of sodium amytal for the lateralisation of cerebral speech dominance: experimental and clinical observations. *J Neurosurg* 1960; 12: 230.

Wang D, Blümcke I, Gui Q, *et al*. Clinico-pathological investigations of Rasmussen encephalitis suggest multifocal disease progression and associated focal cortical dysplasia. *Epileptic Disord* 2013; 15: 32-43.

Wiebe S, Blume WT, Girvin JP, Eliasziw M. A randomized, controlled trial of surgery for temporal-lobe epilepsy. *N Engl J Med* 2001; 345: 311-8.

Wieser HG. ILAE Commission Report. Mesial temporal lobe epilepsy with hippocampal sclerosis. *Epilepsia* 2004; 45: 695-714.

Wieser HG, Ortega M, Friedman A, Yonekawa Y. Long-term seizure outcomes following amygdalohippocampectomy. *J Neurosurg* 2003; 98: 751-63.

Wilson SJ, Baxendale S, Barr W, *et al*. Indications and expectations for neuropsychological assessment in routine epilepsy care: Report of the ILAE Neuropsychology Task Force, Diagnostic Methods Commission, 2013-2017. *Epilepsia* 2015; 56: 674-81.

Wolf HK, Buslei R, Schmidt Kastner R, *et al*. NeuN: a useful neuronal marker for diagnostic histopathology. *J-Histochem-Cytochem* 1996; 44: 1167-71.

Wyler AR, Dohan FC, Schweitzer JB, Berry AD. A grading system for mesial temporal pathology (hippocampal sclerosis): from anterior temporal lobectomy. *J Epilepsy* 1992; 5: 220-5.

Yasuda CL, Morita ME, Alessio A, *et al*. Relationship between environmental factors and gray matter atrophy in refractory MTLE. *Neurology* 2010; 74: 1062-8.

Yilmazer-Hanke DM, Blümcke I, Wolf HK, Wiestler OD. Subregional pathology of the amygdala complex and entorhinal cortex in surgical specimens from patients with pharmaco-resistant temporal lobe epilepsy. *Clin Neuropathol* 1997; 16: 297.

Yilmazer-Hanke DM, Wolf HK, Schramm J, Elger CE, Wiestler OD, Blümcke I. Subregional pathology of the amygdala complex and entorhinal region in surgical specimens from patients with pharmacoresistant temporal lobe epilepsy. *J Neuropathol Exp Neurol* 2000; 59: 907-20.

3. Malformations of cortical development

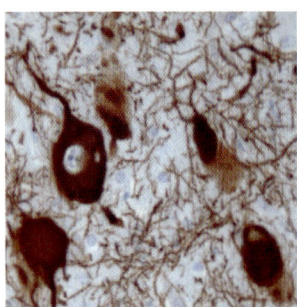

Harvey B. Sarnat, Ingmar Blümcke

Malformations of cortical development (MCD) represent a wide range of cortical lesions resulting from derangements of normal intrauterine developmental processes and involving cells implicated in the formation of the cortical mantle (Barkovich *et al.*, 2012; Marin-Padilla, 1978; Marin-Padilla, 1983; Najm *et al.*, 2014; Rakic, 1972; Ramon y Cajal, 1890; Ramon y Cajal, 1897; Ramon y Cajal, 1909-1911; Sarnat, 1992; Sarnat and Flores-Sarnat, 2002; Sarnat and Flores-Sarnat, 2013). In the past, these malformations have been defined as "neuronal migration disorders"; nevertheless, this term coined by American geneticists is technically inaccurate because neurones are mature cells that do not and cannot migrate, hence "neuroblast migratory disorder" is more suitable. However, both continue to be used. Moreover, since not all the cortical abnormalities have been proven to be due to migratory derangements, the general term of MCD is preferred as a reflection of our improved knowledge on normal and pathological brain development (Aronica *et al.*, 2012; Barkovich *et al.*, 2001; Sarnat and Flores-Sarnat, 2002). MCD are now recognized as a heterogeneous group of focal or diffuse anatomical abnormalities, determined by different causes that develop during crucial periods of cortical ontogenesis and their pathological features thus depend largely on the timing of the defect in the developmental processes, as well as on its causes (Barkovich *et al.*, 2012). It is implicit that the term MCD does not signify that developmental aberrations in the brain are necessarily exclusive to the cerebral cortex, as they often are associated with abnormal development of the hippocampus, cerebellum, basal ganglia and other structures of neural tube origin.

In analyzing congenital malformations of the brain, or indeed of any tissue of the body, distinction must be made between *aetiology* and *pathogenesis*. Genetic mutations or epigenetic insults such as foetal cerebral infarcts denote aetiology. The genotype does not necessarily predict the phenotype, nor does it explain the mechanism of development of tissue architecture and cellular morphology. Pathogenesis implies *mechanism* of tissue morphogenesis, often an aberration of one or more of the defined developmental processes, such as cellular proliferation, lineage, growth, apoptosis, migration, formation of neurites and synaptogenesis. *Neuroembryology* is a term that describes morphogenesis, both macroscopically as in the formation of convolutions of the cortex, and microscopically as in the arrangement of neurones and other cells. Technically, neuroembryology should be restricted to the first six weeks of post-conceptional age, the embryonic period proper in humans, but the term is usually now broadened to encompass the entire prenatal period.

The aetiology of malformative disorders often remains uncertain. Recent molecular biological and genetic studies have greatly expanded our knowledge, however, on brain ontogenesis so that several disorders of cortical development have been recognized and, for some of them, specific causative genetic defects have been identified (Guerrini and Dobyns, 2014; Guerrini *et al.*, 2008; Jamuar *et al.*, 2014). Though brain malformations have been recognized by neuropathologists since the XIXth century, improved imaging techniques, namely high resolution magnetic resonance imaging (MRI), have had a great diagnostic impact in this field, allowing *in vivo* diagnosis of various MCDs and providing correlations between imaging features, neurological deficits, developmental delays, and electro-clinical findings related to epilepsy (Colombo *et al.*, 2009; De Ciantis *et al.*, 2015). Furthermore, new methodological techniques including quantitative image analysis, MR spectroscopy (MRS), functional MRI (fMRI), diffusion tensor imaging (DTI) and fibre tract reconstructions are increasingly available and applicable to clinical practice, especially for the detection of small malformations (Berkovic and Jackson, 2014; Bernasconi and Bernasconi, 2014; Colombo *et al.*, 2009; Huppertz *et al.*, 2005; Jones *et al.*, 2014; Vollmar *et al.*, 2011; Yasuda *et al.*, 2014). These novel technologies will further improve our understanding about the functional relevance of affected cortical areas. Due to abnormal rearrangement of synaptic circuitries, MCDs can be intrinsically epileptogenic, a feature addressed by an increasing number of scientific publications during the last decade (Aronica *et al.*, 2012; Falace *et al.*, 2014; Lozovaya *et al.*, 2014; Yu *et al.*, 2012). The abnormal circuitry may be restricted to the malformed cortical area or may involve adjacent areas anatomically and functionally linked to the disorganized cortex. Due to the intrinsic epileptogenicity of these lesions most of partial epilepsies, previously defined as "cryptogenic" and frequently resistant to pharmacological therapy, are now recognized to be associated with malformative cortical lesions and likely susceptible to surgical therapy. As a consequence, an increasing number of epilepsy patients are surgically treated. Increasing availability of surgical specimens also evokes the interest of neuropathologists (Blümcke *et al.*, 2014; Blümcke and Spreafico, 2012). Their input not only covers a systematic microscopic work-up for diagnosis, but also the possibility to answer basic questions about the pathogenesis of MCDs and related epilepsies. This has been recently made possible by the addition to traditional routine histopathological methods, "new" powerful techniques fruitfully applied to human surgical tissue samples.

A precise incidence of MCDs is not known, but it appears that they are more common, particularly in patients with epilepsy, than was recognized in the pre-MRI era. Furthermore the increasing number of patients admitted for epilepsy surgery has further elucidated the neuropathological incidence of MCD in patients with otherwise unremarkable MRI, often because small lesions are below the resolution of neuroimaging. In large surgical series of patients with intractable epilepsy, the incidence of post-surgical diagnosis of different types of MCDs progressively increased from the early 1990s to the last few years (Lerner *et al.*, 2009; Tassi *et al.*, 2012). Although the statistical incidence of MCD in surgically treated patients varies in different centres, biased by factors such as different methodological approaches, patient selection, and MRI *versus* neuropathological diagnosis, it is estimated that 25%-40% of drug resistant childhood epilepsies are due to MCD and that 75% of patients with MCD will have epilepsy sometime in their life (Leventer *et al.*, 1999).

An increasing number of malformations are described in the current literature and many types and variants can be encountered in clinical practice. MCD represent the 3rd most frequent aetiology (n = 1,067; 19%) in the series of 5,603 surgical specimens reviewed at the German Neuropathology Reference Centre for Epilepsy Surgery (see *Chapter 1, Table I*). These patients

Table I

Clinico-pathological findings in epilepsy patients with cortical malformations

	All cases		Age at Onset	Surgery	Duration Epilepsy	Location FRON	TEMP	MULTI	PAR	OCC	OTHER
FCD II	427	40.0%	4.8	17.8	13.0	54.8%	18.7%	15.7%	5.6%	4.4%	0.7%
FCD I	170	15.9%	8.0	17.8	9.9	22.9%	36.5%	27.1%	5.3%	8.2%	~
mMCD	170	15.9%	9.6	22.6	13.1	31.2%	54.1%	11.8%	0.6%	1.8%	0.6%
FCD NOS	149	14.0%	7.2	21.0	13.7	26.8%	44.3%	12.1%	8.7%	7.4%	0.7%
PMG	51	4.8%	2.6	8.4	5.8	25.5%	23.5%	47.1%	3.9%	~	~
Tuber (TSC)	48	4.5%	1.3	7.7	6.4	54.2%	14.6%	12.5%	10.4%	8.3%	~
HME	34	3.2%	0.0	1.1	1.1	~	11.8%	88.2%	~	~	~
HET	15	1.4%	8.2	20.7	12.5	6.7%	26.7%	53.3%	13.3%	~	~
HAM	3	0.3%	1.3	28.0	26.7	~	33.3%	~	~	~	66.7%
TOTAL	1,067		6.0	17.7	11.6	38.1%	30.7%	20.5%	5.2%	4.8%	0.7%

Summary of 1,067 patients with intractable epilepsies and histopathologically confirmed malformations of cortical development. The data were obtained from the German Neuropathology reference centre for epilepsy surgery. FCD: focal cortical dysplasia; mMCD: mild malformations of cortical development (according to Palmini *et al.* 2004); HME: hemimegalencephaly; PMG: polymicrogyria; HET: nodular heterotopia; NOS: not otherwise specified; HAM: hamartoma, incl. hypothalamic hamartoma; age at onset and surgery: mean (in years); duration of epilepsy: mean (in years); location: frontal (FRON), temporal (TEMP), multilobar (MULTI), parietal (PAR) and occipital (OCC).

had a mean onset of their epilepsy at age 6 years and submitted to surgery at age 17. However, when reviewing only children (defined by age < 18 years), MCDs represent the most frequent cause with 37% of these 1,609 specimens. Seizure onset was at 1.8 years and surgery performed at 6.8 years of age (see *Table III* in chapter 8).

Some malformations have a clear pattern of inheritance, while others are almost exclusively sporadic; the genetic underpinnings of these malformations are increasingly being defined such that by now, more than 30 causative genes have been identified (Guerrini and Dobyns, 2014; Guerrini *et al.*, 2008; Jamuar *et al.*, 2014). Environmental causes, such as intrauterine infections, trauma and vascular-ischaemic events, also could be determinants for the generation of cortical malformations. Abnormal cortical development represents a major cause of epilepsy and severe malformations manifest with profound developmental delay and early onset seizures. Mild malformations may be detected after seizure onset at various ages in otherwise healthy individuals. There is no general consensus on these complex structural abnormalities and the current nomenclature is not uniform and, therefore, often misleading. Thus formulating a classification scheme for MCD is difficult and despite many efforts, it is widely recognized that classifications utilized in the current literature are far from satisfactory (Barkovich *et al.*, 2012; Barkovich *et al.*, 2001; Barkovich *et al.*, 2005). Indeed a particular defect in corticogenesis may give rise to more than one morphological subcategory of MCD and conversely a morphological subtype of MCD may result from multiple different mechanisms. Due to the complexity of the central nervous system (CNS) and to continuous progress in different fields of neurosciences, a unified and comprehensive classification is far from being formulated and needs continued debate. Any scheme must be flexible enough to be changed from time to time to accommodate with new data and revised interpretations.

Neuropathology has had a great impact in this aspect and careful analysis of neuropathological material, especially with the aid of new diagnostic methodologies, allowed the distinction and categorization of different forms of MCD. Differences amongst malformations previously grouped together have been revealed by high resolution MRI, while correlations between morphologically recognized malformations and electro-clinical findings have provided the basis for new classification schemes. Recent advances, particularly those derived from genetic analyses, highlight the need for more integrated and complex approaches to clarify MCD. A combined morphological and genetic scheme referring to malformations of the entire brain has been proposed, while Barkovich and co-workers have developed a new classification, specifically addressed to MCD, based on major stages at which cortical development is affected (Barkovich *et al.*, 2012; Barkovich *et al.*, 2005). The categories are based on known developmental steps, pathological features, genetics (when possible), and neuroimaging features. Since focal cortical dysplasias (FCD) are among the most frequent epileptogenic malformations, particularly susceptible to surgical treatment, a need for a specific classification of these abnormalities was envisaged. Based on combined neuroimaging, electro-clinical and neuropathological findings, different classifications of FCD have been proposed (Barkovich *et al.*, 2005; Mischel *et al.*, 1995; Palmini *et al.*, 2004; Tassi *et al.*, 2002). In light of the latest data however, including post-surgical outcome, a new consensus classification has been proposed by an ad hoc task force of the International League Against Epilepsy (ILAE) Diagnostic Methods Commission (Blümcke *et al.*, 2011).

It is already evident that the success of seizure control is better in FCD II than in FCD I (Najm *et al.*, 2014), despite the more severe histopathological appearance of FCD II because of the cellular dysmorphism and cytomegaly and the association with mTOR and tau abnormalities. One reason may be that FCD II is more focal, hence total resection is feasible in most cases, whereas some epileptogenic dysplastic cortex is left behind in many cases of FCD I (Krsek *et al.*, 2009). Aetiology remains, however, an important predictor for long-term seizure control after epilepsy surgery (Jehi *et al.*, 2015). When neuropathological criteria are not strictly applied for classification (Blümcke and Coras, 2013), reported outcome will continue to show large variability and contradiction between individual surgical series (Blümcke *et al.*, 2009; Fauser *et al.*, 2015; Krsek *et al.*, 2009).

The neuroembryologic basis of human cortical development and its various malformations

Columns are fatally attractive. To Western eyes reared on classical and neoclassical forms, they seem an existential necessity of the built world.
N.M. da Costa and K.A.C. Martin (2010)

Perhaps our human obsession with columns begins with the primordial columnar architecture of our foetal cerebral cortex.
H.B. Sarnat (2015)

To understand the pathogenesis of FCD, one must be familiar with the progressive development of the cerebral cortex during foetal life. A background of neuroembryology is primordial to neuropathological interpretation of surgical resections of epileptic foci in infants, children and adults, particularly if the lesion is developmental in nature. In the context of genetic aetiology and neuroembryology, the anatomical features and pathogenesis of the focal cortical dysplasias can be understood as dynamic aberrant processes of development rather than simply described as static resulting lesions. The epileptogenesis of such lesions also can be approached in terms of synaptic circuitry, imbalance of excitatory and inhibitory synaptic influences, neurotransmitter ratios and other physiological features that may also be reflected in electroencephalographic (EEG) recordings. Microscopically, immunoreactivities provide insight beyond what can be gleaned from interpretation of simple histological stains alone.

Gestational age (weeks)	Morphogenic process
3.5	Closure of the anterior neuropore; formation of the prosencephalic vesicle
4.5	Interhemispheric fissure divides prosencephalon into paired telencephalic hemispheres; cerebral mantle (ventricular to pial surface) consists of 2 layers: ventricular zone of neuroepithelium and marginal zone
5	Neuroblast migration from ganglionic eminence (ventricular zone) into marginal zone to form pre-plate plexus; continued tangential migration from ganglionic eminence
6	Formation of radial glial fibres from sub-ventricular zone extending to pial surface
7	First wave of radial migratory neuroblasts along radial glia from sub-ventricular zone into middle of marginal zone to form the cortical plate, also separating the superficial part of marginal zone as the molecular zone (future layer 1 of cortex) and sub-plate zone deep to cortical plate; first axons of anterior and hippocampal commissures cross midline
8-16	Continued waves of radial migratory neuroblasts, the most recent arrivals to the surface of the cortical plate and the earlier arrivals deeper into cortical plate (inside-out arrangement); 90% of neuroblast migration complete by 16 weeks; most radial migratory cells from sub-ventricular zone after 16 weeks become cortical protoplasmic astrocytes
10	Pioneer axons of corpus callosum traverse midline, their cells of origin are pyramidal neurones of future cortical layer 3
14	First synapses in deep molecular zone and subplate zone
8-22	Micro-columnar histological architecture of cortical plate
22	Superimposition of tangential (horizontal) lamination of cortical plate, which eventually predominates; synaptogenesis begins in cortical plate, initially in deep tangential layers
32-early post-natal period	Retraction of radial glial processes no longer needed to guide migratory cells; most become fibrillary astrocytes of white matter; continued cytological maturation of cortical neurones and synapse formation

Table II

Summary of events in morphogenesis and maturation of the human cerebral cortex. Age refers to post-conceptional weeks of gestation

The cerebral mantle or pallium of the human embryo at 4-6 weeks gestation consists of two concentric zones between the ventricular and pial surfaces and then four concentric zones in the foetus at 7-8 weeks. The two zones before 7 weeks are the ventricular zone of neuroepithelium, with proliferating cells at the ventricular surface where ependymal is not yet differentiated, and the more peripheral marginal zone that contains scattered neurons that form a pre-plate plexus before the first wave of radial migratory neuroblasts occurs (Duckett and Pearse, 1968; Marin-Padilla, 1978, Marin-Padilla, 1983; Marín-Padilla, 2011; Sarnat, 1992; Sarnat and Flores-Sarnat, 2002). Beginning at about 7 weeks, post-mitotic neuroblasts initiate a radial migration from the ventricular zone. In the superficial layer of the ventricular zone, specialized radial glial cells form, each projecting a long, thin process radially to span the entire cerebral mantle to terminate at its pial surface (Rakic, 1972). This sub-ventricular zone consists of post-mitotic neuroepithelial cells, radial glial cells and pre-migratory neuroblasts. It also is known as the germinal matrix, not technically correct because it does not include proliferative cells, but the term has become traditional in usage. Migratory neuroblasts attach to the outsides of radial glial fibres to form a row of distally moving cells into the middle of the marginal zone, where they form the cortical plate, leaving the most superficial part of the marginal zone as the molecular layer, later to become layer 1 of the mature horizontally laminated cortex, and the part deep to the cortical plate as the subplate zone, a transitory foetal structure later incorporated into the deep cortical laminae. An intermediate zone lies between the sub-ventricular zone and the sub-plate zone.

To summarize, the four concentric zones of the foetal cerebral mantle after 7 weeks gestations are, from the ventricle outward: 1) the ventricular (proliferative neuroepithelium); 2) sub-ventricular (post-mitotic, pre-migratory neuroblasts and glioblasts and radial glial cells); 3) intermediate zone (future subcortical white matter, traversed by radial glial fibres and their migratory neuroblasts); and 4) the cortical plate together with the molecular layer and sub-plate (former marginal zone).

• Radial migration and the origin of micro-columnar neocortical architecture

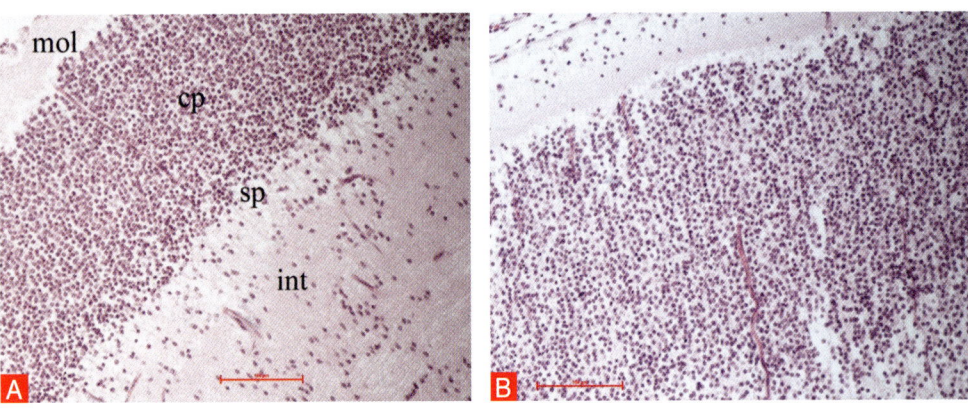

Figure 1

Microscopic findings in human cortical development

Cortical plate of foetuses of A) 9 weeks and B) 15 weeks gestation. The cortical plate (cp) forms in the middle of the previous marginal zone, leaving a superficial molecular layer (mol) and a deep subplate zone (sp). Migratory neuroblasts are seen in the intermediate zone (int), the future sub-cortical white matter.

The initial architecture (i.e. arrangement of neurones) within the foetal cortical plate is radial micro-columnar until mid-gestation (Figure 1). After 22 weeks the histological pattern of a tangential or horizontal lamination becomes evident, initially superimposed upon the radial micro-columnar pattern and eventually predominates. Even in the normal mature neocortex of adults, however, some evidence of the earlier radial pattern persists, particularly in areas where the cortex bends, in the depths of sulci and the crowns of gyri. The term micro-columnar denotes a single row of cells arranged perpendicular to the pial surface, whereas columnar refers more to a radial column of clustered cells or a mixed radial aggregate of neurones, glial cells, dendritic bundles and vertical synaptic layers. In ischaemia of the foetal brain, radial glial fibres tend to approach the radially oriented arterioles and thus perivascular columns of migratory cells are demonstrated.

Because the immature neurones of the cortical plate have sparse cytoplasm and a paucity of neuropil between them, the architecture may be difficult to discern in young foetuses, but a micro-columnar architecture predominates throughout the first half of gestation, the more mature tangential (horizontal) histological layering becoming superimposed and eventually dominating after 22 weeks gestation. Nevertheless, horizontal layer-specific protein markers can identify a tangential primordium even before it becomes histologically evident. This foetal pattern of micro-columnar architecture of the cortex thus may be regarded as a maturational arrest when it appears as a feature of FCD Ia in the postnatal period and in older children and adults. NeuN, a late marker of neuronal maturation, is not yet reactive in cortical neurones during the first half of gestation, hence cannot be applied to early foetal cortex.

As the cerebral mantle grows, there is a corresponding growth in length of the radial glial fibres (Schmechel and Rakic, 1979), as well as curving of these fibres with the formation of the telencephalic flexure and, later, with development of sulci and gyri (*Figure 2*). Radial glial cells do not normally proliferate after mid-gestation (Schmechel and Rakic, 1979), but have the potential to do so under certain pathological conditions. Radial glial cells retain many properties of resident stem cells, expressing primitive proteins such as vimentin and nestin and, if injury occurs in the foetal cortical plate, they are capable of differentiating as new neurones to replace those lost, a regenerative process unique to the foetal brain. When neuroblast and glioblast migration is nearly complete, from about 32 weeks gestation into the early postnatal weeks, the long, slender radial glial fibres retract from the pial surface and their cells of origin mainly mature as fibrillary astrocytes of the white matter.

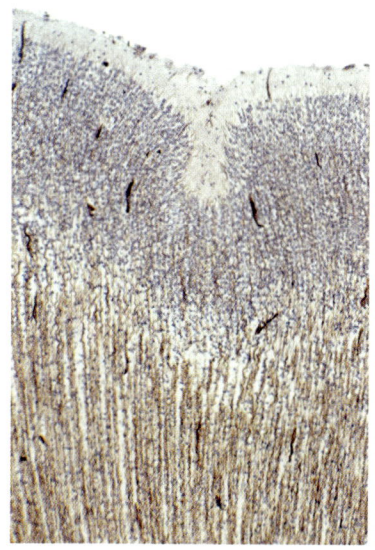

Figure 2

Early formation of a sulcus

Cerebral cortex of a 24-week foetus, showing early formation of a sulcus. The radial glial fibres, here demonstrated by brown vimentin immunoreactivity, curve around the developing sulcus. Haematoxylin counterstain for cellular nuclei.

Polypeptides as cell adhesion molecules in the extra-cellular matrix between the membranes of the radial glial fibre and the migratory neurones are needed to enable attachment of neuroepithelial cells to the radial glial fibre at the proximal end (Anton *et al.*, 1996). Disadhesion molecules are required at the distal end of the journey. Antibodies against these molecules cause retraction of the leading process of the migratory cell, changes in microtubular organization and, finally, detachment of the cell from the radial glial fibre (Reisin and Colombo, 2002). This detachment mechanism within the cortical plate enables the inverse gradient of organization of the micro-columns, so that more recent arrivals on the same radial glial fibre can bypass the earlier arrived neuroblasts; when migratory cells are prevented from detaching, the organization of the cortical plate is disrupted (Reisin and Colombo, 2002).

Vertically oriented glial septa form between the micro-columns; these glial cells have an intimate relation with the adjacent neuroblast and may facilitate the development of membrane receptors and ion channels of the immature neuronal membrane, as well as serving to isolate neighbouring columns (Ciceri *et al.*, 2013; Costa and Hedin-Pereira, 2010; Reisin and Colombo, 2002). Another unique type of astrocyte, the comet cell, is associated with the Cajal-Retzius neurones and also plays an important role in maintenance and repair of the glia limitans at the pial surface of the cortex (Ramon y Cajal, 1890).

• Role of Cajal-Retzius and sub-plate neurones

About 20% of neurones of the cortical plate arrive not by radial migration but rather by tangential migration from the lateral ganglionic eminence, a specialized region of the germinal matrix overlying the head of the caudate nucleus and extending posteriorly (Bayer and Altman, 1990; Lavdas *et al.*, 1999; Marín-Padilla, 1998; Rakic, 1995; Ulfig, 2001). These cells become inhibitory GABAergic inter-neurones and are distributed in all horizontal layers of the mature cortex, though they predominate in the superficial layers. The ganglionic eminence also is the origin of the Cajal-Retzius neurones of the pre-plate plexus and of neurones of the sub-plate zone, preceding the arrival of the first wave of radial neuroblast migrations (Marin-Padilla, 1978; Marin-Padilla, 1983; Marín-Padilla, 1998). The large bipolar and multi-polar Cajal-Retzius neurones, with their long axons extending parallel to the pial surface, were first described in the 1890s (Ramon y Cajal, 1890; Ramon y Cajal, 1897; Retzius, 1891; Retzius, 1894) and confirmed by much later investigators (Frotscher, 1997; Sarnat and Flores-Sarnat,

2002). Their long horizontal axons give rise to multiple collateral axons that extend ventrally into all depths of the cortical plate. They provide the first intrinsic cortical synaptic circuits with dendrites from neurones in deep parts of the cortical plate, many of which ascend radially to the molecular layer for synaptic contact (Marin-Padilla, 1978). Cajal-Retzius neurones express the gene *Reelin* (*RELN; Reln*), important in mediating the initial micro-columnar organization of the cortical plate (Frotscher, 1997; Nishikawa *et al.*, 2002; Schmechel and Rakic, 1979). The *reeler* mouse is a mutant model exhibiting failure of the normal "inside-out" pattern of neocortical formation (Dernoncourt *et al.*, 1991; Falconer, 1951). It displays disruption of vertical columnar structure of the neocortex, demonstrating the importance of Reln and Cajal-Retzius neurones for micro-columnar, as well as for later horizontal lamination (Nishikawa *et al.*, 2002). Early foetal alcohol exposure also alters cortical columnar organization and may account for cortical visual impairment in infants with foetal alcohol syndrome (Medina *et al.*, 2005). In the developing hippocampus, *Reelin* signalling attracts newly generated neurones toward their terminal destination and is particularly essential for horizontal lamination of granular neurones of the dentate gyrus (Zhao *et al.*, 2004). Deficiency of *Reelin* causes granule cell dispersion from the dentate gyrus in hippocampi of epileptic patients (Haas and Frotscher, 2010; Kobow *et al.*, 2009). Reelin also is essential for the centripetal migration of the external granular layer of the cerebellar cortex. Another gene primordial in the reorganization and maturation of the foetal cortical plate is GPR56 that programmes a family of cell-adhesion G-protein-coupled receptors with a large extracellular domain to regulate the integrity of the pial membrane and cortical lamination; defective expression of GPR56 results in polymicrogyria with abnormal microscopical lamination (Bahi-Buisson *et al.*, 2010; Li *et al.*, 2008).

Cajal-Retzius neurones are GABAergic and strongly immuno-reactive for calcium-binding proteins such as calretinin (Allendoerfer and Shatz, 1994, Imamoto *et al.*, 1994; Marty *et al.*, 1996; Sarnat, 2013; Ulfig, 2002; Verney and Derer, 1995). Brain-derived neurotrophic factor (BDNF) regulates the calretinin content of Cajal-Retzius neurones, but is not necessary for their survival (Marty *et al.*, 1996). It was once thought that Cajal-Retzius neurones were transitory cells that disappeared during maturation, because they are frequent in mid-gestational foetal brains, less in term neonates and rarely encountered in adult brains. It is now known that they do not undergo apoptosis, degenerate or disappear; because they do not proliferate after embryonic and early foetal life, they simply become sparse because of volumetric dilution with growth of the brain (Martin *et al.*, 1999; Sanides and Sas, 1970). They are more prominent in the molecular zone in polymicrogyric cortex (Eriksson *et al.*, 2001) and hippocampal sclerosis (Blümcke *et al.*, 1996; Blümcke *et al.*, 1999).

The sub-plate zone also is critical in the initial organization and maturation of the cortical plate, including its micro-columnar architecture in the first half of gestation. This zone is histologically most evident between 13 and 34 weeks gestation (Allendoerfer and Shatz, 1994; Kostovic and Jovanov-Milosevic, 2008; Rakic, 1972), but most prominent shortly after mid-gestation, thereafter regressing as its neurones become incorporated into layer 6. A primordial sub-plate zone already is formed, however, at the time of the initial appearance of the cortical plate at 7 weeks, when the first radial migration to the middle of the marginal layer begins (*Figure 1*). Its neurones are GABAergic and strongly reactive with anti-calretinin and anti-parvalbumin antibodies, as with Cajal-Retzius neurones (Belichenko *et al.*, 1995; Imamoto *et al.*, 1994; Sarnat, 2013; Sarnat, 2015; Ulfig, 2002; Verney and Derer, 1995). They have extensive dendritic and axonal ramifications that enable an electrical discharge rate exceeding 40 Hz, enabling them to function as important amplifying units with the developing neocortical circuitry (Luhmann *et al.*, 2009). Prominent gap junction coupling in the subplate and cortical plate elicit 10-20 Hz oscillations in the local columnar network (Luhmann *et al.*, 2009). The early maturation of sub-plate neurones and their numerous neurites account for the large amount of neuropil in the sub-plate, by contrast with sparse neuropil in the overlying cortical plate. The spontaneous early intrinsic electrical activity in the subplate subserves a framework for development of cortical columnar architecture (McConnell *et al.*, 1989).

Subplate neurones are generally oriented perpendicular to the surface of the brain, contrasting with the horizontal orientation of Cajal-Retzius neurones. They emit transitory pioneer axons for the incipient internal capsule that later guide the permanent long projection axons from pyramidal neurones in layers 5 and 6 (McConnell *et al.*, 1989; McConnell *et al.*, 1994). Subplate pioneer axones from the cingulate cortical plate also provide pioneer axones of the corpus callosum at 25-32 weeks gestation to guide permanent axones of small pyramidal neurones in layer 3 (deAzevedo *et al.*, 1997). Afferent thalamo-cortical axones may be an extrinsic factor influencing columnar organization during corticogenesis (Hubel and Wiesel, 1972; Li *et al.*, 2013; McConnell *et al.*, 1994; Rockland, 2002). Blockade of glutamate receptors of cortical plate synapses interferes with development of thalamo-cortical projections and columnar architecture (Fox *et al.*, 1996).

The arrangement of the cortical plate in the first half of gestation, mediated by radial migration and organized by Cajal-Retzius and sub-plate neurones, thus is a multi-columnar architecture without tangential (*i.e.* horizontal) layering yet evident histologically. The first recognition of this radial architecture was made by Golgi impregnations by Ramón y Cajal (Ramon y Cajal, 1881; Ramon y Cajal, 1909-1911) and by Lorente de Nó (Lorente de Nó, 1934), but further defined by Mountcastle (Mountcastle, 1997), who elaborated the concept of functional micro-columns because of his integration of neuroanatomical and neurophysiological data (see below). Microcolumns in focal cortical dysplasias are best demonstrated by NeuN immunoreactivity, but NeuN is a late maturational marker and is not expressed in neurones of the cortical plate during the first and early second trimesters, so histological stains such as H&E are usually employed; antibodies against MAP2, an early neuronal marker also can be used (Sarnat, 2013).

• Dendritic bundles in micro-columns

Micro-columns involve not only the arrangement of immature neuronal somata, but also columns of their ascending dendrites. These dendritic bundles do not extend through the full thickness of the cortex, but rather exhibit intra- and inter-areal variations within and between columns (Molliver *et al.*, 1973). The perpendicular extensions of these radial dendritic bundles laterally to adjacent columns during the first half of gestation is most pronounced and longest from the superficial cortical plate, the future layer 2, even though the granular neurones of layer 2 are from the last waves of radial migration. Perhaps their relation to a mainly afferent rather than a mainly efferent lamina of pyramidal neurones is the principal reason. In mouse somato-sensory cortex, connections between pyramidal neurones of layer 5 form independently of apical dendritic bundling (Cameron and Rakic, 1994). Despite dendritic arborization, chemical synapses are not formed in the cortical plate until about 22 weeks gestation as shown by synaptophysin reactivity (Sarnat *et al.*, 2010). Synapses can be demonstrated by transmission electron microscopy in the molecular and sub-plate zones at their junctions with the cortical plate as early as 14 weeks gestation, but not in the cortical plate itself (Molliver *et al.*, 1973). In early stages, local neuronal networks are organized in the cortex by non-synaptic gap junctions that form a columnar syncytium (McConnell *et al.*, 1994).

Vertically oriented glial septa form between the micro-columns; these glial cells have an intimate relation with the adjacent neuroblast and may facilitate the development of membrane receptors and ion channels of the immature neuronal membrane, as well as serving to isolate neighbouring columns (Ciceri *et al.*, 2013; Costa and Hedin-Pereira, 2010; Reisin and Colombo, 2002). Another unique type of astrocyte, the comet cell, is associated with the Cajal-Retzius neurones and also plays an important role in maintenance and repair of the glia limitans at the pial surface of the cortex (Ramon y Cajal, 1890).

• Tangential/horizontal cortical lamination

In the second half of gestation, the familiar horizontal layering becomes superimposed on the micro-columnar architecture and becomes the predominant histological pattern by 30 weeks. Ascending dendrites of cortical neurones are not confined exclusively to their respective micro-columns, but have lateral growth as well to begin to interconnect adjacent micro-columns, which helps establish the tangential or horizontal lamination. Neuronal maturation in each horizontal layer also helps to distinguish the layers, pyramidal cells forming layers 3, 5 and 6 and granular neurones forming layers 2 and 4. Synaptic layers also can be demonstrated between cellular horizontal laminae in the cortex, but vertical lamination of synapses is not seen in the first half of gestation because there are no synapses in the cortical plate, hence no synaptic vesicle reactivity of synaptophysin. The horizontal synaptic layering is evident from about 24 to 35 weeks gestation, but after that time synaptophysin reactivity becomes so uniform throughout the grey matter of the cerebral cortex that the synaptic layers no longer show sufficient contrast to be distinguished from synaptic vesicular reactivity around neurones and neuropil in the cellular layers. Neuronal lineage may already be tentatively programmed in pre-migratory neuroblasts in the sub-ventricular zone, so that later, neuronal differentiation within the cortical plate corresponds to horizontal laminar more than the earlier radial microcolumnar organization even before tangential lamination is histologically evident, and may be altered in FCD (Arai *et al.*, 2012; Costa and Hedin-Pereira, 2010; Hadjivassiliou *et al.*, 2010; Hevner, 2007; Rossini *et al.*, 2011; Sakakibara *et al.*, 2012; Sanes and Yamagata, 1999). Excitatory projection neurones may be amenable to directed reprogramming of their class-specific features to enable enhanced cortical plasticity in the mature brain (Lodato *et al.*, 2015). Input from the thalamus appears to have minimal influence on initial reorganization of the cortex, but may be essential for other aspects of maturation (Rakic, 2002). Thalamic input to developing cortex helps organize the cortical plate into topographic zones in the rostro-caudal gradient of the longitudinal axis (Finlay and Uchiyama, 2015).

Tangential migration of GABAergic inhibitory interneurones of the cortical plate, arriving from the ganglionic eminence, begins soon after the cortical plate forms, though the Cajal-Retzius and subplate neurones are evidence of earlier migrations from that site. At mid-gestation, about 5% of cortical neurones are calretinin-reactive and by term about 12% of total cortical neurones are reactive. Other calcium-binding proteins, particularly parvalbumin, react for the remaining 8% of interneurones. This subset of GABAergic cortical interneurones reactive for parvalbumin is unique because they inhibit other inhibitory interneurones rather than inhibiting excitatory cortical neurones from radial migrations as do the calretinin-reactive interneurones (Gentet *et al.*, 2012; Kepecs and Fishell, 2014; Lee *et al.*, 2012; Lovett-Barron *et al.*, 2012; Pfeffer *et al.*, 2013; Pi *et al.*, 2013). Whereas calretinin is a good marker of the majority (80%) of GABAergic inhibitory interneurons in the cerebral cortex, parvalbumin is a specific marker of a subpopulation of these GABAergic interneurons (Andressen *et al.*, 1993) that suppress somatostatin and specialize in disinhibitory control, mediated by inhibiting other inhibitory interneurons (Kepecs and Fishell, 2014). A wide range of specialized variability of GABAergic inhibitory interneurones is increasingly recognized (Katzel *et al.*, 2011), as well as the columnar and horizontal laminar extents of their synaptic relations with excitatory neurones of the cerebral cortex (Powell and Mountcastle, 1959).

• Functions of columnar cortical architecture

How the micro-columns function in the human foetus in the first half of gestation is poorly understood, particularly in the absence of intrinsic synapses in the cortical plate. Functional columns in the mature cortex were defined by Rakic as "neurones within a given column that are stereotypically interconnected in the vertical dimension, share extrinsic connectivity and hence act as basic units subserving a set of common functions" (Feldmeyer *et al.*, 2013; Lovett-Barron *et al.*, 2012). Functional columns in the mature cerebral cortex were first defined by Powell and Mountcastle (Powell and Mountcastle, 1959) and shortly thereafter in the 1981 Nobel Prize-winning studies by Hubel and Wiesel (Hubel and Wiesel, 1969; Hubel and Wiesel, 1972; Hubel *et al.*, 1977) in the visual cortex of the cat, and even more precisely in the monkey. Their studies confirmed and expanded the concept of functional visual orientation columns in striate cortex of the adult, despite the distinctive histological pattern of horizontal lamination with a prominent layer 4 that is uniquely subdivided into two laminae only in occipital striate cortex. Local columnar micro-circuits also have been demonstrated in somato-sensory cortex to subserve the vibrissae (i.e. whiskers) of animals such as cats and rodents that rely upon this sensory input to ambulate in the dark (Rakic, 2000). Motor cortex also exhibits a columnar organization, based on electrophysiological evidence (Sato *et al.*, 2008). Mountcastle defined the concept of intracortical columnar "modules" with linkages between them and with variable subsets based upon different extrinsic connections (Mountcastle, 1997). Rakic complemented this concept by showing that the radial unit hypothesis of expansion of neocortical surface area (by more than a thousand-fold, without a corresponding increase in cortical thickness) during mammalian evolution and human ontogenesis can be explained by columnar architecture (Rakic, 2000); regulator genes programme the timing (onset, rate and duration) and mode (symmetrical *vs.* asymmetrical) of cell division in the ventricular zone that determines the number of cortical cells at maturity (Keil *et al.*, 2010). Despite considerable enlargement of the primary visual cortex in the cat, the spacing between columns is largely preserved, but a growth-induced reorganization that renders the columns more "zig-zag" occurs, representing a dynamical instability (Horton and Adams, 2005). There are regional differences in the functional columns as the cortex differentiates, for example between the insular and somatosensory cortex, so that columnar information processing may not be uniform across different cortical areas (Mischel *et al.*, 1995). Functional columns in both developing and mature sensory cortex are often termed "barrels" by neurophysiologists.

Despite the large volume of anatomical evidence of columnar architecture in early development and electrophysiological columnar organization of the cortex at maturity, some investigators remain reserved or even sceptical of the importance of functional columns or barrels (da Costa and Martin, 2010; Horton and Adams, 2005). Rockland and Ichinohe questioned whether the columnar dendritic bundles they helped describe really correspond to functional columns (Rockland and Ichinohe, 2004).

Focal cortical dysplasia (FCD)

Taylor and colleagues were first in 1971 to describe neuropathological features of FCD in surgical specimens of 10 epilepsy patients (Taylor *et al.*, 1971). They reported, as the most evident microscopic feature, the disruption of the normal cortical lamination by the presence of "large aberrant neurones", as well as the presence of "grotesque cells" in both cortex and subcortical white matter (Taylor *et al.*, 1971). The authors suggested that these aberrant ("exotic") populations of nerve cells may underlie the clinical manifestations of certain forms of focal epilepsy and also discuss the similarities with the neuropathological features of cortical lesions in patients with tuberous sclerosis complex (TSC), emphasizing the possibility of a *forme fruste* of TSC (Taylor *et al.*, 1971). Before the comprehensive description provided by Taylor and colleagues, few autopsy cases of focal cerebral gliosis with giant nerve cells in patients with intractable epilepsy had been reported and interpreted as a congenital condition of unknown aetiology and pathogenesis (Crome, 1957). Already in 1896, Lombroso and Roncoroni reported focal cytoarchitectural cortical malformations reminiscent of the *Taylor-Type* FCD in patients with epilepsy (reviewed in (Chio *et al.*, 2003). Since these first reports, it has become clear that different histopathological features can be encountered in clinical practice and that the morphological spectrum of FCD is broad, including FCD variants with architectural and cytoarchitectural abnormalities.

FCD may represent an isolated lesion, although cortical dyslamination can also be detected adjacent to hippocampal sclerosis, glio-neuronal tumours, vascular malformations, as well as adjacent to a large variety of lesions acquired either early during brain development or later during brain maturation (Blümcke, 2009). During the past 15 years, different FCD classification systems have been proposed (Barkovich *et al.*, 2012; Barkovich *et al.*, 2005; Mischel *et al.*, 1995; Palmini *et al.*, 2004; Tassi *et al.*, 2002). The classification published by Palmini in 2004 was the consensus report of an international workshop and was mainly based on histopathological features, sub-classifying the FCD into Type I and Type II categories. Palmini's FCD Type I referred to alterations in cortical lamination for Type Ia, with additional cytoarchitectural abnormalities found in Type Ib; Palmini's FCD Type II referred to FCD including both cortical dyslamination and cellular abnormalities (equivalent to the *Taylor-Type* FCD), such as the presence of dysplastic (dysmorphic) neurones (Type IIa) and with balloon cells in addition (Type IIb). During the past 6 years this classification system has been extensively used as a basis for several scientific reports (Sisodiya *et al.*, 2009; Spreafico and Blümcke, 2010), but failed to provide consistent associations with clinical and neuroradiological features. Furthermore, the prediction of postsurgical seizure control remained ambiguous, particularly for FCD Type I (Blümcke *et al.*, 2009; Krsek *et al.*, 2008; Lerner *et al.*, 2009; Spreafico and Blümcke, 2010). This variability may possibly reflect inconsistent histological diagnoses, especially for Type I FCDs, which in the Palmini's classification included different entities (*i.e.*, isolated and associated FCD variants).

Accordingly, a recent study reported excellent interobserver concordance for the neuropathological diagnosis of FCD Type II, but relatively poor inter- and intra-observer agreement for the type I subtypes (Chamberlain *et al.*, 2009). These findings suggested the need to refine neuropathological diagnostic criteria of FCD subtypes to achieve improved reproducibility and enhanced insight into the clinico-pathological correlations of FCD subtypes. A task force of the ILAE has therefore generated a new consensus classification of FCD subtypes based on histopathological features and representing the basis for prospective clinical studies addressing the epileptogenicity of different FCD variants (Blümcke *et al.*, 2011). Its histopathological reliability also was tested by a large and comprehensive intra- and inter-rater agreement (Coras *et al.*, 2012).

Table III

ILAE consensus neuropathological classification system for FCDs

The three-tiered ILAE classification system for focal cortical dysplasias (FCD) distinguishes isolated forms (FCD Type I and II) from those cortical layer abnormalities associated with another principal lesion (FCD Type III)

FCD Type I (isolated)	Focal cortical dysplasia with abnormal radial cortical organization (FCD Ia)	Focal cortical dysplasia with abnormal tangential cortical lamination (FCD Ib)	Focal cortical dysplasia with abnormal radial and tangential cortical organization (FCD Ic)
FCD Type II (isolated)	Focal cortical dysplasia with dysmorphic neurones (FCD IIa)		Focal cortical dysplasia with dysmorphic neurones and balloon cells (FCD IIb)
FCD Type III (associated with principal lesion)	Cortical lamination abnormalities in the temporal lobe associated with hippocampal sclerosis (FCD IIIa)	Cortical lamination abnormalities adjacent to a glial or glio-neuronal tumour (FCD IIIb)	Cortical lamination abnormalities adjacent to vascular malformation (FCD IIIc)	Cortical lamination abnormalities adjacent to any other lesion acquired during early life, *e.g.*, trauma, ischemic injury, encephalitis (FCD IIId)

FCD Type III (not otherwise specified, NOS): if clinically/radiologically suspected principal lesion is not available for microscopic inspection.

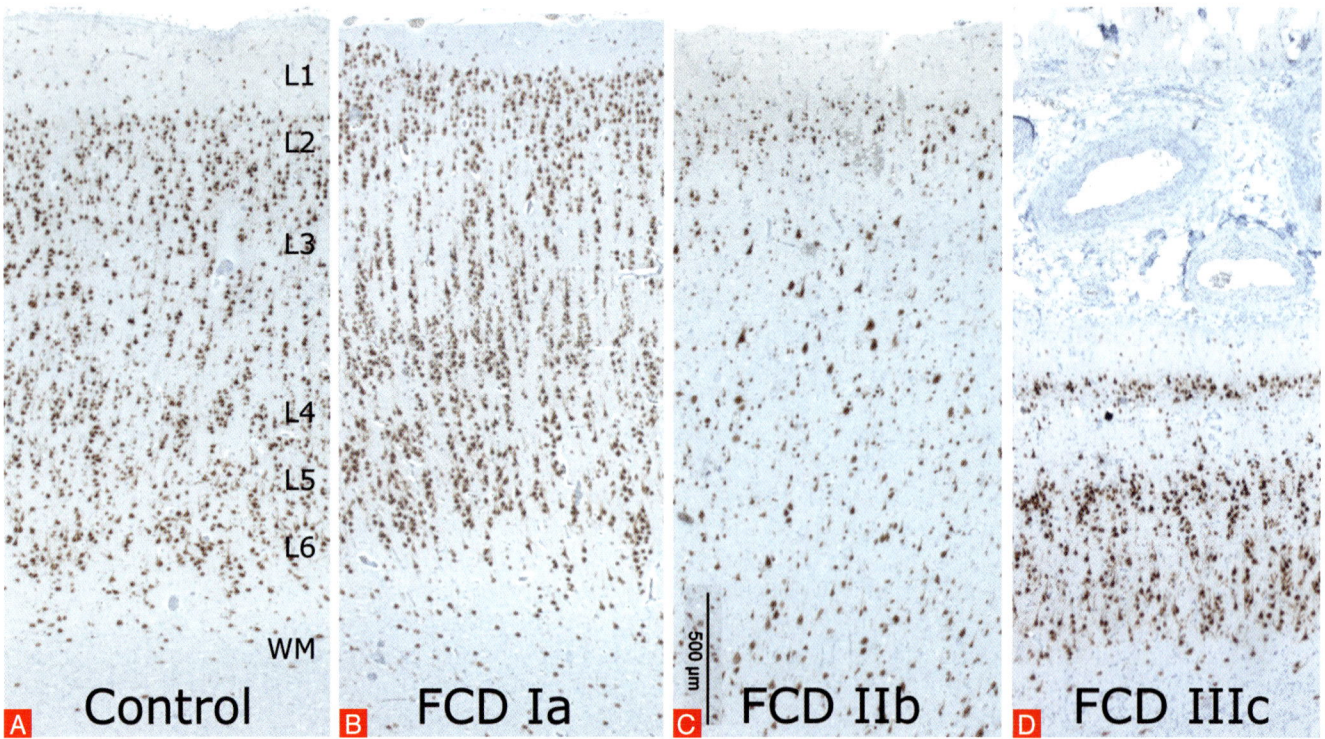

Figure 3

Histopathological signatures of ILAE FCD subtypes.

NeuN immunoreactivity in human neocortical brain specimens obtained from epilepsy surgery (L1-L6: cortical layering; WM: white matter). Note that each FCD subtype can be classified by its distinct architectural signature. Refer to specific paragraphs below for detailed description of FCD I, II and III subtypes.

• FCD ILAE Type I

The ILAE classification system of FCD consists of a three-tiered system, including both isolated and associated FCD variants (Blümcke *et al.*, 2011). FCD Type I refers to isolated forms of FCD, characterized by an abnormal cortical layering, which may affect one or multiple lobes and is often observed in young patients with severe epilepsy and psychomotor retardation (Blümcke *et al.*, 2010; Krsek *et al.*, 2009; Tassi *et al.*, 2010). The new ILAE classification includes three FCD Type I subtypes, according to the pattern of cortical dyslamination (*Table III*). FCD Type Ia is characterized by abnormal radial migration (*Figure 3*), as well as neuronal maturation with immature small diameter neurones organized into micro-columns, resembling the micro-columnar organization pattern described during the early stages of cortical development (Blümcke *et al.*, 2011, Rakic and Lombroso, 1998). However, the diagnosis of this FCD subtype requires particular attention when studying specimens of temporal polar cortex, including areas that tend to maintain a columnar appearance (Ding *et al.*, 2009). In addition to the micro-columnar organization, increased numbers of heterotopic neurones are often observed and hypertrophic neurones can also be encountered outside layer 5 (Blümcke *et al.*, 2011). FCD Type Ib is characterized by abnormal cortical layering affecting the 6-layered tangential organization of the neocortex and including a large spectrum of histopathological features ranging from alterations of the entire neocortical architecture to a more subtle abnormal layering involving specific layers, such as layer 2 or layer 4 or both (Blümcke *et al.*, 2011). Also in this FCD subtypes heterotopic neurones in white matter and hypertrophic neurones (outside layer 5) can be encountered, as well as normal neurones with disoriented dendrites (Blümcke *et al.*, 2011). FCD Type Ic refers to isolated lesions characterized by abnormal cortical layering affecting both radial and tangential cortical organization (Blümcke *et al.*, 2011). Immunocytochemical analysis using antibodies directed against NeuN (Neuronal nuclear antigen) can improve the visualization of the cortical layer abnormalities characteristics of the FCD type I subtypes; heterotopic neurones within the white matter can be visualized using NeuN or MAP2 (microtubule-associated protein 2) immunohistochemistry (Blümcke *et al.*, 2011).

FCD ILAE Type Ia in the context of foetal cortical development

FCD Ia is the most frequent subtype of type I. It is characterized by a histological pattern of the cerebral cortex as radial micro-columnar architecture rather than horizontal lamination of neurones and synaptic layers, the mature cortical pattern. FCD1a can be regarded as a maturational arrest at mid-gestation, before the histological transition from micro-columnar to tangential (horizontal) lamination. The radial pattern is abnormal because of the age of the patient and persistence of the foetal pattern (Sarnat and Flores-Sarnat, 2013).

Another pattern often seen in FCD Ia, at times in adjacent gyri of the same brain that exhibits micro-columnar architecture, is lack of any identifiable organization, neither radial nor horizontal. Neurones have disoriented neurites, are often displaced in the wrong layers and each horizontal layer has an abnormal mixture of neuronal types. From a developmental perspective, this lack of cortical architecture may be secondary to failure of migratory neuroblasts to detach from their radial glial guide fibres within the cortical plate, so that later arrivals cannot bypass the earlier arrivals. This defect could be related to defective extra-cellular dis-adhesion molecules (Anton *et al.*, 1996).

The reason for a focal arrest in maturation and failure of transition from radial micro-columnar to tangential or horizontal laminar architecture is unclear. The great majority of FCD type 1 cases are sporadic, but familial cases are now described, raising the question of a possible genetic origin in some that express a Mendelian trait and perhaps in others in which a novel genetic mutation appears not present in earlier generations (Leventer *et al.*, 2014).

Maturational arrest of the cortical organization of the first half of gestation also can occur in a more generalized cortical distribution in some genetic mutations and chromosomopathies, such as DiGeorge syndrome (22q11.1 locus), and in some systemic inborn metabolic diseases beginning in foetal life, such as methylmalonic acidaemia (Sarnat and Flores-Sarnat, 2013). These cases are genetic defects, generally germline mutations.

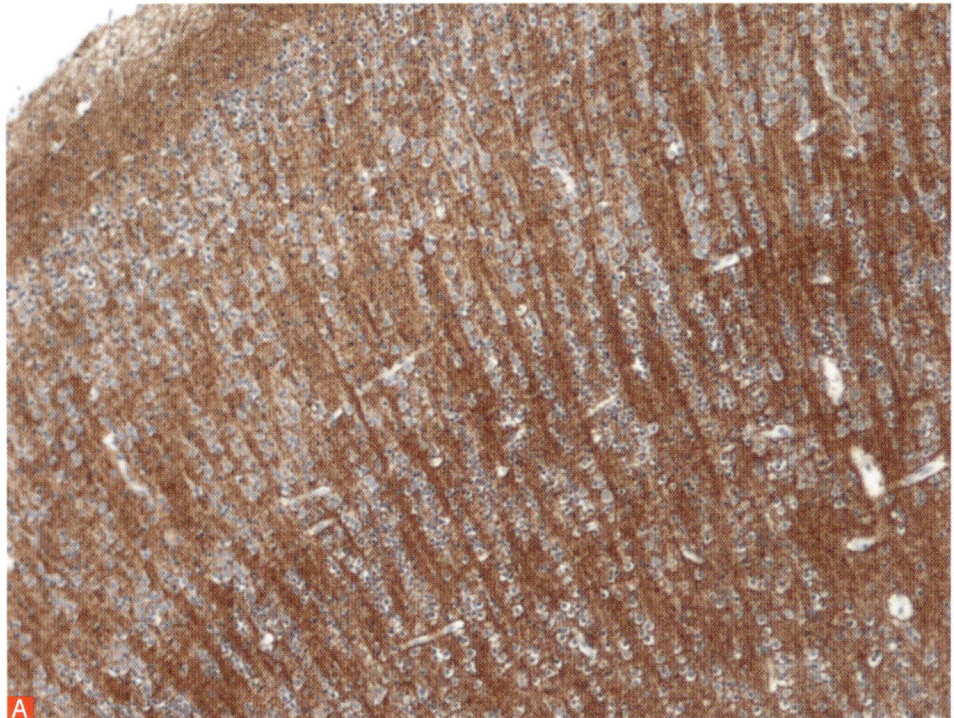

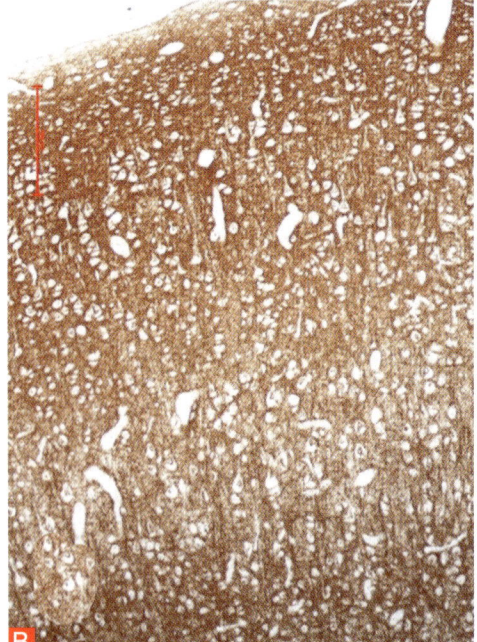
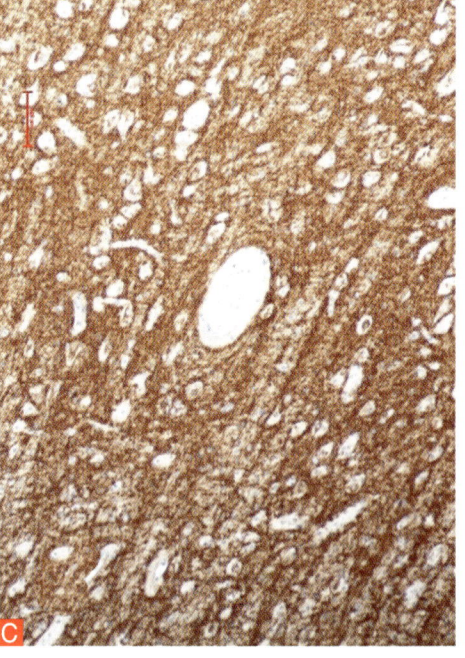

Figure 4

Synaptophysin immunoreactivity in FCD Type I

A) Frontal neocortex of a 6-week-old male infant, born at 34 weeks gestation, with DiGeorge syndrome. Vertical sheets of synapses are seen between the micro-columns of neurones, a feature found in all lobes of the neocortex. This orientation of synaptic layering is abnormal. **(B, C)** Frontal neocortex of an 8-year-old girl with FCD Ia at the site of the epileptic focus. Some micro-columns of neurones (appear white) are seen, but they are not well organized. Radial synaptic layers can be detected between them. After infancy these radial synaptic layers are sometimes difficult to discern because of more uniform synaptic vesicle reactivity throughout the cortical neuropil. Synaptophysin immunoreactivity is weaker in the middle layers of cortex in this case, another feature of maturational delay.

Synaptophysin demonstrates that in FCD Type 1a and also in generalized non-focal Type 1 associated with genetic and metabolic disorders, vertical synaptic layers occur between the micro-columns of neurones. This synaptic pattern never is found in normal mature cerebral cortex (Sarnat and Flores-Sarnat, 2013) (*Figure 4A*). Radial synaptic columns are not seen in normal foetal cortex in the first half of gestation because synapses do not form in the cortical plate before the second half of gestation.

FCD ILAE Type Ib in the context of foetal cortical development

Several forms of abnormal horizontal lamination are described in focal cortical dysplasias. In one form, layer 3 is selectively depleted of neurones and the sparsely populated remaining neurones are calretinin-reactive, indicating a disturbance of radial, but not of tangential, neuroblast migration during neocortical development (Spreafico and Blümcke, 2010).

Another form is identified immunohistochemically by zones of cortex, particularly involving the superficial layers, in which neurones lack NeuN expression; in surrounding cortical regions NeuN is normally expressed in all layers. These NeuN deficient neurones appear histologically normal without cellular loss or degenerative changes (Beaumont et al., 2012). This unique pattern can be explained as a developmental phosphorylation and subsequent activation of mitogen-activated protein kinases (MAPK; not to be confused with MAP as an abbreviation of microtubule-associated proteins). Such kinases are associated also with phosphorylation of immediate early gene transcription factors, in particular c-AMP-response element binding protein (CREB) (Edelmayer et al., 2014). CREB and Fox1 are related transcription factors that are essential for such non-neurological metabolic processes as the regulation of hepatic gluconeogenesis as well as their function in the nervous system. NeuN is programmed by *Fox3*, a member of the *Fox1* gene family of regulatory splicing factors (Beaumont et al., 2012; Dent et al., 2010; Kim et al., 2009). Phosphorylation of its transcription factor may suppress NeuN expression in the nucleoplasm of mature neurones, specifically the well-demarcated populations of granular neurones in layer 2 and small pyramidal neurons of layer 3 (Beaumont et al., 2012). In FCD Ib, a disorder of tangential (horizontal) lamination, NeuN reactivity is lost in zones of the cortex that specifically involves layer 4 most severely; this distribution is synchronous with increased ERK/CREB signaling in layers 2 and 3 which activates plasticity genes involved in spike generation in these superficial laminae (Barkmeier et al., 2012; Beaumont et al., 2012).

In many FCD Ib lesions, GABAergic interneurons arriving to the cortical plate by tangential migration and labeled by calretinin immunoreactivity, may be well preserved or even more numerous than expected because of selective loss of neurons that arrived, or should have arrived, by radial migration that changes the ratio of the two populations. The same is found in the hippocampus in the presence of sclerosis of Ammon's horn in epileptic children: calretinin-reactive neurones are normal in number but pyramidal neurons that are not calretinin-reactive are reduced (Blümcke et al., 1996; Blümcke et al., 1999). Despite a relative increase in inhibitory influence of these GABAergic neurones, most patients continue to have seizures, a physiological phenomenon not yet fully understood.

FCD ILAE Type Ic in the context of foetal cortical development

Though the ILAE classification scheme also has specified a mixed form of architectural abnormalities, including radial (FCD Ia) and tangential (FCD Ib) patterns, a mixed form with equally distributed abnormalities of tangential and vertical cortical organization has only rarely come to our attention during microscopic examination of 5,603 cases submitted to the German Neuropathology Reference Centre for Epilepsy Surgery. We are aware of recent reports describing this entity as most frequent FCD subtype in MRI-negative patients suffering from epilepsy (Wang et al., 2013). To the best of our knowledge, different thresholds in the assessment of abnormalities in cortical architecture from normal variants may account for this discrepancy. Such differentiation may be even more difficult when not systematically applying recommended immunoreactivities such as NeuN. However, a combination of both radial and tangential architectural abnormalities is frequently encountered in FCD associated with vascular or other acquired lesions during early life, *i.e.* FCD IIIc and IIId variants.

• FCD ILAE Type II

FCD Type II refers to an isolated malformation characterized by disrupted cortical lamination and cytological abnormalities and (as in the previous Palmini classification system), includes two subtypes, FCD Type IIa (with dysmorphic neurons, but without balloon cells) and FCD Type IIb (with dysmorphic neurons and balloon cells; *Table III*). The cortical dyslamination in FCD Type II is often pronounced, without any recognizable layers (except for Layer 1). In addition, blurring of the grey/white matter junction often is observed due to increased heterotopic neurones in white matter. Dysmorphic neurons in FCD Type II can be identified in routine H&E and cresyl violet (Nissl-staining) staining. However, since they accumulate neurofilament proteins (phosphorylated and non-phosphorylated) in their cell bodies, antibodies directed against these proteins (2F11 or SMI32) may be useful to detect dysmorphic neurones, showing their abnormal shape, size, and orientation. Balloon cells (histologically identical to giant cells in tubers of TSC patients) can be detected in routine H&E; however, vimentin and the splice variant of GFAP, GFAP-δ, may represent helpful markers for the demonstration of balloon cells in FCD specimens (Boer et al., 2010, Lamparello et al., 2007, Martinian et al., 2009). In addition, some balloon cells also express the class II CD34 epitope (Fauser et al., 2004) and the adhesion molecule on glia (AMOG) (Boer et al., 2010). Reduction of myelin staining, particularly evident in FCD IIb, can be visualized using Luxol-Fast Blue or Klüver-Barrera staining (Blümcke et al., 2011, Muhlebner et al., 2012).

The histopathological characteristics and classification of the various types of FCDs are defined and can be identified in microscopic sections of cerebral cortical brain tissue resected in the surgical treatment of refractory epileptic foci (Krsek et al., 2008; Krsek et al., 2009; Mischel et al., 1995; Palmini et al., 2004; Sarnat and Flores-Sarnat, 2013; Spreafico and Blümcke, 2010). The criteria are now established by a consensus of an international consortium of neuropathologists with special interest and experience in epilepsy surgery (Blümcke et al., 2011) and confirmed by independent blind review (Coras et al., 2012). These criteria have now been adopted by the International League Against Epilepsy (ILAE) and the Consortium has evolved to become an official Task Force or "Commission on Neuropathology" of the ILAE.

FCD ILAE Type II in the context of foetal cortical development

FCD II differs neuropathologically from types I and III mainly in showing cellular dysmorphism in addition to abnormal architecture of neuronal arrangement within the cortex. The pathogenesis is substantially different. In cortical lesions of type II, normal-appearing neurones are adjacent to others that exhibit abnormal morphology, cellular growth, orientation and position within the cortical plate. These neurones are described as *megalocytic* because of their excessively large size and *dysmorphic* because of abnormal shape of the soma and neurites and often displacement of the nucleus to the periphery of the cytoplasm. Bi-nucleated neurones also may be seen. Subtype IIb differs from IIa by the additional presence of *balloon cells*. At times, the abnormal cells in FCD IIa and IIb also exhibit a micro-columnar cortical architecture similar to FCD Ia.

The aetiology of FCD II is post-zygotic somatic mutation of some, but not all, undifferentiated cells of the neuroepithelium (mosaicism), so that clones of normal neuroblasts from unaffected cells and clones of abnormal neuroblasts from affected neuroepithelial cells are mixed (Poduri et al., 2013). Post-zygotic genetic mutations differ substantially from germline mutations that occur at the time of fertilization, in which all cells of the body exhibit the mutated genotype though not necessarily phenotypical expression. An example is DiGeorge syndrome, associated with a generalized radial micro-columnar architecture resembling FCD Ia but involving all neocortical lobes and regions (Sarnat and Flores-Sarnat, 2013).

The cellular dysmorphism and abnormal growth of neurones in FCD IIa and IIb indicates a very early disorder of cellular lineage and differentiation, likely involving subcellular cytoskeletal proteins or microtubules, as with tuberous sclerosis complex (TSC) and hemimegalencephaly (HME). Tau is one of many microtubule-associated proteins that is upregulated in an abnormally phosphorylated form not only in several adult neurodegenerative diseases (Mackenzie et al., 2011) but also in infantile tauopathies, which include TSC, HME, FCD II and ganglioglioma, a tumour with neuronal dysplasia and astrocytic neoplasia. All of these "infantile tauopathies" are disorders of the mTOR signalling pathway (Crino, 2007; Crino, 2011; Sarnat et al., 2012; Sarnat and Flores-Sarnat, 2015). Several members of the mTOR signalling pathway have been already identified to carry somatic mutations (D'Gama et al., 2015; Guerrini and Dobyns, 2014; Jamuar et al., 2014), amongst which DEPDC5 (disheveled, Egl-10 and pleckstrin domain containing protein) appear to play a prominent role in FCD Type II (Baulac et al., 2015; D'Gama et al., 2015). These mutations were shown to disinhibit mTOR signalling (Dibbens et al., 2013; Ishida et al., 2013), thereby promoting cell growth and proliferation. Availability of selective pharmacologic mTOR antagonists renders this pathway interesting and also accessible for novel therapeutic strategies (Krueger et al., 2010).

In contrast, a reported infection with human papilloma viruses (HPV16) transmitting the high-risk oncogene E6 (Chen et al., 2012; Liu et al., 2013) in patients with FCD IIb could not be confirmed (Coras et al., 2015; Thom et al., 2015). HPV16-E6 is a potent activator of mTOR signalling (Spangle and Munger, 2010), and elicited thereby interest in epilepsy research. However, several clinico-pathological observations in FCD IIb make a HPV infection less likely: 1) FCD IIb were never reported to occur at multiple sites in one brain, which may be envisaged after viral infection of neuroepithelial precursor cells; 2) there is no report on malignant transformation of FCD IIb into cancer, despite the carcinogenic risk of E6 and E7 oncoproteins of high-risk HPV types; 3) patient's mothers were never reported to carry HPV infections. This also leads to the entirely open question of the mode of HPV transmission into the brain, and we concluded also from published literature, that transplacental transmission of HPV16 has not yet been proven (Coras *et al.*, 2015).

Balloon cells characterize FCD IIb but not IIa, though both subtypes show cellular dysplasia. The pathogenesis of balloon cells, also typically found in TSC and HME, is incompletely understood, but they often show mixed cellular lineage, expressing both glial and neuronal proteins as well as strong expression of primitive cellular proteins such as vimentin and nestin. Balloon cells also exhibit intense expression of the heat-shock protein α-B-crystallin, which also serves as a metabolic immunocytochemical marker of epileptic foci in tissue sections (Sarnat and Flores-Sarnat, 2009).

Over-expressed phosphorylated tau in the developing brain is quite different from that of mature, and especially the aging, brain. Rather than causing neuronal degeneration and loss, presenting clinically as dementia but not usually epilepsy, upregulated tau in embryonic and foetal brains causes abnormal cellular differentiation, migration, synapse formation and function that result in cortical malformations, such as tubers, the severe dysplasias of HME and FCD II. Microtubules are essential for neuronal maturation in terms of polarity, growth, morphology, migration and expression of specific proteins as specified times during cytological maturation (Rakic *et al.*, 1996). The dysmorphic, megalocytic neurones in FCD II may be a fundamental disorder of microtubules from the earliest time of neuronal differentiation. Microtubules even form the fine strands of the mitotic spindle during cellular division. Evidence is emerging that there is cellular injury and degeneration in some cells in FCD II, perhaps providing a linkage between effects of tau and other factors at the two extremes of life (Iyer *et al.*, 2014; Kovacs *et al.*, 2014).

• FCD ILAE Type III

A major advance of the 2011 classification is represented by the FCD Type III category where FCD is combined with other potentially epileptogenic pathologies (Blümcke *et al.*, 2011; Sisodiya, 2011). FCD type III consists of four different subtypes: IIIa associated with hippocampal sclerosis (HS); IIIb associated with tumours; IIIc associated with vascular malformations; IIId associated with any other lesion acquired during early life (*Table III*). The histopathological features of FCD type III subtypes may be similar to those detected in FCD I, with alterations in architectural (cortical dyslamination) and/or cytoarchitectural composition of the neocortex (hypertrophic neurones), however distinct patterns can be identified in specific variants, such as FCD IIIa. In approx. 10% of surgical specimens of patients with HS, the temporal cortex shows an abnormal band of small and clustered "granular" neurones in the outer part of layer 2 (Garbelli *et al.*, 2006; Thom *et al.*, 2009). In addition, small "lentiform" nodular heterotopia have been reported in a subset of patients with HS. Immunocytochemical analysis using antibodies directed against NeuN, MAP2 and neurofilament proteins can improve the visualization of architectural and/or cytoarchitectural alterations of the cortex. Additional antibodies directed against CD34, p53, mutant IDH1, and Ki-67 can also be helpful in the evaluation of FCD IIIb, to exclude neocortex infiltrated by neoplastic cells that should not be diagnosed as FCD (Blümcke *et al.*, 2014). Cellular abnormalities in FCD III variants can include hypertrophic neuronal phenotypes which may be difficult to distinguish from those observed in FCD Type II. However, such cells may be the result from ongoing brain plasticity adjacent to pathogenic brain lesions, such as Sturge-Weber syndrome, and should be regarded, therefore, as FCD IIIc (Wang *et al.*, 2014). FCD Type IIId includes a large spectrum of early cerebral insults, such as middle cerebral artery occlusion at mid-gestation. The margin of a porencephalic cyst is cerebral tissue exposed to prolonged ischaemia, enough to arrest further development but not so severe to result in frank ischaemic necrosis. These margins often exhibit micro-columnar architecture with transition to normal tangential or horizontal lamination (Sarnat and Flores-Sarnat, 2013). Other examples include early onset Rasmussen encephalitis with cortical layer and cytological abnormalities classified as FCD IIId (Wang *et al.*, 2013). However, the molecular aetiopathology of Type III FCDs remains to be clarified. Post-migratory pathomechanisms have been proposed that eventually contribute to a picture previously described as progressive cortical dysplasia in infancy (Marin-Padilla *et al.*, 2002, Spreafico, 2010). However, we cannot exclude that some histopathological alterations entirely result from reactive or degenerative changes secondary to long epilepsy duration. A prominent example may be thus of TLE with MRI visible temporo-polar atrophy and grey/white matter blurring. It has been often discussed as imaging feature of FCD in patients with HS. However, systematic neuropathological investigations have clarified that these imaging features (also detectable by *ex vivo* 7T MRI) correlate with secondary white matter degeneration instead of any cortical layer abnormality (Garbelli *et al.*, 2012).

Are developmental cortical dysplasias epileptogenic?

Severe epilepsy is the presenting and most prominent symptom of all focal cortical dysplasias (Najm *et al.*, 2014). Epilepsy is the reason for neurological investigation with EEG and MRI to confirm the diagnosis. Refractory epilepsy is the main reason for surgical resections that lead to neuropathological confirmation and classification of the FCD. The question thus posed of whether FCDs are epileptogenic would seem evident. In generalized Type I cortical dysplasias associated with metabolic and genetic disease, the incidence of epilepsy also is high; in DiGeorge syndrome with a 22q11.1 mutation, the risk of epilepsy is more than 7 times higher than in an age-matched control population.

If radial micro-columnar cortical architecture is a normal transitory stage of development, why do young foetuses not have seizures? Synapse formation in the cortical plate begins at 22 weeks gestation, hence it would be physiologically impossible to have cortically-generated seizures in the first half of gestation, but other cytological developmental processes, particularly those related to the maturation of individual neurones themselves, also would not favour epileptogenesis (Sarnat *et al.*, 2010). Some investigators of animal models of human epilepsies suggest that it is the zone surrounding the FCD, and not from within the FCD itself, that seizures arise (Schwartzkroin and Wenzel, 2012) and some investigators of human epilepsies also pose this question (Bourgeois, 2005). This is confirmed in the zones surrounding foetal infarcts, tumours, vascular malformations and other lesions of FCD Type III, but the question of the microscopic site of origin of seizures in FCD Types I and II remains incompletely resolved. Certainly the epileptogenesis of generalized persistent radial micro-columnar architecture cannot be ascribed to adjacent zones of more normal cortex.

The activation of mTOR pathways in FCD II, HME and TSC may provide clues to a therapeutic approach. Suppression of mTOR activation (*e.g.* everolimus) results in improved control of pre-existing epilepsy in a murine model of cortical dysplasia (Nguyen *et al.*, 2015). Treatment with mTOR inhibitors of neonates and even of late-gestation foetuses with HME has been suggested on theoretical grounds (Sarnat *et al.*, 2012). However, implementation of mTOR inhibitors into clinical practise for treatment of epilepsies awaits further studies and randomized prospective trials.

Up-regulation of tau in FCD II, TSC and HME, all highly epileptic conditions, has already been mentioned. Some authors query whether the tau over-expression itself might be a factor promoting epilepsy or, conversely, whether intractable epilepsy favours tau up-regulation (Xi *et al.*, 2011). Up-regulation of tau is not likely induced by epileptic activity at that focus because FCD I and other epileptic foci do not exhibit tau expression and late-onset adult tauopathies are not epileptogenic. The recent development of tau-labelled tracers for positron emission tomography (PET) for use in the diagnosis of Alzheimer disease in the elderly (Li *et al.*, 2015) might have application in living patients with infantile tauopathies as well.

The role of myelination in the pathogenesis of epilepsy resulting from FCDs is unclear. The neonatal and early infantile cerebral cortex and subcortical white matter are not yet myelinated, except for large pyramidal cell axons (corona radiata) projecting into the internal capsule. MRI lesions of FCD II are reported to resolve with the maturation of myelination (Eltze *et al.*, 2005). A reduction in myelinated axons in white matter of FCD II in mature brain, rather than dysmyelination, correlates with decreased neurofilaments in those axones, but may be influenced by duration of seizures (Shepherd *et al.*, 2013). Our own studies revealed decreased numbers of oligodendrocytes with abnormal cytological configuration in FCD Type IIb lesions characterized by severe loss of myelination and increased numbers of balloon cells (Muhlebner *et al.*, 2012). Impact and contribution of oligodendrogliogenesis and myelination in white matter changes awaits, therefore, further clarification.

• Tissue markers of neuronal maturation

Many of the histochemical stains and immunocytochemical reactivities used in neuropathology to identify cellular lineage in tumours, for example, also can be applied to immature brain to denote the maturation of various developmental processes, such as synaptogenesis, or the expression of neuronal proteins (Sarnat, 2013; Sarnat, 2015). Some are markers of *immaturity*, expressed early and then disappear with maturation, such as vimentin and nestin, but most are markers of *maturity*, appearing only after a particular stage of cellular differentiation, such as NeuN, synaptophysin and parvalbumin. Still others are expressed both in primitive neuroepithelial cells and also in mature neurones, but regress in cells of glial lineage, for example many of the microtubule-associated proteins (Blümcke *et al.*, 2001). Other features for classification of developmental tissue markers is the nature of the molecule demonstrated, water-solubility, whether a cytoskeletal element and subcellular site (i.e. nuclear, cytoplasmic, plasma membrane) and specificity for particular types of neurones. The soluble calcium-binding molecules (*e.g.* parvalbumin; calretinin; calbindin D28k) selectively identify GABAergic inhibitory interneurones (Andressen *et al.*, 1993). Luxol fast blue myelin stain, developed by Klüver and Barrera (Klüver and Barrera, 1953) can be effectively used to demonstrate onset and sequences of myelination in tissue sections at autopsy (Gilles, 1976; Rorke and Riggs, 1969), or myelin basic protein may be applied immunohistochemically.

These special techniques that denote maturation can be effectively applied to resections of epileptogenic focal cortical dysplasias, not only to help recognize cellular lineage in the case of dysmorphic neurones in particular, but also to determine maturational arrest. Even if radial micro-columnar architecture predominates histologically, as in FCD Ia, the neurones do mature and express NeuN and other markers of maturation, but the distribution of synaptic layers may persist in abnormal orientation as shown by synaptophysin (*Figure 4*), and the number and distribution of neocortical GABAergic inhibitory interneurones can be demonstrated by calretinin.

Metabolic tissue markers of epileptic foci

From the late 3rd trimester and the neonatal period to maturity, epileptic foci in brain tissue identified neurophysiologically before and during surgery can be correlated with certain features that serve as markers of those foci. Examples of metabolic markers of epileptic foci, including those associated with FCD of all types, are: 1) the small heat shock protein α-B-crystallin that can be demonstrated in formalin-fixed, paraffin sections by immunocytochemistry, often showing a gradient of diminishing reactivity at 2.5-3.0 cm away from the electrophysiological focus of paroxysmal activity (Sarnat and Flores-Sarnat, 2009); 2) mitochondrial respiratory chain "oxidative" enzymes that can be demonstrated in frozen sections by histochemistry or in paraffin sections by immunocytochemistry in tissue sections. Scattered neurones exhibit hyper-intense mitochondrial enzymatic activity, accompanied by a proliferation of mitochondria demonstrated ultra-structurally. It is proposed that these neurones are hyper-metabolic because they are "epileptic" with almost continuous discharges (Sarnat *et al.*, 2011). In FCD II, the zone of seizure onset exhibits a deficit of cytochrome-c-oxidase (mitochondrial respiratory chain complex IV) as determined by biochemical assay of small frozen tissue homogenates (Miles *et al.*, 2015); 3) foetal and postnatal brains with TSC also can exhibit inflammatory markers even during development, which may denote the later development of an epileptic focus (Prabowo *et al.*, 2013). Such inflammatory markers might also be expressed in HME and FCD II, but to date the evidence is insufficient to draw conclusions.

Mild malformation of cortical development (mMCD)

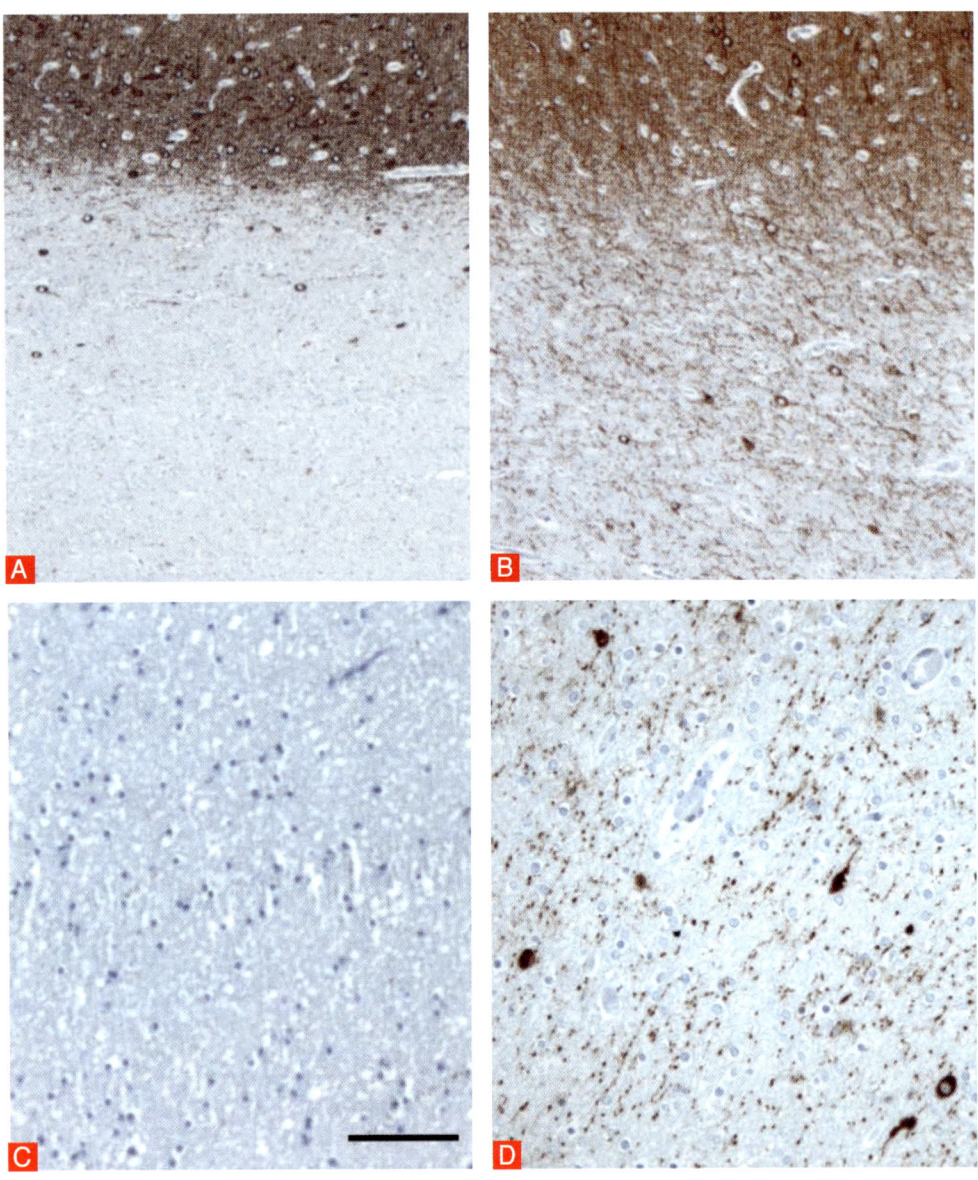

Figure 5

Abundant heterotopic neurones in white matter (mMCD Type II)

Grey/white matter boundary (as shown by anti-MAP2 staining) is sharply demarcated in controls **a)**, but severely blurred in an epilepsy surgery specimen of otherwise normal cortical architecture **(b)**; **c)** Deep white matter neurones are rarely detectable at a distance > 500 μm apart from the grey matter border in controls, but frequently encountered in epilepsy surgery specimens **(d)**. Scale bar in c = 100 μm, applies also to **a–d**. Modified from Muhlebner et al., 2011.

The terminology of "mMCD" was coined in Palmini's FCD classification from 2004 (Palmini et al., 2004) to describe abundance of heterotopic neurones occurring either in Layer 1 of the neocortex (mMCD Type I) or in subcortical white matter (mMCD Type II). It has to be mentioned here, however, that neither pathogenic mechanisms nor impact for epileptogenicity was shown yet and this diagnosis should be considered only when any other structural lesion has been ruled out (Blümcke and Muhlebner, 2011; Blümcke et al., 2011).

Heterotopic neurones in layer 1 were first described as microdysgenesis in post-mortem brains from patients with primary generalized epilepsies (Meencke and Janz, 1984; Meencke and Veith, 1999). However, the term of microdysgenesis already was abandoned by Palmini in 2004 and also is not used by the ILAE classification for FCDs (Blümcke et al., 2011). In our experience with surgical epilepsy specimens, persistence of layer 1 neurones is a rare condition and should be classified hitherto as mMCD Type I.

In contrast to the very rare finding of mMCD Type I, heterotopic neurones in white matter can be observed in many epilepsy surgery specimens in the absence of any other structural lesion and classify as mMCD Type II (Blümcke et al., 2011).

However, they also represent a physiological feature of the temporal lobe even in adult brain specimens (Chun and Shatz, 1989; Emery et al., 1997; Hardiman et al., 1988; Hildebrandt et al., 2005; Muhlebner et al., 2012; Rojiani et al., 1996; Thom et al., 2001). It is therefore difficult to establish a reliable threshold for differentiation from normal variance (Muhlebner et al., 2012). As an example, more than 20 heterotopic white matter neurones per high-power field at 20x objective magnification (mm²) is likely a pathological finding in epilepsy surgery specimens, compared to age-matched controls from the temporal lobe (approx. 10 neurones per mm²) or extra-temporal localization (< 10 neurones per mm²) (Hildebrandt *et al.*, 2005). Immunohistochemistry is helpful to identify such neurones and we recommend antibodies directed against the neuronal microtubule associated protein 2 (MAP2) and synaptophysin, as they also highlight the amount of heterotopic neuropil (*Figure 5*).

The boundary between grey and white matter is of particular interest for clinical investigation, and MRI studies often describe a compromized interface between cortex and white matter (Colombo *et al.*, 2009; Schijns *et al.*, 2011). The structural nature of altered MRI signal intensities remains, however, uncertain and may result not only from abundant heterotopic neurones and their neuropil but also from altered and decreased myelination densities. Yet, we can only speculate about the origin of heterotopic neuronal profiles in epilepsy surgery samples. They may derive from resting adult stem/precursor cells, as recent neurodevelopmental studies provide evidence for neurogenic radial glia in the outer subventricular zone of human neocortex (Hansen *et al.*, 2010), a region that will turn into white matter at later maturation stages. Persistence of subplate neurones

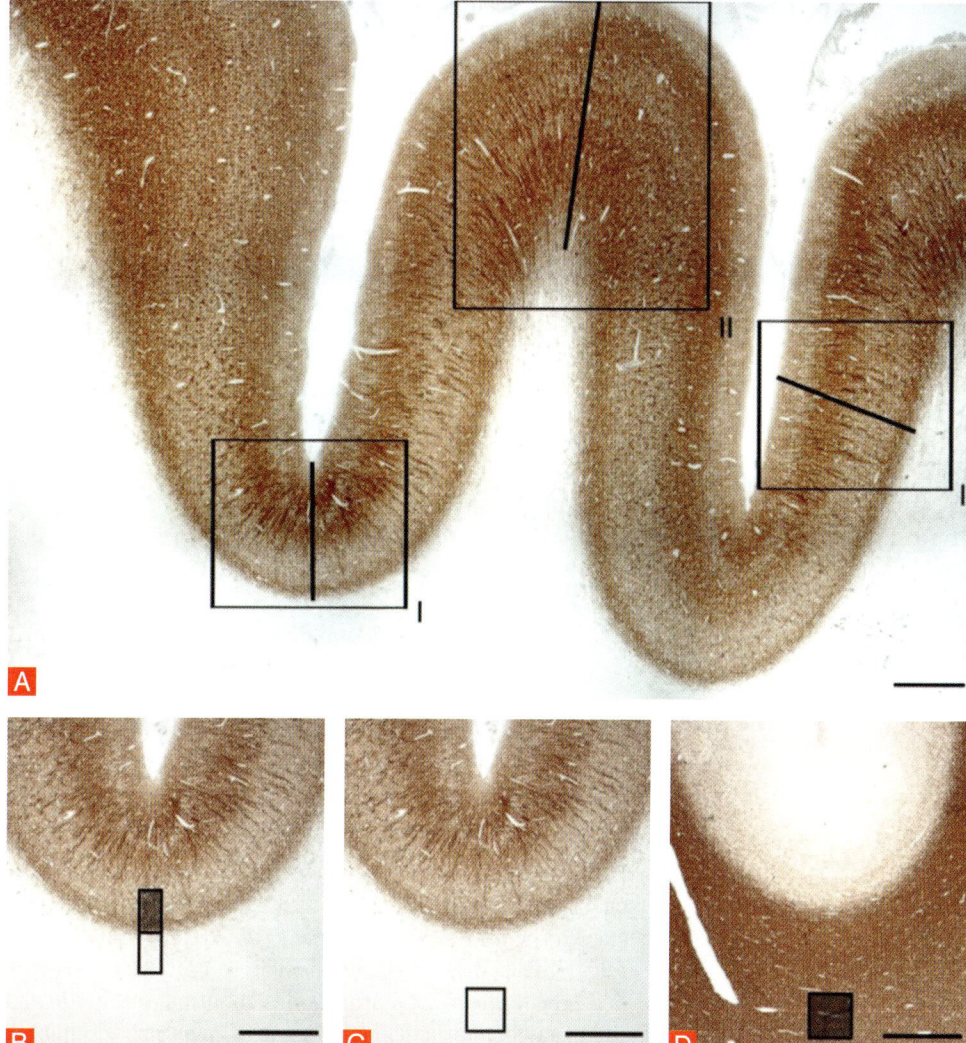

Figure 6

Definition of ROI for examining neocortex and white matter in epilepsy surgery specimens

a) Anti-MAP2 staining of the frontal cortex in a 42 year old male autopsy control. Rectangles referred to three regions of interest (ROI): I: "bottom of sulcus"; II: "crown of gyrus"; III: "intermediate zone". **b)** Assessment of the grey-white matter border. **c)** Assessment of "deep white matter" more than 500 μm apart from the grey matter border. **d)** Anti-CNPase staining to specifically contrast the white matter compartment. Scale bars in a-d = 1,000 μm. Modified from Muhlebner *et al.*, 2011.

from foetal life seems unlikely because the great majority of foetal subplate neurones are highly reactive with anti-calretinin antibodies in both the rat (Fonseca *et al.*, 1995) and human (Ulfig, 2002) and, in our experience, only a minority of subcortical white matter neurones in epilepsy surgery specimens react to this antibody. The functional impact of aberrantly located white matter neurons to seizure susceptible neuronal networks is another controversial issue, as seizure initiation from white matter location is not very well documented (Loup *et al.*, 2009).

Hemimegalencephaly (HME)

Hemimegalencephaly (HME) is a hamartomatous malformation that principally involves a portion or the totality of only one cerebral hemisphere and, rarely, the ipsilateral cerebellar hemisphere and brainstem. It is one of the most epileptogenic cerebral malformations. The enlarged hemisphere, now known as hemimegalencephaly, was first described almost two centuries ago by Sims (Sims, 1835). Imaging features of HME, in both isolated and syndromic forms, are typically characterized by an enlarged cerebral hemisphere with abnormal gyral pattern, thickened cortex and white matter abnormalities, with loss of grey/white matter differentiation, on the enlarged side (Flores-Sarnat, 2002; Kalifa et al., 1987; Nakahashi et al., 2009; Yagishita et al., 1998). Though seem with the greatest detail by MRI, it also can be diagnosed by CT and even by foetal and neonatal ultrasonography and by prenatal foetal MRI.

For many years HME was regarded as one of the most enigmatic of congenital brain malformations because of this asymmetry. The reason is now disclosed by recent genetic studies. HME is a post-zygotic somatic mutation of the neuroepithelium (Jamuar and Walsh, 2014; Poduri et al., 2012), similar to tuberous sclerosis complex (Kwiatkowski and Manning, 2014) and is unlike a germline mutation that occur at the time of conception, in which every cell of the body expresses the same mutation even if genotype and phenotype do not always correspond.

HME may be isolated or be a component of a more systemic disorder, especially in various neurocutaneous syndromes but epidermal nevus syndrome in particular and with highest frequency (Cusmai et al., 1990; Flores-Sarnat, 2002; Flores-Sarnat, 2013; Sakuta et al., 1991). The defective gene in isolated HME is *AKT3* (Jamuar and Walsh; 2014, Poduri et al.; 2012) and in Proteus syndrome it is AKT1 (Lindhurst et al., 2011), a related member of the same family. The tuberous sclerosis genes, *TSC1* and *TSC2*, are not involved in HME unless associated with TSC, but HME and TSC share a common metabolic defect in activation of the mTOR signalling pathway (Crino, 2011; Crino et al., 2006; Sarnat et al., 2012) and both disorders, as well as FCD II also exhibit up-regulation of abnormal phosphorylated tau protein in neurons, their neurites and neuropil (Sarnat et al., 2012). Tau is one of many microtubule-associated proteins. In adult neurodegenerative diseases with dementia its accumulation is associated with neuronal loss, but in immature neuroepithelial cells and neuroblasts, it causes disruption of microtubules that are important for cellular polarity, growth, morphology and synapse formation, hence the dysmorphic and megalocytic neurones. Unlike adult tauopathies, in HME and FCD II it is not accompanied by other abnormal proteins such as ubiquitin, β-amyloid and TDP43.

The histopathological findings in the involved brain tissue in HME are characterized not only by disorganization of cortical and subcortical architecture, but also by dysmorphic and megalocytic neurones as well (Arai et al., 2012; Flores-Sarnat et al., 2003; Robain et al., 1988; Takashima et al., 1991), very similar to cortical tubers in tuberous sclerosis complex and to FCD Type II. Neuronal maturation is abnormal (Arai et al., 2012; Flores-Sarnat et al., 2003) and there may be mixed cellular lineage of neuronal and glial proteins expressed in the same cells (Flores-Sarnat et al., 2003). Balloon cells are found in some cases (Flores-Sarnat et al., 2003; Salamon et al., 2006) and absent in others, particularly in foetuses (Boer et al., 2007; Salamon et al., 2006). The cerebral cortex is often severely dyslaminated and disorganized, including fused adjacent gyri. The distribution of layer-specific markers within the cortex is altered (Arai et al., 2012). The white matter is hypertrophic, due in part to greatly enlarged axons with relatively thin myelin sheaths, and in part to gliosis (Kato et al. 1996; (Flores-Sarnat et al., 2003). Scattered dysmorphic neurons occasionally are found in the contralateral "normal" cerebral hemisphere (Sarnat et al., 2012; Sato et al., 2007). The diagnosis of HME, whether isolated or systemic, can be established in the neonatal period and infancy by neuroimaging (Flores-Sarnat, 2002; Kalifa et al., 1987; Nakahashi et al., 2009; Yagishita et al., 1998) and prenatal diagnosis is now feasible by foetal ultrasound and MRI (Sarnat et al., 2012). Hemispherectomy or major resections of hemimegalencephalic brain tissue for refractory epilepsy are performed often now in most major epilepsy centres, so that neuropathological examination is no longer limited to post-mortem tissue. Another neurosurgical approach is "functional hemispherectomy" in which the dysplastic hemisphere is isolated by severing its connections with the rest of the brain but without physically removing a large volume of brain tissue.

• FCD ILAE Type II and HME probably are the same malformation with differences in timing of mitotic cycles

Focal cortical dysplasia type II (FCD II) and hemimegalencephaly (HME) share many fundamental characteristics: both are non-neoplastic disorders of cellular growth, lineage, differentiation and migration. Both additionally form defective cerebral architecture. Both are disturbances of microtubules with over-expression of abnormally phosphorylated forms of the microtubule-associated protein tau. Both are disturbances of the mTOR signalling pathway (Crino, 2011; Crino and Becker, 2006; Crino *et al.*, 2002; Sarnat *et al.*, 2012; Tsai *et al.*, 2014). They share these characteristics with tuberous sclerosis complex (TSC). Both FCD2 and HME are post-zygotic somatic, not germline, mosaicisms. A principal difference between FCD2 and HME is the size and extent of the resulting cerebral lesions. FCD2 often is a "transmantle dysplasia" between the ventricular wall and the cerebral cortex, extending either as a thin line or an expanding cone with its apex at the ventricular surface and a broader base at the grey/white matter junction or extending into the cerebral cortex. Dysplastic neurones may exhibit abnormal timing of expression of certain proteins, which define the type of neuron and each of which normally appears in early, intermediate or late stages of neuronal differentiation and maturation. For example, neuronal nuclear antigen (NeuN) is expressed in dysplastic as well as in normal neurons as a late marker, but chromogranin-A (CgrA) is expressed only in normally maturing, but not in dysplastic, neurones (Sarnat, 2013).

Different timing may explain the relation of these two different malformations in which different temporal onsets of the spontaneous mutations within the periventricular neuroepithelium yields very different phenotypes. The periventricular neuroepithelium has been calculated undergo 10 mitotic cycles in the rat and 33 cycles in the human, to produce all of the neurones of the cerebral cortex, the cellular proliferation being exponential (Caviness *et al.*, 1981). The time of the mitotic cycle can determine the extent and in part the site of hamartomatous malformations. *Table IV* shows the arbitrary estimated cycles and the types of malformations that might be expected for FCD2 and HME. If the mosaic somatic mutation occurs in a late cycle, the lesion would be smaller and more restricted in distribution than mutations that occur during earlier cycles. The earliest mitotic cycles of somatic mutation might also involve the neuroepithelium of the 4th ventricle and rhombic lip of Hiss. The lesions are unilateral or asymmetrical because the mutation occurs focally in one or a few local neuroepithelial cells on one side only.

Table IV

Hypothesis
Focal cortical dysplasia type 2 (FCD2) and hemimegalencephaly (HME) are the same disorder, the difference being *timing*: in which of the 33 mitotic cycles of the periventricular neuroepithelium the post-zygotic somatic mosaic mutation first occurred.
Adapted from Sarnat, 2015, Sarnat *et al.*, 2015

Mitotic cycle (estimated)	Malformation
4-5	Total HME, involving an entire cerebral hemisphere and also the ipsilateral half of the cerebellum and brainstem
10-11	HME involving all telencephalic and diencephalic structures of one hemisphere
16-17	HME involving part of one hemisphere
28-29	FCD2, wider extent, involving 2 or more gyri
31-32	FCD2, small, restricted to one gyrus

The earliest mitotic cycle involvement often produces mosaicism not only in the brain but in skin, heart, bone and other organs. Examples are tuberous sclerosis complex and epidermal nevus syndrome including Proteus and CLOVES syndromes. Many of these multi-systemic manifestations are mediated by mutations in neural crest cells before or during their migrations.

Timing of onset of somatic mosaicism in undifferentiated neuroepithelial cells still in the mitotic cycle thus provides an explanation of distinct cerebral malformations depending upon the stage of development. Such a hypothesis implicates different timing of onset as the main factor distinguishing FCD2 and HME. HME involving only a part of one hemisphere and sparing other portions (D'Agostino *et al.*, 2004; Kwa *et al.*, 1995; Nakahashi *et al.*, 2009) thus are not novel malformations or syndromes as first proposed, but rather are part of the continuum depending upon which mitotic cycle was first affected by the somatic mutation.

The tetrad of neuropathological features that define this group of malformations is: 1) post-zygotic somatic mosaicism; 2) histologically dysplastic and megalocytic neurons; 3) activation of the mTOR signalling pathway; and 4) up-regulation of the microtubule-associated protein tau, in a pathological phosphorylated form. The term "infantile tauopathies" has been proposed for the 4 identified hamartomatous diseases in this category: TSC, HME, focal cortical dysplasia IIb and ganglioglioma, a mixed lesion with dysplastic neurones and neoplastic glial cells (Sarnat and Flores-Sarnat, 2015). Tauopathies traditionally designate a group of adult-onset neurodegenerative diseases with dementia, but not epilepsy, as the principal clinical presentation. They also often involve the deposition of abnormal protein products such as β-amyloid precursors and expression of α-synuclein, ubiquitin and TDP-43, products not demonstrated in infantile tauopathies, hence it is a partly semantic question of how narrow or broad the definition of tauopathy should be and some neuropathologists might reject the concept of "infantile tauopathies".

Timing of the onset of genetic expression during ontogenesis is as primary as the onset of morphogenesis. Developmental delay and maturational arrest are well recognized since first conceptualized by Esquirol (Esquirol, 1818) and Cruveilhier (Cruveilhier, 1828), but the demonstration in brain malformations of precociousness in developmental processes is a relatively recent recognition. Precocious cortical synaptogenesis in the foetus may result in an early development of epileptic circuitry and post-natal severe infantile epilepsies, including infantile spasms or West syndrome (Sarnat and Flores-Sarnat, 2013; Sarnat and Flores-Sarnat, 2015).

Cortical tubers in tuberous sclerosis complex (TSC)

Tuberous sclerosis complex (TSC) is an autosomal dominant, multi-systemic disorder that results from mutations in the *TSC1* or *TSC2* genes (ECTS, 1993; van Slegtenhorst *et al.*, 1997). Central nervous system (CNS) involvement is common in TSC and the neurological manifestations of TSC are the most disabling including: developmental delay, neurobehavioral abnormalities such as autism, and severe epilepsy (Bolton, 2004; Curatolo *et al.*, 2002). Although a clear genotype-phenotype correlation has not been established, the majority of studies suggest that patients with mutations in *TSC2* have a more severe neurological phenotype (Au *et al.*, 2007; Dabora *et al.*, 2001; Nellist *et al.*, 2005). Complex structural brain abnormalities are believed to underlie the neurological symptoms of TSC patients. Neuropathological examination of post-mortem and surgical TSC brains specimens reveals three major lesions: subependymal nodules, subependymal giant cell astrocytomas (SEGAs), and non-neoplastic cortical tubers (DiMario, 2004; Mizuguchi and Takashima, 2001). However, recent advances in neuroimaging allow the detection of more subtle structural brain abnormalities present throughout the brain, that are believed to contribute to the complex neurological features of TSC (DiMario, 2004; Griffiths *et al.*, 2011; Luat *et al.*, 2007).

Subependymal nodules (SENs) represent small, usually multiple, benign proliferative lesions lining the ventricular system that are believed to develop in foetal life and to be asymptomatic; microscopically. SENs often contain calcifications and are mainly composed of glial cells with variable morphology (plump or elongated glial cells), sometimes including small clusters of giant cells (Boer *et al.*, 2008; Grajkowska *et al.*, 2010; Mizuguchi and Takashima, 2001). SENs may grow and develop into SEGAs, which are low-grade, slow-growing tumours that arise from the periventricular region and can cause obstructive hydrocephalus, particularly if located at the foramen of Monro (Adriaensen *et al.*, 2009; Grajkowska *et al.*, 2010; Mizuguchi and Takashima, 2001). Cortical tubers are focal developmental malformations detected, as single or multiple lesions, in more than 80% of patients with TSC (for reviews see (Crino *et al.*, 2006; Orlova and Crino, 2010). Several cases have been reported with prenatal detection of CNS lesions (Chen *et al.*, 2006; Glenn and Barkovich, 2006; Wortmann *et al.*, 2008) and with histopathological confirmation of tubers as early as 20 weeks gestation (Park *et al.*, 1997), indicating that tubers form during embryonic brain development, probably between weeks 9 and 20 of human gestation. Cortical tubers display cortical dyslamination with different cell types, including dysmorphic neurones, reactive astrocytes and giant cells (Boer *et al.*, 2008; Grajkowska *et al.*, 2010; Mizuguchi and Takashima, 2001; Zurolo *et al.*, 2011). There is no obvious cytological difference between the dysmorphic neurones observed in tubers of TSC patients and those detected in specimens of patients with FCD IIa/b or HME. Similarly, the giant cells in TSC are histologically identical to balloon cells detected in FCD IIb (large cell body and opalescent glassy eosinophilic cytoplasm). Such cells have been shown to express both neuronal and immature glial markers, suggesting a failure to differentiate prior to migration into the cortex (Boer *et al.*, 2009; Crino *et al.*, 1996; Lee *et al.*, 2003; Talos *et al.*, 2008); for a review see (Orlova and Crino, 2010).

A growing body of evidence suggests that cortical tubers are not static lesions, but are instead highly dynamic, exhibiting evolving features over time. Recently, the cystic evolution of tubers has gained interest due to its strong association, in approximately 50% of patients, with a *TSC2* genetic mutation and with a more aggressive seizure phenotype (Chu-Shore *et al.*, 2009). Cyst-like tubers possibly represent the end-stage of a large spectrum of degenerative changes, affecting the white matter. An additional study suggests that astrogliosis in tubers is a dynamic process as well, with progression of astrocytes from "reactive" to "gliotic", supporting the hypothesis that tubers are dynamic lesions (Sosunov *et al.*, 2008). The identification of the *TSC1* and *TSC2* genes has facilitated our understanding of the molecular mechanisms involved in the development of malformative and neoplastic lesions in TSC brain. Loss of function mutations results in a constitutive activation of the mTOR cascade, which play a critical role in the regulation of cell growth and proliferation (Chan *et al.*, 2004; Kwiatkowski, 2003; Orlova and Crino, 2010). Several studies have provided evidence of cell-specific activation of the mTOR pathway in tubers, showing that dysmorphic neurones and giant cells are strongly immunoreactive for the phosphorylated isoform of p70S6 kinase1 and ribosomal protein S6 (pS6) (Baybis *et al.*, 2004; Boer *et al.*, 2009; Miyata *et al.*, 2004; Orlova and Crino, 2010; Talos *et al.*, 2008). Expression of activated (phosphorylated) components of the mTOR pathway, such as pS6 now permits the analysis of the cellular components of tubers not simply on the basis of their morphology, but on the basis of the specific pathogenetic defect underlying the development of these lesions. Interestingly, recent observations in foetal brain indicate that mTOR hyperactivation represents an early event in the pathogenesis of tuber formation and is strictly linked to cytoarchitectural features characteristic of tubers (Crino and Aronica unpublished observations).

Many TSC-associated tumours show loss of heterozygosity (LOH) at either the *TSC1* or *TSC2* locus (Al-Saleem *et al.*, 1998; Chan *et al.*, 2004; Green *et al.*, 1994). There is still debate about whether this "two-hit" hypothesis explains tuber formation (Jozwiak and Jozwiak, 2005; Qin *et al.*, 2010). A recent study, by sequencing *TSC1* and *TSC2* in micro-dissected pS6-immune-labelled giant cells, identified in 5 out of 6 tuber specimens, a somatic mutation in single giant cells that was not detected in whole tuber sections or leukocyte DNA, suggesting that a single somatic inactivating mutations may represent a mechanism underlying the formation of tubers adjacent to morphologically normal cortex (Crino *et al.*, 2010). Histologically normal-appearing perituberal cortex may show dysregulation of mTOR signalling and aberrant synaptic connectivity enabling intrinsic epileptogenicity (Ruppe *et al.*, 2014).

White matter heterotopia

Heterotopia are cells displaced within their organ of origin (*e.g.* brain), whereas *ectopia* are cells displaced outside their organ of origin (*e.g.* isolated neurones in the leptomeninges) (Sarnat, 2000; Sarnat and Flores-Sarnat, 2004). Both heterotopia and ectopia are already plural forms of their Greek derivatives; hence the addition of an "s" at the end of the word is redundant and is incorrect English. White matter neurones are found in normal brains at all ages, particularly in the temporal lobes. In FCD the number of these heterotopic neurones is often excessive. Quantitative criteria are being developed to objectively determine how many of such neurones are too many in each lobe of the brain. As single cells, heterotopic neurones appear "isolated" in histological stains such as haematoxylin-eosin or Nissl stains, but synaptophysin immunoreactivity demonstrates that they indeed are in synaptic contact with other white matter neurones and also with the overlying cortex, hence they have the potential to contribute to epileptic circuitry (Sarnat *et al.*, 2010). White matter neurons usually exhibit synaptophysin reactivity in their axons, as well as within terminal axons at their somatic membrane. This reactivity within axons is characteristic of immature neurones and represents axonal transport of the synaptophysin molecules from the somatic cytoplasm where they are produced to the axonal terminal where they will be assembled into synaptic vesicular membranes, but axonal synaptophysin reactivity then disappears with neuronal maturation. Heterotopic white matter neurones thus appear in sharp contrast with the non-reactive long axons that constitute most of the white matter volume. Synaptophysin well labels the network of connections between subcortical white matter neurones in FCD in a manner not done by histological stains, such as H&E, or neuronal somatic markers, such as MAP2 or neuronal nuclear markers such as NeuN. Numerous white matter neurones near to the bottom of the cortical plate help explain a lack of sharp grey/white matter demarcation in MRI in FCD and also some other lesions of white matter demonstrated by imaging in epilepsy, with distinction between types of lesions (Campos et al., 2015). If heterotopic neurones cluster together in the white matter, they may form nodules large enough to detect by MRI, but scattered single white matter neurones can only be identified neuropathologically. At times nodules of heterotopic neurones are large enough to be identified prenatally in foetal MRI (Glenn et al., 2012).

Histopathologically, white matter heterotopic neurones may be identified by histological stains (e.g. H&E) or Nissl stains (e.g. cresyl-violet) and are labelled by the general immunocytochemical neuronal markers (e.g. NeuN; SMI-32; MAP2; neuron-specific enolase). Calcium-binding markers (e.g. calretinin; parvalbumin) specifically identifies those that arrived by tangential migration. Synaptophysin is particularly useful, not only as a neuronal marker, but because it offers clues to synaptic circuitry because the axones of sub-cortical white matter neurones are reactive, in addition to the synaptic vesicles in axonal terminals surrounding the somata of these heterotopic neurones, offering good contrast to the long axones comprising most of the white matter in which these cells are embedded and that do not express synaptophysin except in immature foetal brain (Sarnat, 2013; Sarnat, 2015). The normal white matter neurones in mature brain are located near to the cortex and their axones generally are parallel to the bottom surface of the cortex. In epilepsy due to FCD, the number of white matter neurones not only is numerically increased, but they lie deeper within the subcortical white matter, as well as near to the cortex, and synaptophysin often shows a complex and dense network of connections between individual heterotopic neurones and their axones extending perpendicular to and entering the cortex, where they can make synaptic contact with cortical neurones, hence contributing to epileptic circuitry.

• Nodular heterotopia (NH)

Nodular heterotopia refers to clustering of heterotopic neurones into aggregates that are large enough to resolve in neuroimaging and to identify macroscopically by neuropathological inspection. There are three principal sites of such heterotopia: 1) the periventricular region; 2) the centrum semiovale and other subcortical white matter; and 3) forming dysplastic nodules within the cortical plate and especially in the molecular zone. Heterotopic neurones in the cortex are displaced and disoriented neurones in the wrong location, such as large pyramidal cells in the most superficial part of the cortical plate. Heterotopic nodules in the cortex are difficult to discern from focal areas of focal dysgenesis as occurs in FCD I, but there often are neurones displaced in to the molecular zone (Ramos et al., 2014). Such layer 1 heterotopic neurones can be distinguished from resident Cajal-Retzius cells because they have nuclei strongly reactive for NeuN and are not reactive for calretinin, the reverse of expected Cajal-Retzius reactivities (Sarnat, 2013; Sarnat and Flores-Sarnat, 2002). The term *grey matter heterotopia* may be misleading because it refers to heterotopic clustering of neurones into nodules comprising grey matter, rather than their location within cortical grey matter.

Periventricular nodules (e.g. *Filamin-1* mutations) are composed of neurones that have matured *in situ* because they could not attach to radial glial fibres for migration. Sub-ependymal nodules contain both neurones and glial cells and do not generally mineralize, thus differing from the often calcified periventricular nodules in TSC which are composed exclusively of glial cells not mixed with neurones. The nodules may be confined to the occipital horn or the trigone region including the temporal horn, or may be more extensive and also involve the frontal horns of the lateral ventricles. Abnormalities of gyration of the overlying cortex, particularly focal or generalized polymicrogyria, are frequent but not invariable. Diffuse NH also is associated with many of the severe genetic neuroblast migratory disorders with pachygyria, lissencephaly or schizencephaly.

The causes of periventricular nodular heterotopia are many, but they often are a marker of chromosomopathies, particularly if bilateral, and may be associated with a large variety of chromosomal translocations and deletions (Abe *et al.*, 2014; Balci *et al.*, 2007; Conti *et al.*, 2014; Descartes *et al.*, 2011; Ferland *et al.*, 2006; Grosso *et al.*, 2008; Kiehl *et al.*, 2009; Sheen *et al.*, 2003; Shiba *et al.*, 2013; So *et al.*, 2014). The most frequent genetic mutation is the *Filamin-A* (*FLNA*) mutation, an X-linked dominant cause of bilateral periventricular nodular heterotopia (Fox *et al.*, 1998; Parrini *et al.*, 2006), which accounts for a female predominance. Germline mosaicism may be demonstrated in this X-linked form, important for genetic counselling (LaPointe *et al.*, 2014). Periventricular NH is reported in patients with SCN1A gene mutation, a known genetic cause of epilepsy (Barba *et al.*, 2014). Periventricular nodular heterotopia usually are associated with many other brain malformations in addition to cortical dysplasias and subcortical white matter heterotopia, such as agenesis or dysgenesis of the corpus callosum, cerebellar cortical dysgenesis and even spinal cord malformation (Barba *et al.*, 2014; Pardoe *et al.*, 2015; Pisano *et al.*, 2012; Shiba *et al.*, 2013).

Subcortical laminar heterotopia are sheets of neurones that could not complete their migration, sometimes alternatively called *band heterotopia* or *double cortex*, though this layer of neurones within the white matter does not fulfill the histological criteria of a true cortex, so that this latter term should be avoided even though the most frequent gene that is mutated in this disorder carries the unfortunate name *Doublecortin (DCX)*.

In all cases, the nodules consist of masses of neurones, with well-defined boundaries, surrounded by white matter fibres some of which infiltrate the nodules suggesting a functional connection between the nodules and the overlying cortex. Neuropathological investigations report that all of the nodules, regardless of their size and number (single or multiple), lobe, and depth of location (subependymal and/or subcortical) have similar morphological and immunocytochemical characteristics. The nodules contain pyramidal cells as well as all of the subtypes of inhibitory inter-neurones of normal morphology. Interestingly, the presence of cell-free zones with small vessels, reminiscent of the molecular layer, and glial cells, with radiating fibers similar to radial pattern of superficial gliosis, was described suggesting a rudimentary laminar pattern within the nodules. In addition small *Reelin*-immunoreactive neurones within the cell-free zone were identified, mirroring their normal location in the molecular layer of the overlying cortex. This peculiar organization was further confirmed by studies performed by analyzing the expression patterns of 3 layer-specific genes (Ror β, ER81, and Nurr1) in tissues from patients with subcortical NH and demonstrating the prevalent expression of neurones belonging to layer VI and layer V in the external border of the nodules, with those belonging to layer IV in a more internal region.

The hypothesis that in subcortical nodular heterotopia, some of the Cajal-Retzius, *Reelin*-secreting, cells remain displaced within the sub-plate during early stages of cortical development and that these cells, wrongly located in this transient layer, attract migrating neurones into a heterotopic position leading to the formation of a heterotopic malformation with a rudimentary laminar organization was postulated. This hypothesis was indirectly supported by demonstrating that ectopically expressed *Reelin* in developing mouse cortex is able to determine subcortical nodular aggregates with laminar organization similar to those observed in human pathology. Evidence refuting the hypothesis that white matter heterotopia are due to persistence of the foetal sub-plate zone is that most sub-plate neurones are strongly express calretinin, whereas the neurones in heterotopia contain only a few scattered calretinin-reactive neurones. Another mechanism in some cases may be that neuroepithelial cells fail to attach to their intended radial glial fibre for migration, hence they remain in their original periventricular location and mature as neurones in situ that cluster to form nodules.

Though MRI frequently suggests a polymicrogyric cortex overlying the nodular heterotopia, recent neuropathological data reported abnormal gyration but without histological abnormalities consistent with the typical four layered or unlayered polymicrogyria. However various degrees of cortical laminar disorganization similar to those observed in FCD has been described with reduced expression of calcium-binding proteins suggesting an impairment of the GABAergic system. In other cases, a normal cortical organization can be found although cortical disruption can be noted in areas where nodules invade the cortex. When nodular heterotopia involves the temporal lobe, hippocampal sclerosis may also be present. Amongst the different types of nodular heterotopia (NH), the number of bilateral and unilateral cases are approximately equal and bilateral symmetrical NH account for about one third of bilateral cases (Aronica et al., 2012). Periventricular nodule excitability in an animal model causes c-fos activation in organo-typical hippocampal slices, but the nodules are not responsible for enhanced excitability in the cortex or, presumably, for initiation of seizures (Doisy et al., 2015).

Clinical correlates with periventricular nodular heterotopia are mainly epilepsy, developmental delay and intellectual impairment. The clinical spectrum is difficult to assess, however, because of commonly associated other cerebral malformations, both cortical and subcortical, and a high incidence of chromosomal and other genetic disease (Raymond et al., 1994; Srour et al., 2011; Watrin et al., 2015). Isolated periventricular NH usually lack synaptic connections with the distant cortex, hence are not inherently epileptogenic, unlike white matter and cortical grey matter heterotopia. They may be associated with focal cortical dysplasia, however, which is epileptogenic. If connections with overlying cortex are established, however, some children with isolated periventricular NH do indeed have epilepsy even without cortical dysplasia (Christodoulou et al., 2013).

Types of epilepsies vary greatly, ranging from infantile spasms and other severe infantile seizure disorders, to generalized major motor seizures, to focal simple or focal complex dyscognitive seizures. In isolated unilateral periventricular nodular heterotopia of the temporo-occipital region, there may be no clinical neurological or intellectual deficits; many such patients do not have epilepsy or even an abnormal EEG, the heterotopia discovered as an incidental finding if MRI is performed for another reason, such as head trauma, in both children and adults.

The prevalence of NH has not been ascertained in the general population or patients with epilepsy, but diagnosis by MRI has been reported in 13%-20% of large series of epileptic patients with malformations of cortical development.

Polymicrogyria, including schizencephaly and opercular syndrome

Polymicrogyria (PMG) is a cortical malformation characterized by an excessive number of small irregular gyri separated by shallow sulci leading to an irregular cortical surface with a lumpy aspect (Aronica et al., 2012). Microscopically, the polymicrogyria that forms the grey matter lining of the cleft, as with polymicrogyria in general, exhibits several distinctive histopathological patterns. All appear to arise in early stages of cortical malformation with disruption of the cortical surface due to pial defects that enable over-migration, thickening and duplication of the pial collagen layers and increased leptomeningeal vascularity (Squier & Jansen, 2014). One of the most frequent, but not invariable, features is the fusion of the molecular zone of adjacent microgyri without an intervening pial membrane or arachnoidal tissue. Pial cells are neural crest derivatives and migrate from ventral to dorsal over the developing forebrain, also producing several signalling factors important for neuronal positioning within the cortical plate (Squier & Jansen, 2014). The distribution and orientation of synaptic activity may be altered. PMG can be localized to a single gyrus or can involve a portion of one hemisphere or be bilateral, with or without asymmetry. PMG may be confused with "thickened cortex" in imaging studies when CT scan or low field MRI are performed but, if appropriate age related protocols are used with high resolution MRI, it can be reliably differentiated from other malformations of cortical development and be recognized by the presence of numerous cortical gyrations even in the absence of irregular grey/white matter junctions.

The extent and location of PMG in different brain regions can determine a variety of specific syndromes with a wide range of clinical manifestations, from severe encephalopathy with intractable epilepsy to only selective impairment of cognitive function. Several malformation syndromes have been described such as bilateral perisylvian or opercular, bilateral parasagittal parieto-occipital, bilateral frontal, and unilateral perisylvian or multilobar types. However, the most common form of PMG is represented by the bilateral perisylvian PMG characterized by distinct clinico-pathological features and frequent familial recurrence. The best technique for identifying polymicrogyria in the living patient is MRI and it can be demonstrated even in late prenatal life by foetal MRI (Herman-Sucharska et al., 2009).

Various patterns of inheritance have been described for the different subtypes of polymicrogyria (Guerreiro et al., 2000). Perisylvian PMG and schizencephaly is associated with high frequency with septo-optic-pituitary dysplasia. It also is seen as a highly epileptogenic *perisylvian syndrome* without other cerebral malformations, as in the case shown in *Figure 7*. The perisylvian syndrome is identified by MRI as PMG involving both lips (frontal and temporal) of the Sylvian fissure and by EEG with localization of the paroxysmal activity to the region of the Sylvian fissure, usually bilaterally. Both lips of the Sylvian fissure are involved because they both are derived from the ventral surface of the initial telencephalic hemisphere, which bends with formation of the telencephalic flexure; this also explains how genes following a ventro-dorsal gradient in the vertical axis of the neural tube would involve both lips but not the dorsal surface of the hemisphere (Sarnat, 2000, Sarnat and Flores-Sarnat, 2004).

Yakovlev and Wadsworth (1946) made a sharp distinction between the "open-lip" and "closed-lip" varieties, depending upon the degree of separation of the lips of the operculum, and present-day neuroradiologists continue to report these two types of schizencephaly because they are so evident on neuroimaging (Yakovlev and Wadsworth, 1946). The diagnosis of schizencephaly can be made prenatally by foetal MRI (Denis et al., 2001). There is little difference, however, in terms of clinical presentation, severity of epilepsy, cognitive impairment or prognosis, and the histopathological features of the cortex bordering the Sylvian fissure also are similar in both open and closed-lip forms. One difference is that closed-lip

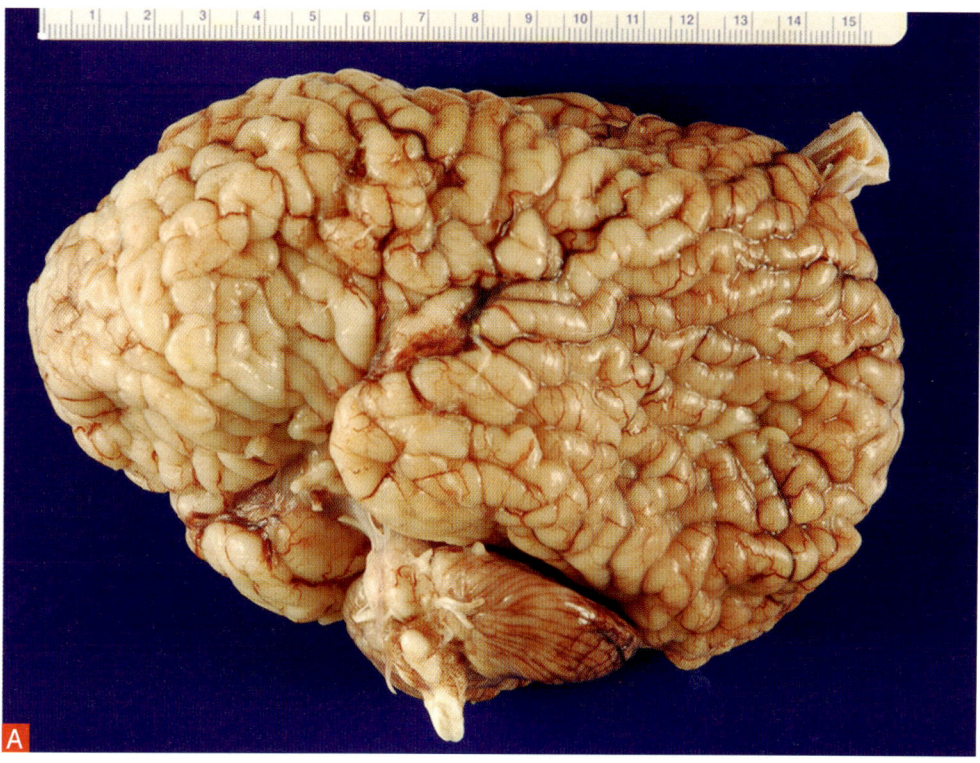
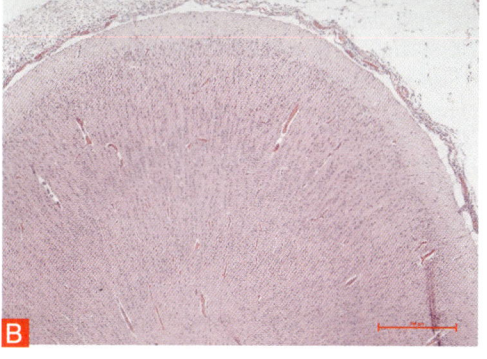
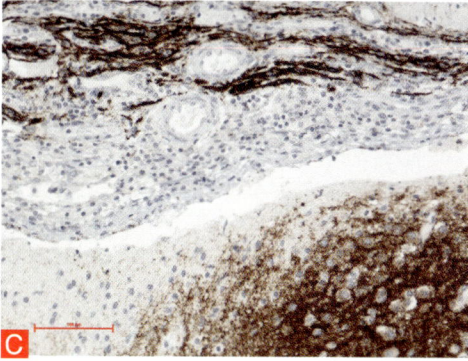

Figure 7

Neuropathology findings in polymicrogyria

A term neonate with bilateral schizencephaly or perisylvian polymicrogyria. **A.** The architecture of the cerebral cortex is disorganized. Many small, almost nodular gyri are identified, some fused to adjacent gyri by continuity of their molecular zones without intervening sulci (see also Chapter 7, *Figure 27*). **B.** Microscopically, a micro-columnar architecture is identified resembling FCD Type I. The molecular zone exhibits intense synaptophysin immuno-reactivity. Synaptophysin is non-uniformly distributed within the cortical grey matter and synaptic layers with various orientations are demonstrated, some radial and others tangential. Ectopic synaptophysin immuno-reactivity is seen in the leptomeninges (**C**).

schizencephaly is less frequently complicated by hydrocephalus than the open-lip form. Most textbook traditionally classify schizencephaly as a neuroblast migratory disorder, but evidence is sparse that this is the primary mechanism of pathogenesis.

No individual genes have been linked to any of the bilateral forms with isolated polymicrogyria. In familial schizencephaly with perisylvian PMG, the homeobox *EMX2* gene was implicated initially (Brunelli *et al.*, 1996; Granata *et al.*, 1997), but more comprehensive genotyping of a larger series of cases failed to confirm mutations of this gene (Tietjen *et al.*, 2007). Despite extensive genetic studies of affected patients, no single consistent mutation has been demonstrated, though several different mutated genes have been demonstrated (Jansen & Andermann, 2005; Squier & Jansen, 2014). Similarly, a large cohort of schizencephaly patients had sequencing performed of candidate genes associated with septo-optic-pituitary dysplasia (*LHX2, HESX1, SOX2*) because the association of these two malformations (Polizzi *et al.*, 2006), but no pathogenic mutations were found (Mellado *et al.*, 2010). A mutation in *MECP2* was observed in a male patient with bilateral perisylvian disorder and severe neonatal encephalopathy. A hybrid genetic-MRI approach led to the identification of the homeobox gene *PAX6* as a factor, in which mutations can result in unilateral polymicrogyria (Mitchell *et al.*, 2003). As observed frequently for other types of cortical malformations, polymicrogyria may be part of multiple congenital anomaly syndromes and is frequently observed in the vicinity of encephaloclastic lesions, such as some cases of schizencephaly (Caraballo *et al.*, 2004; Guerrini and Filippi, 2005). Post-natal MRI follow-up of polymicrogyric cortex in preterm infants provides evidence of encephaloclastic lesions similar to periventricular leukomalacia, suggesting ischaemic injury as a basis (Inder *et al.*, 1999).

PMG also can be epigenetic, secondary to exogenic causes such as infections including cytomegaly, toxoplasmosis, rubeola, as well as to impaired hemodynamic disturbances, particularly referred to the perfusion area of the middle cerebral artery, and thus easily confused with porencephaly. Though PMG is frequently associated with epileptic syndromes, mechanisms of epileptogenesis related to PMG are not entirely understood. In an experimental model in which microgyri are generated by a freezing insult, it was demonstrated that functional abnormalities extend beyond the anatomical malformation (Jacobs *et al.*, 1999, Redecker *et al.*, 2000). These data corroborate observations in humans revealing that the cortex surrounding the PMG is also involved in epileptogenesis and suggest that surgical resection restricted to the polymicrogyric area may not be sufficient to substantially attenuate or abolish recurrent epileptic seizures (Sisodiya, 2000; Sisodiya, 2004). Polymicrogyria is, however, not inevitably associated with epilepsy, and it may present as developmental delay or congenital hemiparesis in a minority of cases.

In PMG, the gyri are atypically organized with abnormalities of the physiological laminar cytoarchitectural structure. Although a variety of intermediate neuropathological phenotypes exist, two main histological types are observed: an unlayered and a four-layered types. In unlayered PMG, the molecular layer is continuous and does not follow convolutional profiles. Neurones have a radial distribution without any laminar organization (Ferrer, 1984). By contrast, the four-layered PMG shows a laminar structure composed by a molecular layer, outer neuronal layer, nerve fibre layer and inner neuronal layer. Apparently, the third layer (nerve fibres) results from cellular necrosis. Occasionally, in the neuronal cell layers, granular as well as pyramidal neurones can be observed, resembling residuals of the normal six-layer cortical architecture. This subtype of malformation is thought to be the result of perfusion failure, occurring between the 20th and 24th weeks of gestation, leading to intracortical laminar necrosis with consequent late migration disorder and post-migratory overturning of cortical organization. These two histopathological subtypes do not necessarily have a distinct origin, as both may coexist in contiguous cortical regions (Bird and Gilles, 1987, Guerrini, 2005).

Generalized (non-focal) cortical dysplasias

There are a large number of generalized cerebral cortical dysplasias associated with specific genetic mutations that are mostly neuroblast migratory disorders. They are characterized by abnormal convolutions of the cortex or lack of gyration and thus are now easily diagnosed by neuroimaging. MRI often shows abnormal thickening of the cortex and poor demarcation of cortical grey and sub-cortical white matter. Histopathological patterns vary widely. In lissencephaly 1 (Miller-Dieker syndrome; *LIS1* micro-deletion at 17q13.3) there is a 4-layer cortex, but in lissencephaly 2 (Walker-Warburg syndrome; Fukuyama muscular dystrophy; muscle-eye-brain disease of Santavuori), by contrast, the histological pattern of the cortex is very disorganized but is not the 4 layers of lissencephaly 1 nor does it correspond to any of the patterns seen in FCD I or II. In holoprosencephaly, the cortex at the midline and in the para-median zone is nodular rather than laminar and the laminar cortex of the more lateral zones (following a medio-lateral gradient) also is abnormal. These cortical dysplasias are almost all epileptogenic, but because they are not *focal* cortical dysplasias and are not amenable to surgical treatment, they are beyond the scope of this monograph.

References

Abe Y, Kikuchi A, Kobayashi S, et al. Xq26.1-26.2 gain identified on array comparative genomic hybridization in bilateral periventricular nodular heterotopia with overlying polymicrogyria. *Dev Med Child Neurol* 2014; 56: 1221-4.

Adriaensen ME, Schaefer-Prokop CM, Stijnen T, Duyndam DA, Zonnenberg BA, Prokop M. Prevalence of subependymal giant cell tumors in patients with tuberous sclerosis and a review of the literature. *Eur J Neurol* 2009; 16: 691-6.

Al-Saleem T, Wessner LL, Scheithauer BW, et al. Malignant tumors of the kidney, brain, and soft tissues in children and young adults with the tuberous sclerosis complex. *Cancer* 1998; 83: 2208-16.

Allendoerfer KL, Shatz CJ. The subplate, a transient neocortical structure: its role in the development of connections between thalamus and cortex. *Annu Rev Neurosci* 1994; 17: 185-218.

Andressen C, Blümcke I, Celio MR. Calcium-binding proteins: selective markers of nerve cells. *Cell Tiss Res* 1993; 271: 181-208.

Anton ES, Cameron RS, Rakic P. Role of neuron-glial junctional domain proteins in the maintenance and termination of neuronal migration across the embryonic cerebral wall. *J Neurosci* 1996; 16: 2283-93.

Arai A, Saito T, Hanai S, et al. Abnormal maturation and differentiation of neocortical neurons in epileptogenic cortical malformation: unique distribution of layer-specific marker cells of focal cortical dysplasia and hemimegalencephaly. *Brain Res* 2012; 27: 89-97.

Aronica E, Becker AJ, Spreafico R. Malformations of cortical development. *Brain Pathol* 2012; 22: 380-401.

Au KS, Williams AT, Roach ES, et al. Genotype/phenotype correlation in 325 individuals referred for a diagnosis of tuberous sclerosis complex in the United States. *Genet Med* 2007; 9: 88-100.

Bahi-Buisson N, Poirier K, Boddaert N, et al. GPR56-related bilateral frontoparietal polymicrogyria: further evidence for an overlap with the cobblestone complex. *Brain* 2010; 133: 3194-209.

Balci S, Unal A, Engiz O, et al. Bilateral periventricular nodular heterotopia, severe learning disability, and epilepsy in a male patient with 46,XY,der(19)t(X;19) (q11.1-11.2;p13.3). *Dev Med Child Neurol* 2007; 49: 219-24.

Barba C, Parrini E, Coras R, et al. Co-occurring malformations of cortical development and SCN1A gene mutations. *Epilepsia* 2014; 55: 1009-19.

Barkmeier DT, Senador D, Leclercq K, et al. Electrical, molecular and behavioral effects of interictal spiking in the rat. *Neurobiol Dis* 2012; 47: 92-101.

Barkovich AJ, Guerrini R, Kuzniecky RI, Jackson GD, Dobyns WB. A developmental and genetic classification for malformations of cortical development: update 2012. *Brain* 2012; 135: 1348-69.

Barkovich AJ, Kuzniecky RI, Jackson GD, Guerrini R, Dobyns WB. Classification system for malformations of cortical development: update 2001. *Neurology* 2001; 57: 2168-78.

Barkovich AJ, Kuzniecky RI, Jackson GD, Guerrini R, Dobyns WB. A developmental and genetic classification for malformations of cortical development. *Neurology* 2005; 65: 1873-87.

Baulac S, Ishida S, Marsan E, et al. Familial focal epilepsy with focal cortical dysplasia due to DEPDC5 mutations. *Ann Neurol* 2015; 77: 675-83.

Baybis M, Yu J, Lee A, et al. mTOR cascade activation distinguishes tubers from focal cortical dysplasia. *Ann Neurol* 2004; 56: 478-87.

Bayer SA, Altman J. Development of layer I and the subplate in the rat neocortex. *Exp Neurol* 1990; 107: 48-62.

Beaumont TL, Yao B, Shah A, Kapatos G, Loeb JA. Layer-specific CREB target gene induction in human neocortical epilepsy. *J Neurosci* 2012; 32: 14389-401.

Belichenko PV, Vogt-Weisenhorn DM, Myklossy J, Celio MR. Calretinin-positive Cajal-Retzius cells persist in the adult human neocortex. *Neuroreport* 1995; 6: 1869-74.

Berkovic SF, Jackson GD. "Idiopathic" no more! Abnormal interaction of large-scale brain networks in generalized epilepsy. *Brain* 2014; 137: 2400-2.

Bernasconi N, Bernasconi A. Epilepsy: Imaging the epileptic brain-time for new standards. *Nature reviews Neurology* 2014; 10 (3): 133-4.

Bird CR, Gilles FH. Type I schizencephaly: CT and neuropathologic findings. *Am J Neuroradiol* 1987; 8: 451-4.

Blümcke I. Neuropathology of focal epilepsies: a critical review. *Epilepsy Behav* 2009; 15: 34-9.

Blümcke I, Aronica E, Urbach H, Alexopoulos A, Gonzalez-Martinez JA. A neuropathology-based approach to epilepsy surgery in brain tumors and proposal for a new terminology use for long-term epilepsy-associated brain tumors. *Acta Neuropathol* 2014; 128: 39-54.

Blümcke I, Beck H, Nitsch R, et al. Preservation of calretinin-immunoreactive neurons in the hippocampus of epilepsy patients with Ammon's horn sclerosis. *J Neuropathol Exp Neurol* 1996; 55: 329-41.

Blümcke I, Beck H, Suter B, et al. An increase of hippocampal calretinin-immunoreactive neurons correlates with early febrile seizures in temporal lobe epilepsy. *Acta Neuropathol* 1999; 97: 31-9.

Blümcke I, Becker AJ, Normann S, et al. Distinct expression pattern of microtubule-associated protein-2 in human oligodendrogliomas and glial precursor cells. *J Neuropathol Exp Neurol* 2001; 60: 984-93.

Blümcke I, Coras R. The curse of in silico transformation from Palmini's into the ILAE classification system of focal cortical dysplasia: a critical comment. *Epilepsia* 2013; 54: 1506-7.

Blümcke I, Muhlebner A. Neuropathological work-up of focal cortical dysplasias using the new ILAE consensus classification system – practical guideline article invited by the Euro-CNS Research Committee. *Clin Neuropathol* 2011; 30: 164-77.

Blümcke I, Pieper T, Pauli E, et al. A distinct variant of focal cortical dysplasia type I characterised by magnetic resonance imaging and neuropathological examination in children with severe epilepsies. *Epileptic Disord* 2010; 12: 172-80.

Blümcke I, Russo GL, Najm I, Palmini A. Pathology-based approach to epilepsy surgery. *Acta Neuropathol* 2014; 128: 1-3.

Blümcke I, Spreafico R. Cause matters: a neuropathological challenge to human epilepsies. *Brain Pathol* 2012; 22: 347-9.

Blümcke I, Thom M, Aronica E, et al. The clinico-pathological spectrum of Focal Cortical Dysplasias: a consensus classification proposed by an ad hoc Task Force of the ILAE Diagnostic Methods Commission. *Epilepsia* 2011; 52: 158-74.

Blümcke I, Vinters HV, Armstrong D, Aronica E, Thom M, Spreafico R. Malformations of cortical development and epilepsies. *Epileptic Disord* 2009; 11: 181-93.

Boer K, Lucassen PJ, Spliet WG, et al. Doublecortin-like (DCL) expression in focal cortical dysplasia and cortical tubers. *Epilepsia* 2009; 50: 2629-37.

Boer K, Middeldorp J, Spliet WG, et al. Immunohistochemical characterization of the out-of frame splice variants GFAP Delta164/Deltaexon 6 in focal lesions associated with chronic epilepsy. *Epilepsy Res* 2010; 90: 99-109.

Boer K, Spliet WG, van Rijen PC, Jansen FE, Aronica E. Expression patterns of AMOG in developing human cortex and malformations of cortical development. *Epilepsy Res* 2010; 91: 84-93.

Boer K, Troost D, Jansen F, et al. Clinicopathological and immunohistochemical findings in an autopsy case of tuberous sclerosis complex. *Neuropathology* 2008; 28: 577-90.

Boer K, Troost D, Spliet WG, Redeker S, Crino PB, Aronica E. A neuropathological study of two autopsy cases of syndromic hemimegalencephaly. *Neuropathol Appl Neurobiol* 2007; 33: 455-70.

Bolton PF. Neuroepileptic correlates of autistic symptomatology in tuberous sclerosis. *Dev Disabil Res Rev* 2004; 10: 126-31.

Bourgeois JP. [Brain synaptogenesis and epigenesis]. *Médecine Sciences* 2005; 21: 428-33.

Brunelli S, Faiella A, Capra V, et al. Germline mutations in the homeobox gene EMX2 in patients with severe schizencephaly. *Nat Genet* 1996; 12: 94-6.

Cameron RS, Rakic P. Identification of membrane proteins that comprise the plasmalemmal junction between migrating neurons and radial glial cells. *J Neurosci* 1994; 14: 3139-55.

Campos BM, Coan AC, Beltramini GC, et al. White matter abnormalities associate with type and localization of focal epileptogenic lesions. *Epilepsia* 2015; 56: 125-32.

Caraballo RH, Cersosimo RO, Fejerman N. Unilateral closed-lip schizencephaly and epilepsy: a comparison with cases of unilateral polymicrogyria. *Brain Dev* 2004; 26: 151-7.

Caviness VS, Jr., Pinto-Lord MC, Evrand P. *The Development of Laminated Patterns in the Mammalian Neocortex*. New York: Raven Press, 1981.

Chamberlain WA, Cohen ML, Gyure KA, et al. Interobserver and intraobserver reproducibility in focal cortical dysplasia (malformations of cortical development). *Epilepsia* 2009; 50: 2593-8.

Chan JA, Zhang H, Roberts PS, et al. Pathogenesis of tuberous sclerosis subependymal giant cell astrocytomas: biallelic inactivation of TSC1 or TSC2 leads to mTOR activation. *J Neuropathol Exp Neurol* 2004; 63: 1236-42.

Chen CP, Su YN, Hung CC, Shih JC, Wang W. Novel mutation in the *TSC2* gene associated with prenatally diagnosed cardiac rhabdomyomas and cerebral tuberous sclerosis. *J Formos Med Assoc* 2006; 105: 599-603.

Chen J, Tsai V, Parker WE, Aronica E, Baybis M, Crino PB. Detection of human papillomavirus in human focal cortical dysplasia type IIB. *Ann Neurol* 2012; 72: 881-92.

Chio A, Spreafico R, Avanzini G, Ghiglione P, Vercellino M, Mutani R. Cesare Lombroso, cortical dysplasia, and epilepsy: keen findings and odd theories. *Neurology* 2003; 61: 1412-6.

Christodoulou JA, Barnard ME, Del Tufo SN, et al. Integration of gray matter nodules into functional cortical circuits in periventricular heterotopia. *Epilepsy Behav* 2013; 29: 400-6.

Chu-Shore CJ, Frosch MP, Grant PE, Thiele EA. Progressive multifocal cystlike cortical tubers in tuberous sclerosis complex: Clinical and neuropathologic findings. *Epilepsia* 2009; 50: 2648-51.

Chun JJ, Shatz CJ. Interstitial cells of the adult neocortical white matter are the remnant of the early generated subplate neuron population. *J Comp Neurol* 1989; 282: 555-69.

Ciceri G, Dehorter N, Sols I, Huang ZJ, Maravall M, Marin O. Lineage-specific laminar organization of cortical GABAergic interneurons. *Nat Neurosci* 2013; 16: 1199-210.

Colombo N, Salamon N, Raybaud C, Ozkara C, Barkovich AJ. Imaging of malformations of cortical development. *Epileptic Disord* 2009; 11: 194-205.

Conti V, Pantaleo M, Barba C, et al. Focal dysplasia of the cerebral cortex and infantile spasms associated with somatic 1q21.1-q44 duplication including the AKT3 gene. *Clinical Genet* 2014 [Epub ahead of print].

Coras R, de Boer OJ, Armstrong D, et al. Good interobserver and intraobserver agreement in the evaluation of the new ILAE classification of focal cortical dysplasias. *Epilepsia* 2012; 53: 1341-8.

Coras R, Korn K, Bien CG, et al. No evidence for human papillomavirus infection in focal cortical dysplasia IIb. *Ann Neurol* 2015; 77: 312-9.

Costa MR, Hedin-Pereira C. Does cell lineage in the developing cerebral cortex contribute to its columnar organization? *Front Neuroanat* 2010; 4: 26.

Crino PB. Focal brain malformations: a spectrum of disorders along the mTOR cascade. *Novartis Found Symp* 2007; 288: 260-72; discussion 72-81.

Crino PB. mTOR: A pathogenic signaling pathway in developmental brain malformations. *Trends Mol Med* 2011; 17: 734-42.

Crino PB, Aronica E, Baltuch G, Nathanson KL. Biallelic *TSC* gene inactivation in tuberous sclerosis complex. *Neurology* 2010; 74: 1716-23.

Crino PB, Becker AJ. Gene profiling in temporal lobe epilepsy tissue and dysplastic lesions. *Epilepsia* 2006; 47: 1608-16.

Crino PB, Miyata H, Vinters HV. Neurodevelopmental disorders as a cause of seizures. neuropathologic, genetic and mechanistic considerations. *Brain Pathol* 2002; 12: 212-33.

Crino PB, Nathanson KL, Henske EP. The tuberous sclerosis complex. *N Engl J Med* 2006; 355: 1345-56.

Crino PB, Trojanowski JQ, Dichter MA, Eberwine J. Embryonic neuronal markers in tuberous sclerosis: single-cell molecular pathology. *Proc Natl Acad Sci USA* 1996; 93: 14152-7.

Crome L. Infantile cerebral gliosis with giant nerve cells. *J Neurol Neurosurg Psychiatry* 1957; 20: 117-24.

Cruveilhier J. *Maladies du cerveau*. Paris, 1928.

Curatolo P, Verdecchia M, Bombardieri R. Tuberous sclerosis complex: a review of neurological aspects. *Eur J Paediatr Neurol* 2002; 6: 15-23.

Cusmai R, Curatolo P, Mangano S, Cheminal R, Echenne B. Hemimegalencephaly and neurofibromatosis. *Neuropediatrics* 1990; 21: 179-82.

D'Agostino MD, Bastos A, Piras C, et al. Posterior quadrantic dysplasia or hemi-hemimegalencephaly: a characteristic brain malformation. *Neurology* 2004; 62: 2214-20.

D'Gama AM, Geng Y, Couto JA, et al. Mammalian target of rapamycin pathway mutations cause hemimegalencephaly and focal cortical dysplasia. *Ann Neurol* 2015; Jan 19 [Epub ahead of print].

da Costa NM, Martin KA. Whose cortical column would that be? *Front Neuroanat* 2010; 4: 16.

Dabora SL, Jozwiak S, Franz DN, et al. Mutational analysis in a cohort of 224 tuberous sclerosis patients indicates increased severity of TSC2, compared with TSC1, disease in multiple organs. *Am J Hum Genet* 2001; 68: 64-80.

De Ciantis A, Barkovich AJ, Cosottini M, et al. Ultra-high-field MR imaging in polymicrogyria and epilepsy. *AJNR Am J Neuroradiol* 2015; 36: 309-16.

deAzevedo LC, Hedin-Pereira C, Lent R. Callosal neurons in the cingulate cortical plate and subplate of human fetuses. *J Comp Neurol* 1997; 386: 60-70.

Denis D, Maugey-Laulom B, Carles D, Pedespan JM, Brun M, Chateil JF. Prenatal diagnosis of schizencephaly by fetal magnetic resonance imaging. *Fetal Diagn Ther* 2001; 16: 354-9.

Dent MA, Segura-Anaya E, Alva-Medina J, Aranda-Anzaldo A. NeuN/Fox-3 is an intrinsic component of the neuronal nuclear matrix. *FEBS letters* 2010; 584: 2767-71.

Dernoncourt C, Ruelle D, Goffinet AM. Estimation of genetic distances between "reeler" and nearby loci on mouse chromosome 5. *Genomics* 1991; 11: 1167-9.

Descartes M, Mikhail FM, Franklin JC, McGrath TM, Bebin M. Monosomy1p36.3 and trisomy 19p13.3 in a child with periventricular nodular heterotopia. *Pediatr Neurol* 2011; 45: 274-8.

Dibbens LM, de Vries B, Donatello S, et al. Mutations in DEPDC5 cause familial focal epilepsy with variable foci. *Nat Genet* 2013; 45: 546-51.

DiMario FJ, Jr. Brain abnormalities in tuberous sclerosis complex. *J Child Neurol* 2004; 19: 650-7.

Ding SL, Van Hoesen GW, Cassell MD, Poremba A. Parcellation of human temporal polar cortex: a combined analysis of multiple cytoarchitectonic, chemoarchitectonic, and pathological markers. *J Comp Neurol* 2009; 514: 595-623.

Doisy ET, Wenzel HJ, Mu Y, Nguyen DV, Schwartzkroin PA. Nodule excitability in an animal model of periventricular nodular heterotopia: c-fos activation in organotypic hippocampal slices. *Epilepsia* 2015; Mar 6 [Epub ahead of print].

Duckett S, Pearse AGE. The cells of Cajal-Retzius in the developing human brain. *J Anat* 1968; 102: 183-7.

ECTS C. Identification and characterization of the tuberous sclerosis gene on chromosome 16. The European Chromosome 16 Tuberous Sclerosis Consortium. *Cell* 1993; 75: 1305-15.

Edelmayer RM, Brederson JD, Jarvis MF, Bitner RS. Biochemical and pharmacological assessment of MAP-kinase signaling along pain pathways in experimental rodent models: a potential tool for the discovery of novel antinociceptive therapeutics. *Biochem Pharmacol* 2014; 87: 390-8.

Eltze CM, Chong WK, Bhate S, Harding B, Neville BG, Cross JH. Taylor-type focal cortical dysplasia in infants: some MRI lesions almost disappear with maturation of myelination. *Epilepsia* 2005; 46: 1988-92.

Emery JA, Roper SN, Rojiani AM. White matter neuronal heterotopia in temporal lobe epilepsy: a morphometric and immunohistochemical study. *J Neuropathol Exp Neurol* 1997; 56: 1276-82.

Eriksson SH, Thom M, Heffernan J, *et al.* Persistent reelin-expressing Cajal-Retzius cells in polymicrogyria. *Brain* 2001; 124: 1350-61.

Esquirol E. *Idiotie*. Paris: CLF Panckoucke, 1818.

Falace A, Buhler E, Fadda M, *et al.* TBC1D24 regulates neuronal migration and maturation through modulation of the ARF6-dependent pathway. *Proc Natl Acad Sci USA* 2014; 111: 2337-42.

Falconer DS. Two new mutants, "trembler" and "reeler", with neurological actions in the house mouse (Mus musculus L.). *J Genet* 1951; 50: 192-201.

Fauser S, Becker A, Schulze-Bonhage A, *et al.* CD34-immunoreactive balloon cells in cortical malformations. *Acta Neuropathol* 2004; 108: 272-8.

Fauser S, Essang C, Altenmuller DM, *et al.* Long-term seizure outcome in 211 patients with focal cortical dysplasia. *Epilepsia* 2015; 56: 66-76.

Feldmeyer D, Brecht M, Helmchen F, *et al.* Barrel cortex function. *Prog Neurobiol* 2013; 103: 3-27.

Ferland RJ, Gaitanis JN, Apse K, Tantravahi U, Walsh CA, Sheen VL. Periventricular nodular heterotopia and Williams syndrome. *Am J Med Genet* 2006; 140: 1305-11.

Ferrer I. A Golgi analysis of unlayered polymicrogyria. *Acta Neuropathol* 1984; 65: 69-76.

Finlay BL, Uchiyama R. Developmental mechanisms channeling cortical evolution. *Trends Neurosci* 2015; 38: 69-76.

Flores-Sarnat L. Hemimegalencephaly: part 1. Genetic, clinical, and imaging aspects. *J Child Neurol* 2002; 17: 373-84; discussion 84.

Flores Sarnat L. *Epidermal Nevus Syndrome*. Edinburgh, London, NY, Toronto: Elsevier, 2013.

Flores-Sarnat L, Sarnat HB, Davila-Gutierrez G, Alvarez A. Hemimegalencephaly: part 2. Neuropathology suggests a disorder of cellular lineage. *J Child Neurol* 2003; 18: 776-85.

Fonseca M, Delrio JA, Martinez A, Gomez S, Soriano E. Development of calretinin immunoreactivity in the neocortex of the rat. *J Comp Neurol* 1995; 361: 177-92.

Fox JW, Lamperti ED, Eksioglu YZ, *et al.* Mutations in filamin 1 prevent migration of cerebral cortical neurons in human periventricular heterotopia. *Neuron* 1998; 21: 1315-25.

Fox K, Schlaggar BL, Glazewski S, O'Leary DD. Glutamate receptor blockade at cortical synapses disrupts development of thalamocortical and columnar organization in somatosensory cortex. *Proc Natl Acad Sci USA* 1996; 93: 5584-9.

Frotscher M. Dual role of Cajal-Retzius cells and reelin in cortical development. *Cell Tissue Res* 1997; 290: 315-22.

Garbelli R, Meroni A, Magnaghi G, *et al.* Architectural (Type IA) focal cortical dysplasia and parvalbumin immunostaining in temporal lobe epilepsy. *Epilepsia* 2006; 47: 1074-8.

Garbelli R, Milesi G, Medici V, *et al.* Blurring in patients with temporal lobe epilepsy: clinical, high-field imaging and ultrastructural study. *Brain* 2012; 135: 2337-49.

Gentet LJ, Kremer Y, Taniguchi H, Huang ZJ, Staiger JF, Petersen CC. Unique functional properties of somatostatin-expressing GABAergic neurons in mouse barrel cortex. *Nat Neurosci* 2012; 15: 607-12.

Gilles FH. Myelination in the neonatal brain. *Hum Pathol* 1976; 7: 244-8.

Glenn OA, Barkovich AJ. Magnetic resonance imaging of the fetal brain and spine: an increasingly important tool in prenatal diagnosis, part 1. *AJNR Am J Neuroradiol* 2006; 27: 1604-11.

Glenn OA, Cuneo AA, Barkovich AJ, Hashemi Z, Bartha AI, Xu D. Malformations of cortical development: diagnostic accuracy of fetal MR imaging. *Radiology* 2012; 263: 843-55.

Grajkowska W, Kotulska K, Jurkiewicz E, Matyja E. Brain lesions in tuberous sclerosis complex. Review. *Folia Neuropathol* 2010; 48: 139-49.

Granata T, Farina L, Faiella A, *et al.* Familial schizencephaly associated with EMX2 mutation. *Neurology* 1997; 48: 1403-6.

Green AJ, Smith M, Yates JR. Loss of heterozygosity on chromosome 16p13.3 in hamartomas from tuberous sclerosis patients. *Nat Genet* 1994; 6: 193-6.

Griffiths PD, Batty R, Warren D, *et al.* The use of MR imaging and spectroscopy of the brain in children investigated for developmental delay: what is the most appropriate imaging strategy? *Eur Radiol* 2011; 21: 1820-30.

Grosso S, Fichera M, Galesi O, *et al.* Bilateral periventricular nodular heterotopia and lissencephaly in an infant with unbalanced t(12;17)(q24.31; p13.3) translocation. *Dev Med Child Neurol* 2008; 50: 473-6.

Guerreiro MM, Andermann E, Guerrini R, *et al.* Familial perisylvian polymicrogyria: a new familial syndrome of cortical maldevelopment. *Ann Neurol* 2000; 48: 39-48.

Guerrini R. Genetic malformations of the cerebral cortex and epilepsy. *Epilepsia* 2005; 46 (Suppl 1): 32-7.

Guerrini R, Dobyns WB. Malformations of cortical development: clinical features and genetic causes. *Lancet Neurol* 2014; 13: 710-26.

Guerrini R, Dobyns WB, Barkovich AJ. Abnormal development of the human cerebral cortex: genetics, functional consequences and treatment options. *Trends Neurosci* 2008; 31: 154-62.

Guerrini R, Filippi T. Neuronal migration disorders, genetics, and epileptogenesis. *J Child Neurol* 2005; 20: 287-99.

Haas CA, Frotscher M. Reelin deficiency causes granule cell dispersion in epilepsy. *Exp Brain Res* 2010; 200: 141-9.

Hadjivassiliou G, Martinian L, Squier W, *et al.* The application of cortical layer markers in the evaluation of cortical dysplasias in epilepsy. *Acta Neuropathol* 2010; 120: 517-28.

Hansen DV, Lui JH, Parker PR, Kriegstein AR. Neurogenic radial glia in the outer subventricular zone of human neocortex. *Nature* 2010; 464: 554-61.

Hardiman O, Burke T, Phillips J, *et al.* Microdysgenesis in resected temporal neocortex: incidence and clinical significance in focal epilepsy. *Neurology* 1988; 38: 1041-7.

Herman-Sucharska I, Bekiesinska-Figatowska M, Urbanik A. Fetal central nervous system malformations on MR images. *Brain Dev* 2009; 31: 185-99.

Hevner RF. Layer-specific markers as probes for neuron type identity in human neocortex and malformations of cortical development. *J Neuropathol Exp Neurol* 2007; 66: 101-9.

Hildebrandt M, Pieper T, Winkler P, Kolodziejczyk D, Holthausen H, Blümcke I. Neuropathological spectrum of cortical dysplasia in children with severe focal epilepsies. *Acta Neuropathol* 2005; 110: 1-11.

Horton JC, Adams DL. The cortical column: a structure without a function. *Philos Trans R Soc Lond B Biol Sci* 2005; 360: 837-62.

Hubel DH, Wiesel TN. Anatomical demonstration of columns in the monkey striate cortex. *Nature* 1969; 221: 747-50.

Hubel DH, Wiesel TN. Laminar and columnar distribution of geniculo-cortical fibers in the macaque monkey. *J Comp Neurol* 1972; 146: 421-50.

Hubel DH, Wiesel TN, Stryker MP. Orientation columns in macaque monkey visual cortex demonstrated by the 2-deoxyglucose autoradiographic technique. *Nature* 1977; 269: 328-30.

Huppertz HJ, Grimm C, Fauser S, *et al.* Enhanced visualization of blurred gray-white matter junctions in focal cortical dysplasia by voxel-based 3D MRI analysis. *Epilepsy Res* 2005; 67: 35-50.

Imamoto K, Karasawa N, Isomura G, Nagatsu I. Cajal-Retzius neurons identified by GABA immunohistochemistry in layer I of the rat cerebral cortex. *Neurosci Res* 1994; 20: 101-5.

Inder TE, Huppi PS, Zientara GP, et al. The postmigrational development of polymicrogyria documented by magnetic resonance imaging from 31 weeks' postconceptional age. *Ann Neurol* 1999; 45: 798-801.

Ishida S, Picard F, Rudolf G, et al. Mutations of DEPDC5 cause autosomal dominant focal epilepsies. *Nat Genet* 2013; 45: 552-5.

Iyer A, Prabowo A, Anink J, Spliet WG, van Rijen PC, Aronica E. Cell injury and premature neurodegeneration in focal malformations of cortical development. *Brain Pathol* 2014; 24: 1-17.

Jacobs KM, Hwang BJ, Prince DA. Focal epileptogenesis in a rat model of polymicrogyria. *J Neurophysiol* 1999; 81: 159-73.

Jamuar SS, Lam AT, Kircher M, et al. Somatic mutations in cerebral cortical malformations. *N Engl J Med* 2014; 371: 733-43.

Jamuar SS, Walsh CA. Somatic mutations in cerebral cortical malformations. *N Engl J Med* 2014; 371: 2038.

Jansen A, Andermann E. Genetics of the polymicrogyria syndromes. *J Med Genet* 2005; 42: 369-78.

Jehi L, Yardi R, Chagin K, et al. Development and validation of nomograms to provide individualised predictions of seizure outcomes after epilepsy surgery: a retrospective analysis. *Lancet Neurol* 2015; 14: 283-90.

Jones SE, Zhang M, Avitsian R, et al. Functional magnetic resonance imaging networks induced by intracranial stimulation may help defining the epileptogenic zone. *Brain Connect* 4: 286-98.

Jozwiak J, Jozwiak S. Giant cells: contradiction to two-hit model of tuber formation? *Cell Mol Neurobiol* 2005; 25: 795-805.

Kalifa GL, Chiron C, Sellier N, et al. Hemimegalencephaly: MR imaging in five children. *Radiology* 1987; 165: 29-33.

Katzel D, Zemelman BV, Buetfering C, Wolfel M, Miesenbock G. The columnar and laminar organization of inhibitory connections to neocortical excitatory cells. *Nat Neurosci* 2011; 14: 100-7.

Keil W, Schmidt KF, Lowel S, Kaschube M. Reorganization of columnar architecture in the growing visual cortex. *Proc Natl Acad Sci USA* 2010; 107: 12293-8.

Kepecs A, Fishell G. Interneuron cell types are fit to function. *Nature* 2014; 505: 318-26.

Kiehl TR, Chow EW, Mikulis DJ, George SR, Bassett AS. Neuropathologic features in adults with 22q11.2 deletion syndrome. *Cereb Cortex* 2009; 19: 153-64.

Kim KK, Adelstein RS, Kawamoto S. Identification of neuronal nuclei (NeuN) as Fox-3, a new member of the Fox-1 gene family of splicing factors. *J Biol Chem* 2009; 284: 31052-61.

Kluver H, Barrera E. A method for the combined staining of cells and fibers in the nervous system. *J Neuropathol Exp Neurol* 1953; 12: 400-3.

Kobow K, Jeske I, Hildebrandt M, et al. Increased reelin promoter methylation is associated with granule cell dispersion in human temporal lobe epilepsy. *J Neuropathol Exp Neurol* 2009; 68: 356-64.

Kostovic I, Jovanov-Milosevic N. Subplate zone of the human brain: historical perspective and new concepts. *Coll Antropol* 2008; 32 (Suppl 1): 3-8.

Kovacs GG, Adle-Biassette H, Milenkovic I, Cipriani S, van Scheppingen J, Aronica E. Linking pathways in the developing and aging brain with neurodegeneration. *Neuroscience* 2014; 269: 152-72.

Krsek P, Maton B, Jayakar P, et al. Incomplete resection of focal cortical dysplasia is the main predictor of poor postsurgical outcome. *Neurology* 2009; 72: 217-23.

Krsek P, Maton B, Korman B, et al. Different features of histopathological subtypes of pediatric focal cortical dysplasia. *Ann Neurol* 2008; 63: 758-69.

Krsek P, Pieper T, Karlmeier A, et al. Different presurgical characteristics and seizure outcomes in children with focal cortical dysplasia type I or II. *Epilepsia* 2009; 50: 125-37.

Krueger DA, Care MM, Holland K, et al. Everolimus for subependymal giant-cell astrocytomas in tuberous sclerosis. *N Engl J Med* 2010; 363: 1801-11.

Kwa VI, Smitt JH, Verbeeten BW, Barth PG. Epidermal nevus syndrome with isolated enlargement of one temporal lobe: a case report. *Brain Dev* 1995; 17: 122-5.

Kwiatkowski DJ. Tuberous sclerosis: from tubers to mTOR. *Ann Hum Genet* 2003; 67 (Pt 1): 87-96.

Kwiatkowski DJ, Manning BD. Molecular basis of giant cells in tuberous sclerosis complex. *N Engl J Med* 2014; 371: 778-80.

Lamparello P, Baybis M, Pollard J, et al. Developmental lineage of cell types in cortical dysplasia with balloon cells. *Brain* 2007; 130: 2267-76.

LaPointe MM, Spriggs EL, Mhanni AA. Germline mosaicism in X-linked periventricular nodular heterotopia. *BMC Neurol* 2014; 14: 125.

Lavdas AA, Grigoriou M, Pachnis V, Parnavelas JG. The medial ganglionic eminence gives rise to a population of early neurons in the developing cerebral cortex. *J Neurosci* 1999; 19: 7881-8.

Lee A, Maldonado M, Baybis M, et al. Markers of cellular proliferation are expressed in cortical tubers. *Ann Neurol* 2003; 53: 668-73.

Lee SH, Kwan AC, Zhang S, et al. Activation of specific interneurons improves V1 feature selectivity and visual perception. *Nature* 2012; 488: 379-83.

Lerner JT, Salamon N, Hauptman JS, et al. Assessment and surgical outcomes for mild type I and severe type II cortical dysplasia: a critical review and the UCLA experience. *Epilepsia* 2009; 50: 1310-35.

Leventer RJ, Jansen FE, Mandelstam SA, et al. Is focal cortical dysplasia sporadic? Family evidence for genetic susceptibility. *Epilepsia* 2014; 55: e22-6.

Leventer RJ, Phelan EM, Coleman LT, Kean MJ, Jackson GD, Harvey AS. Clinical and imaging features of cortical malformations in childhood. *Neurology* 1999; 53: 715-22.

Li H, Fertuzinhos S, Mohns E, et al. Laminar and columnar development of barrel cortex relies on thalamocortical neurotransmission. *Neuron* 2013; 79: 970-86.

Li S, Jin Z, Koirala S, et al. GPR56 regulates pial basement membrane integrity and cortical lamination. *J Neurosci* 2008; 28: 5817-26.

Li Y, Tsui W, Rusinek H, et al. Cortical laminar binding of PET amyloid and tau tracers in Alzheimer disease. *J Nucl Med* 2015; 56: 270-3.

Lindhurst MJ, Sapp JC, Teer JK, et al. A mosaic activating mutation in AKT1 associated with the Proteus syndrome. *N Engl J Med* 2011; 365: 611-9.

Liu S, Lu L, Cheng X, Xu G, Yang H. Viral infection and focal cortical dysplasia. *Ann Neurol* 2013; 75: 614-6.

Lodato S, Shetty AS, Arlotta P. Cerebral cortex assembly: generating and reprogramming projection neuron diversity. *Trends Neurosci* 2015; 38: 117-25.

Lorente de Nó R. Studies on the structure of the cerebral cortex. II: Continuatiuon of the study of the Ammonic system. *J Psychol Neurol* 1934; 46: 113-77.

Loup F, Picard F, Yonekawa Y, Wieser HG, Fritschy JM. Selective changes in GABAA receptor subtypes in white matter neurons of patients with focal epilepsy. *Brain* 2009; 132: 2449-63.

Lovett-Barron M, Turi GF, Kaifosh P, et al. Regulation of neuronal input transformations by tunable dendritic inhibition. *Nat Neurosci* 2012; 15: 423-30, S1-3.

Lozovaya N, Gataullina S, Tsintsadze T, et al. Selective suppression of excessive GluN2C expression rescues early epilepsy in a tuberous sclerosis murine model. *Nature Comm* 2014; 5: 4563.

Luat AF, Makki M, Chugani HT. Neuroimaging in tuberous sclerosis complex. *Curr Opin Neurol* 2007; 20: 142-50.

Luhmann HJ, Kilb W, Hanganu-Opatz IL. Subplate cells: amplifiers of neuronal activity in the developing cerebral cortex. *Front Neuroanat* 2009; 3: 19.

Mackenzie IR, Neumann M, Cairns NJ, Munoz DG, Isaacs AM. Novel types of frontotemporal lobar degeneration: beyond tau and TDP-43. *J Mol Neurosci* 2011; 45: 402-8.

Marin-Padilla M. Dual origin of the mammalian neocortex and evolution of the cortical plate. *Anat Embryol* 1978; 152: 109-26.

Marin-Padilla M. Structural organization of the human cerebral cortex prior to the appearance of the cortical plate. *Anat Embryol* 1983; 168: 21-40.

Marin-Padilla M. Cajal-Retzius cells and the development of the neocortex. *Trends Neurosci* 1998; 21: 64-71.

Marín-Padilla M. *The Human Brain. Prenatal Development and Structure*. Heidelberg – London – New York: Springer, 2011.

Marin-Padilla M, Parisi JE, Armstrong DL, Sargent SK, Kaplan JA. Shaken infant syndrome: developmental neuropathology, progressive cortical dysplasia, and epilepsy. *Acta Neuropathol* 2002; 103: 321-32.

Martin R, Gutierrez A, Penafiel A, Marin-Padilla M, de la Calle A. Persistence of Cajal-Retzius cells in the adult human cerebral cortex. An immunohistochemical study. *Histol Histopathol* 1999; 14: 487-90.

Martinian L, Boer K, Middeldorp J, et al. Expression patterns of glial fibrillary acidic protein (GFAP)-delta in epilepsy-associated lesional pathologies. *Neuropathol Appl Neurobiol* 35: 394-405.

Marty S, Carroll P, Cellerino A, et al. Brain-derived neurotrophic factor promotes the differentiation of various hippocampal nonpyramidal neurons, including Cajal-Retzius cells, in organotypic slice cultures. *J Neurosci* 1996; 16: 675-87.

McConnell SK, Ghosh A, Shatz CJ. Subplate neurons pioneer the first axon pathway from the cerebral cortex. *Science* 1989; 245: 978-82.

McConnell SK, Ghosh A, Shatz CJ. Subplate pioneers and the formation of descending connections from cerebral cortex. *J Neurosci* 1994; 14: 1892-907.

Medina AE, Krahe TE, Ramoa AS. Early alcohol exposure induces persistent alteration of cortical columnar organization and reduced orientation selectivity in the visual cortex. *J Neurophysiol* 2005; 93: 1317-25.

Meencke HJ, Janz D. Neuropathological findings in primary generalized epilepsy: a study of eight cases. *Epilepsia* 1984; 25: 8-21.

Meencke HJ, Veith G. The relevance of slight migrational disturbances (microdysgenesis) to the etiology of the epilepsies. *Adv Neurol* 1999; 79: 123-31.

Mellado C, Poduri A, Gleason D, et al. Candidate gene sequencing of LHX2, HESX1, and SOX2 in a large schizencephaly cohort. *Am J Med Genet* 2010; 152A: 2736-42.

Miles LL, Greiner HM, Mangano FT, Horn PS, Leach JL, Miles MV. Cytochrome-c-oxidase deficit is associated with the seizure onset zone in young patients with focal cortical dysplasia type II. *Metab Brain Dis* 2015 [Epub ahead of print].

Mischel PS, Nguyen LP, Vinters HV. Cerebral cortical dysplasia associated with pediatric epilepsy. Review of neuropathologic features and proposal for a grading system. *J Neuropathol Exp Neurol* 1995; 54: 137-53.

Mitchell TN, Free SL, Williamson KA, et al. Polymicrogyria and absence of pineal gland due to PAX6 mutation. *Ann Neurol* 2003; 53: 658-63.

Miyata H, Chiang AC, Vinters HV. Insulin signaling pathways in cortical dysplasia and TSC-tubers: tissue microarray analysis. *Ann Neurol* 2004; 56: 510-9.

Mizuguchi M, Takashima S. Neuropathology of tuberous sclerosis. *Brain Dev* 2001; 23: 508-15.

Molliver ME, Kostovic I, van der Loos H. The development of synapses in cerebral cortex of the human fetus. *Brain Res* 1973; 50: 403-7.

Mountcastle VB. The columnar organization of the neocortex. *Brain* 1997; 120: 701-22.

Muhlebner A, Coras R, Kobow K, et al. Neuropathologic measurements in focal cortical dysplasias: validation of the ILAE 2011 classification system and diagnostic implications for MRI. *Acta Neuropathol* 2012; 123: 259-72.

Najm IM, Tassi L, Sarnat HB, Holthausen H, Russo GL. Epilepsies associated with focal cortical dysplasias (FCDs). *Acta Neuropathol* 2014; 128: 5-19.

Nakahashi M, Sato N, Yagishita A, et al. Clinical and imaging characteristics of localized megalencephaly: a retrospective comparison of diffuse hemimegalencephaly and multilobar cortical dysplasia. *Neuroradiology* 2009; 51: 821-30.

Nellist M, Sancak O, Goedbloed MA, et al. Distinct effects of single amino-acid changes to tuberin on the function of the tuberin-hamartin complex. *Eur J Hum G* 2005; 13: 59-68.

Nguyen LH, Brewster AL, Clark ME, et al. mTOR inhibition suppresses established epilepsy in a mouse model of cortical dysplasia. *Epilepsia* 2015; Mar 6 [Epub ahead of print].

Nishikawa S, Goto S, Hamasaki T, Yamada K, Ushio Y. Involvement of reelin and Cajal-Retzius cells in the developmental formation of vertical columnar structures in the cerebral cortex: evidence from the study of mouse presubicular cortex. *Cereb Cortex* 2002; 12: 1024-30.

Orlova KA, Crino PB. The tuberous sclerosis complex. *Ann New York Acad Sci* 2010; 1184: 87-105.

Palmini A, Najm I, Avanzini G, et al. Terminology and classification of the cortical dysplasias. *Neurology* 2004; 62 (6 Suppl 3): S2-8.

Pardoe HR, Mandelstam SA, Hiess RK, Kuzniecky RI, Jackson GD. Quantitative assessment of corpus callosum morphology in periventricular nodular heterotopia. *Epilepsy Res* 2015; 109: 40-7.

Park SH, Pepkowitz SH, Kerfoot C, et al. Tuberous sclerosis in a 20-week gestation fetus: immunohistochemical study. *Acta Neuropathol* 1997; 94: 180-6.

Parrini E, Ramazzotti A, Dobyns WB, et al. Periventricular heterotopia: phenotypic heterogeneity and correlation with Filamin A mutations. *Brain* 2006; 129: 1892-906.

Pfeffer CK, Xue M, He M, Huang ZJ, Scanziani M. Inhibition of inhibition in visual cortex: the logic of connections between molecularly distinct interneurons. *Nat Neurosci* 2013; 16: 1068-76.

Pi HJ, Hangya B, Kvitsiani D, Sanders JI, Huang ZJ, Kepecs A. Cortical interneurons that specialize in disinhibitory control. *Nature* 2013; 503: 521-4.

Pisano T, Barkovich AJ, Leventer RJ, et al. Peritrigonal and temporo-occipital heterotopia with corpus callosum and cerebellar dysgenesis. *Neurology* 2012; 79: 1244-51.

Poduri A, Evrony GD, Cai X, et al. Somatic activation of AKT3 causes hemispheric developmental brain malformations. *Neuron* 2012; 74: 41-8.

Poduri A, Evrony GD, Cai X, Walsh CA. Somatic mutation, genomic variation, and neurological disease. *Science* 2013; 341: 1237758.

Polizzi A, Pavone P, Iannetti P, Manfre L, Ruggieri M. Septo-optic dysplasia complex: a heterogeneous malformation syndrome. *Pediatr Neurol* 2006; 34: 66-71.

Powell TP, Mountcastle VB. Some aspects of the functional organization of the cortex of the postcentral gyrus of the monkey: a correlation of findings obtained in a single unit analysis with cytoarchitecture. *Bull Johns Hopkins Hosp* 1959; 105: 133-62.

Prabowo AS, Anink JJ, Lammens M, et al. Fetal brain lesions in tuberous sclerosis complex: TORC1 activation and inflammation. *Brain Pathol* 2013; 23: 45-59.

Qin W, Chan JA, Vinters HV, et al. Analysis of TSC cortical tubers by deep sequencing of TSC1, TSC2 and KRAS demonstrates that small second-hit mutations in these genes are rare events. *Brain Pathol* 2010; 20: 1096-105.

Rakic P. Mode of cell migration to the superficial layers of fetal monkey neocortex. *J Comp Neurol* 1972; 145: 61-83.

Rakic P. Radial versus tangential migration of neuronal clones in the developing cerebral cortex. *Proc Natl Acad Sci USA* 1995; 92: 11323-7.

Rakic P. Radial unit hypothesis of neocortical expansion. *Novartis Found Symp* 2000; 228: 30-42; discussion: 52.

Rakic P. Evolving concepts of cortical radial and areal specification. *Prog Brain Res* 2002; 136: 265-80.

Rakic P, Knyihar-Csillik E, Csillik B. Polarity of microtubule assemblies during neuronal cell migration. *Proc Natl Acad Sci USA* 1996; 93: 9218-22.

Rakic P, Lombroso PJ. Development of the cerebral cortex: I. Forming the cortical structure. *J Am Acad Child Adolesc Psychiatry* 1998; 37: 116-7.

Ramon y Cajal SR. Sur la structure de l'écorce cérébrale de quelques mammifères. *La Cellule* 1881; 7: 125-76.

Ramon y Cajal SR. Sobre la existencia de células nerviosas especiales de la primera capa de las circunvoluciones cerebrales [On the existence of special nerve cells of the first layer of cerebral convolutions]. *Gaceta Méd Catalana* 1890; 1: 225-8.

Ramon y Cajal SR. Las células de cilindro-eje corto de la capa molecular del cerebro [The cells of the molecular layer of the brain]. *Rev Trimest Microsc* 1897; 2: 104-27.

Ramon y Cajal SR. *L'histologie du système nerveux de l'homme et des vértebrés*. Reprinted in English translation, Histology of the Nervous System of Man and Vertebrates (in 2 volumes) New York, Oxford: Oxford University Press, 1995.

Ramos RL, Siu NY, Brunken WJ, et al. Cellular and axonal constituents of neocortical molecular layer heterotopia. *Dev Neurosci* 2014; 36: 477-89.

Raymond AA, Fish DR, Stevens JM, Sisodiya SM, Alsanjari N, Shorvon SD. Subependymal heterotopia: a distinct neuronal migration disorder associated with epilepsy. *J Neurol Neurosurg Psychiatry* 1994; 57: 1195-202.

Redecker C, Luhmann HJ, Hagemann G, Fritschy JM, Witte OW. Differential downregulation of GABAA receptor subunits in widespread brain regions in the freeze-lesion model of focal cortical malformations. *J Neurosci* 2000; 20: 5045-53.

Reisin HD, Colombo JA. Considerations on the astroglial architecture and the columnar organization of the cerebral cortex. *Cell Mol Neurobiol* 2002; 22: 633-44.

Retzius G. Die Cajalschen Zellen der Grosshirnrinde beim Menschen und bei Säugetieren. *Verh Biol Ver* 1891; 3: 90-103.

Retzius G. Weitere Beiträge zur Kenntnis der Cajalschen Zellen der Grosshirnrinde des Menschen. *Biol Untersuch* 1894; 6: 29-34.

Robain O, Floquet C, Heldt N, Rozenberg F .Hemimegalencephaly: a clinicopathological study of four cases. *Neuropathol Appl Neurobiol* 1988; 14: 125-35.

Rockland KS. Non-uniformity of extrinsic connections and columnar organization. *J Neurocytol* 2002; 31: 247-53.

Rockland KS, Ichinohe N. Some thoughts on cortical minicolumns. *Exp Brain Res* 2004; 158: 265-77.

Rojiani AM, Emery JA, Anderson KJ, Massey JK. Distribution of heterotopic neurons in normal hemispheric white matter: a morphometric analysis. *J Neuropathol Exp Neurol* 1996; 55: 178-83.

Rorke LB, Riggs HE. *Myelination in the Brain of the Newborn*. Philadelphia, Toronto: Lippincott, 1969.

Rossini L, Moroni RF, Tassi L, et al. Altered layer-specific gene expression in cortical samples from patients with temporal lobe epilepsy. *Epilepsia* 2011; 52: 1928-37.

Ruppe V, Dilsiz P, Reiss CS, et al. Developmental brain abnormalities in tuberous sclerosis complex: a comparative tissue analysis of cortical tubers and perituberal cortex. *Epilepsia* 2014; 55: 539-50.

Sakakibara T, Sukigara S, Saito T, et al. Delayed maturation and differentiation of neurons in focal cortical dysplasia with the transmantle sign: analysis of layer-specific marker expression. *J Neuropathol Exp Neurol* 2012; 71: 741-9.

Sakuta R, Aikawa H, Takashima S, Ryo S. Epidermal nevus syndrome with hemimegalencephaly: neuropathological study. *Brain Dev* 1991; 13: 260-5.

Salamon N, Andres M, Chute DJ, et al. Contralateral hemimicrencephaly and clinical-pathological correlations in children with hemimegalencephaly. *Brain* 2006; 129: 352-65.

Sanes JR, Yamagata M. Formation of lamina-specific synaptic connections. *Curr Opin Neurobiol* 1999; 9: 79-87.

Sanides F, Sas E. Persistence of horizontal cells of the Cajal foetal type and of the subpial granular layer in parts of the mammalian paleocortex. *Zeitschrift fur mikroskopisch-anatomischen Forschung* 1970; 82: 570-88.

Sarnat H, Flores-Sarnat L, Crino P, Hader W, Bello-Espinosa L. Hemimegalencephaly: foetal tauopathy with mTOR hyperactivation and neuronal lipidosis. *Folia Neuropathol* 2012; 50: 330-45.

Sarnat HB. *Cerebral Dysgenesis. Embryology and Clinical Expression*. New York: Oxford University Press, 1992.

Sarnat HB. Molecular genetic classification of central nervous system malformations. *J Child Neurol* 2000; 15: 675-87.

Sarnat HB. Clinical neuropathology practice guide 5-2013: markers of neuronal maturation. *Clin Neuropathol* 2013; 32: 340-69.

Sarnat HB. Immunocytochemical markers of neuronal maturation in human diagnostic neuropathology. *Cell Tiss Res* 2015 [Epub ahead of print].

Sarnat HB, Flores-Sarnat L. Cajal-Retzius and subplate neurons: their role in cortical development. *Eur J Paediatr Neurol* 2002; 6: 91-7.

Sarnat HB, Flores-Sarnat L. Molecular genetic and morphologic integration in malformations of the nervous system for etiologic classification. *Semin Pediatr Neurol* 2002; 9: 335-44.

Sarnat HB, Flores-Sarnat L. Integrative classification of morphology and molecular genetics in central nervous system malformations. *Am J Med Genet* 2004; 126A: 386-92.

Sarnat HB, Flores-Sarnat L. Alpha-B-crystallin as a tissue marker of epileptic foci in paediatric resections. *Can J Neurol Sci* 2009; 36: 566-74.

Sarnat HB, Flores-Sarnat L. Neuroembryology and brain malformations: an overview. *Handb Clin Neurol* 2013; 111: 117-28.

Sarnat HB, Flores-Sarnat L. Neuropathology of paediatric epilepsy. In: Dulac O, Lassonde M, Sarnat HB, (eds) *Handbook of Clinical Neurology: Paediatric Neurology*. Edinburgh, London, NY, Toronto: Elsevier, p. 399-416, 2013.

Sarnat HB, Flores-Sarnat L. Radial microcolumnar cortical architecture: maturational arrest or cortical dysplasia? *Pediatr Neurol* 2013; 48: 259-70.

Sarnat HB, Flores-Sarnat L. Infantile tauopathies: hemimegalencephaly; tuberous sclerosis complex; focal cortical dysplasia 2; ganglioglioma. *Brain Dev* 2015; 37: 553-62.

Sarnat HB, Flores-Sarnat L, Hader W, Bello-Espinosa L. Mitochondrial "hypermetabolic" neurons in paediatric epileptic foci. *Can J Neurol Sci* 2011; 38: 909-17.

Sarnat HB, Flores-Sarnat L, Trevenen CL. Synaptophysin immunoreactivity in the human hippocampus and neocortex from 6 to 41 weeks of gestation. *J Neuropathol Exp Neurol* 2010; 69: 234-45.

Sarnat HB, Philippart M, Flores-Sarnat L, Wei XC. Timing in neural development: arrest, delay, precociousness, and temporal determination of malformations. *Pediatr Neurol* 2015; 52: 473-86.

Sato H, Shimanuki Y, Saito M, et al. Differential columnar processing in local circuits of barrel and insular cortices. *J Neurosci* 2008; 28: 3076-89.

Sato N, Yagishita A, Oba H, et al. Hemimegalencephaly: a study of abnormalities occurring outside the involved hemisphere. *AJNR Am J Neuroradiol* 2007; 28: 678-82.

Schijns OE, Bien CG, Majores M, et al. Presence of temporal gray-white matter abnormalities does not influence epilepsy surgery outcome in temporal lobe epilepsy with hippocampal sclerosis. *Neurosurgery* 2011; 68: 98-106; discussion: 7.

Schmechel DE, Rakic P. Arrested proliferation of radial glial cells during midgestation in rhesus monkey. *Nature* 1979; 277: 303-5.

Schwartzkroin PA, Wenzel HJ. Are developmental dysplastic lesions epileptogenic? *Epilepsia* 2012; 53 (Suppl 1): 35-44.

Sheen VL, Wheless JW, Bodell A, et al. Periventricular heterotopia associated with chromosome 5p anomalies. *Neurology* 60: 1033-6.

Shepherd C, Liu J, Goc J, et al. A quantitative study of white matter hypomyelination and oligodendroglial maturation in focal cortical dysplasia type II. *Epilepsia* 2013; 54: 898-908.

Shiba N, Daza RA, Shaffer LG, Barkovich AJ, Dobyns WB, Hevner RF. Neuropathology of brain and spinal malformations in a case of monosomy 1p36. *Acta Neuropathol Comm* 2013; 1: 45.

Sims J. On hypertrophy and atrophy of the brain. *Med Chirurg Transactions* 1835; 19: 315-80.

Sisodiya S. Epilepsy: the new order-classifying focal cortical dysplasias. *Nature Rev Neurol* 2011; 7: 129-30.

Sisodiya SM. Surgery for malformations of cortical development causing epilepsy. *Brain* 2000; 123: 1075-91.

Sisodiya SM. Malformations of cortical development: burdens and insights from important causes of human epilepsy. *Lancet Neurol* 2004; 3: 29-38.

Sisodiya SM, Fauser S, Cross JH, Thom M. Focal cortical dysplasia type II: biological features and clinical perspectives. *Lancet Neurol* 2009; 8: 830-43.

So J, Stockley T, Stavropoulos DJ. Periventricular nodular heterotopia and transverse limb reduction defect in a woman with interstitial 11q24 deletion in the Jacobsen syndrome region. *Am J Med Genet* 2014; 164A: 511-5.

Sosunov AA, Wu X, Weiner HL, et al. Tuberous sclerosis: a primary pathology of astrocytes? *Epilepsia* 2008; 49 (Suppl 2): 53-62.

Spangle JM, Munger K. The human papillomavirus type 16 E6 oncoprotein activates mTORC1 signaling and increases protein synthesis. *J Virol* 2010; 84: 9398-407.

Spreafico R. Are some focal cortical dysplasias post-migratory cortical malformations? *Epileptic Disord* 2010; 12: 169-71.

Spreafico R, Blümcke I. Focal cortical dysplasias: clinical implication of neuropathological classification systems. *Acta Neuropathol* 2010; 120: 359-67.

Squier W, Jansen A. Polymicrogyria: pathology, fetal origins and mechanisms. *Acta Neuropathol Commun* 2014; 2: 80.

Srour M, Rioux MF, Varga C, et al. The clinical spectrum of nodular heterotopias in children: report of 31 patients. *Epilepsia* 2011; 52: 728-37.

Takashima S, Chan F, Becker LE, Kuruta H. Aberrant neuronal development in hemimegalencephaly: immunohistochemical and Golgi studies. *Pediatr Neurol* 1991; 7: 275-80.

Talos DM, Kwiatkowski DJ, Cordero K, Black PM, Jensen FE. Cell-specific alterations of glutamate receptor expression in tuberous sclerosis complex cortical tubers. *Ann Neurol* 2008; 63: 454-65.

Tassi L, Colombo N, Garbelli R, et al. Focal cortical dysplasia: neuropathological subtypes, EEG, neuroimaging and surgical outcome. *Brain* 125: 1719-32.

Tassi L, Garbelli R, Colombo N, *et al.* Type I focal cortical dysplasia: surgical outcome is related to histopathology. *Epileptic Disord* 2010; 12: 181-91.

Tassi L, Garbelli R, Colombo N, *et al.* Electroclinical, MRI and surgical outcomes in 100 epileptic patients with type II FCD. *Epileptic Disord* 2012; 14: 257-66.

Taylor DC, Falconer MA, Bruton CJ, Corsellis JA. Focal dysplasia of the cerebral cortex in epilepsy. *J Neurol Neurosurg Psychiatry* 1971; 34: 369-87.

Thom M, Eriksson S, Martinian L, *et al.* Temporal lobe sclerosis associated with hippocampal sclerosis in temporal lobe epilepsy: neuropathological features. *J Neuropathol Exp Neurol* 2009; 68: 928-38.

Thom M, Liu J, Reeves C, Stopps V, Sisodiya SM. A cautionary note in the interpretation of human papillomavirus E6 immunohistochemistry in focal cortical dysplasia. *Ann Neurol* 2015; 77: 352-3.

Thom M, Sisodiya S, Harkness W, Scaravilli F. Microdysgenesis in temporal lobe epilepsy. A quantitative and immunohistochemical study of white matter neurones. *Brain* 2001; 124: 2299-309.

Tietjen I, Bodell A, Apse K, *et al.* Comprehensive EMX2 genotyping of a large schizencephaly case series. *AmJ M Genet* 2007; 143A: 1313-6.

Tsai V, Parker WE, Orlova KA, *et al.* Fetal brain mTOR signaling activation in tuberous sclerosis complex. *Cereb Cortex* 2014; 24: 315-27.

Ulfig N. Expression of calbindin and calretinin in the human ganglionic eminence. *Pediatr Neurol* 2001; 24: 357-60.

Ulfig N. Calcium-binding proteins in the human developing brain. *Adv Anat Embryol Cell Biol* 2002; 165: III-IX, 1-92.

van Slegtenhorst M, de Hoogt R, Hermans C, *et al.* Identification of the tuberous sclerosis gene TSC1 on chromosome 9q34. *Science* 1997; 277: 805-8.

Verney C, Derer P. Cajal-Retzius neurons in human cerebral cortex at midgestation show immunoreactivity for neurofilament and calcium-binding proteins. *J Comp Neurol* 1995; 359: 144-53.

Vollmar C, O'Muircheartaigh J, Barker GJ, *et al.* Motor system hyperconnectivity in juvenile myoclonic epilepsy: a cognitive functional magnetic resonance imaging study. *Brain* 2011; 134: 1710-9.

Wang D, Blümcke I, Gui Q, *et al.* Clinico-pathological investigations of Rasmussen encephalitis suggest multifocal disease progression and associated focal cortical dysplasia. *Epileptic Disord* 2013; 15: 32-43.

Wang DD, Blümcke I, Coras R, *et al.* Sturge-Weber syndrome is associated with cortical dysplasia ILAE Type IIIc and excessive hypertrophic pyramidal neurons in brain resections for intractable epilepsy. *Brain Pathol* 2014; 25: 248-55.

Wang ZI, Alexopoulos AV, Jones SE, Jaisani Z, Najm IM, Prayson RA. The pathology of magnetic-resonance-imaging-negative epilepsy. *Mod Pathol* 2013; 26: 1051-8.

Watrin F, Manent JB, Cardoso C, Represa A. Causes and consequences of gray matter heterotopia. *CNS Neurosci Ther* 2015; 21: 112-22.

Wortmann SB, Reimer A, Creemers JW, Mullaart RA. Prenatal diagnosis of cerebral lesions in Tuberous sclerosis complex (TSC). Case report and review of the literature. *Eur J Pediatr Neurol* 2008; 12: 123-6.

Xi ZQ, Wang XF, Shu XF, *et al.* Is intractable epilepsy a tauopathy? *Med Hypotheses* 2011; 76: 897-900.

Yagishita A, Arai N, Tamagawa K, Oda M. Hemimegalencephaly: signal changes suggesting abnormal myelination on MRI. *Neuroradiology* 1998; 40: 734-8.

Yakovlev PI, Wadsworth RC. Schizencephalies; a study of the congenital clefts in the cerebral mantle; clefts with hydrocephalus and lips separated. *J Neuropathol Exp Neurol* 1946; 5: 169-206.

Yasuda CL, Guimaraes CA, Guerreiro MM, *et al.* Voxel-based morphometry and intellectual assessment in patients with congenital bilateral perisylvian syndrome. *J Neurol* 2014; 261: 1374-80.

Yu S, Li S, Shu H, *et al.* Upregulated expression of voltage-gated sodium channel Nav1.3 in cortical lesions of patients with focal cortical dysplasia type IIb. *Neuroreport* 2012; 23: 407-11.

Zhao S, Chai X, Forster E, Frotscher M. Reelin is a positional signal for the lamination of dentate granule cells. *Development* 2004; 131: 5117-25.

Zurolo E, Iyer A, Maroso M, *et al.* Activation of Toll-like receptor, RAGE and HMGB1 signalling in malformations of cortical development. *Brain* 134: 1015-32.

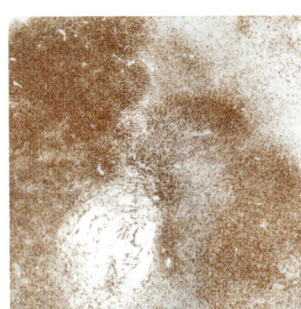

4. Brain tumours associated with early epilepsy onset

Ingmar Blümcke

Any brain tumour can cause sporadic seizures. It is important to recognize the challenging group of brain tumours that manifest with seizure onset during early life (mean age = 16.9 years; *Table I*), and which present with a broad histopathological spectrum of glial and neuronal-glial phenotypes (Wolf and Wiestler, 1993; Blümcke and Wiestler, 2002; Harvey *et al.*, 2008; Piao *et al.*, 2010; Prayson, 2011; Thom *et al.*, 2012; Japp *et al.*, 2013; Blümcke *et al.*, 2014). Another clinical hallmark is their preferential localization in the temporal lobe (73%). As the average duration of epilepsy before surgical treatment was 10.4 years in our series of 1,160 patients collected at the German Neuropathology Reference Centre for Epilepsy Surgery (*see chapter 1, Table I*), we have previously suggested the term "long-term epilepsy associated brain tumours" (Luyken *et al.*, 2003). Due to improved surgical treatment strategies, the term "tumours associated with early epilepsy onset" may be more appropriate and will be used herein. Tumours associated with early epilepsy onset comprise the second largest lesion entity in all patients submitted to epilepsy surgery, whether as adults or children (*see chapter 8, Tables II and III*). By contrast with diffusely infiltrating glial brain tumours, slow tumour growth and low risk for malignant progression is in the range of 1% (Luyken *et al.*, 2004; Thom *et al.*, 2012) and may not necessitate immediate surgical intervention, nor will surgical strategies help achieve long-term seizure control when aimed only at gross tumour resection (Blümcke *et al.*, 2014). A common goal for successful treatment of these patients is the identification of the epileptogenic zone, which may or may not match with the MRI visible lesion (Duncan and de Tisi, 2013; Blümcke *et al.*, 2014). Advanced neurophysiological procedures including invasive EEG recordings are necessary in some patients (Hamer and Hong, 2013; Kennedy and Schuele, 2013; Rosenow and Menzler, 2013). However, weak agreement in the histopathological diagnosis of these tumour entities challenge any meaningful interpretation of published patient series (Thom *et al.*, 2012; Blümcke *et al.*, 2014). A major reason for poor agreement is the large spectrum of morphological variants when reviewing routinely stained haematoxylin and eosin (H&E) sections, sharing one or more of the following features: 1) tumours associated with early epilepsy onset have a histologically variable appearance consisting of dysplastic neuronal and neoplastically transformed glial elements, mostly classified as neuronal-glial tumours by the World Health Organization (WHO) (Louis *et al.*, 2007a; Japp *et al.*, 2013); 2) tumours associated with early epilepsy onset may also present with a diffuse infiltrating oligodendroglia-like cell population, difficult to distinguish from oligodendrogliomas, or between dysembryoplastic neuroepithelial tumour (DNT) and ganglioglioma (GG); 3) the vast majority of these tumours correspond to WHO I (Luyken *et al.*, 2003; Luyken *et al.*, 2004). Reliable guidelines for the identification of tumours that carry a higher risk for recurrence and malignant progression, i.e. atypical ganglioglioma, are not available (Blümcke and Wiestler, 2002; Louis *et al.*, 2007a); 4) these tumours occur predominately in the temporal lobe and present with early seizure onset; 5) these tumours occur during brain development (Blümcke *et al.*, 1999a), and can be associated with focal cortical dysplasia (FCD ILAE Type IIIb) (Blümcke *et al.*, 2011; Palmini *et al.*, 2013), small tumour satellites within adjacent or remote cortex or present with diffuse tumour infiltration. Which tumour entity preferentially follows which of these peculiar patterns, and whether any of these features contribute to enhanced epileptogenicity or ictal onset are yet unanswered questions in need for clarification; 6) tumours associated with early epilepsy onset do not share molecular features typically observed in diffusely infiltrating gliomas, such as IDH1 mutations or 1p/19q deletions (Balss *et al.*, 2008; Parsons *et al.*, 2008; Yan *et al.*, 2009; Ostrom *et al.*, 2013). In contrast, the oncofoetal marker protein CD34 (class II epitope) can be frequently identified (Blümcke *et al.*, 1999b) and developmental genes are likely to be involved (Hoischen *et al.*, 2008). Mutations in B-RAF (Koelsche *et al.*, 2013; Koelsche *et al.*, 2014) or mammalian target of rapamycin (mTOR) signalling (Becker *et al.*, 2001) may be other key features in this group of tumours (Prabowo *et al.*, 2014).

Neuropathological examination and diagnosis rely on microscopic inspection of surgical brain specimens and follow the current WHO classification and grading scale (last revised in 2007) (Louis *et al.*, 2007a). This classification scheme has proven useful for the prediction of the biological behaviour of many malignant gliomas and other CNS tumour entities (Louis *et al.*, 2007b). However, the broad spectrum and variable histomorphological features of tumours associated with early epilepsy onset are not fully recognized within the current WHO grading system and diagnostic criteria remain often vaguely described. Our collection of 1,211 tumour cases includes 18 different entities, with a slight predominance in male patients (*Table I*). Consequently, proper neuropathological evaluation requires diagnostic experience with knowledge of the large spectrum of phenotypic variability. "Over-interpretation" of a tumour's biology and risk of progression may lead to erroneous use of aggressive therapeutic regimens, even though most tumours tend to have a very modest clinical behaviour in the long run without bold risk of recurrence or malignant transformation (Luyken *et al.*, 2004; Thom *et al.*, 2011; Thom *et al.*, 2012). At the same time some tumours with a histologically typical, "benign", neuronal-glial phenotype have been reported to rapidly turn into malignancies (Majores *et al.*, 2008), underscoring the need for reliable biomarkers that could be used to predict the biological behaviour in each patient.

Table I

Summary of brain tumours associated with early epilepsy onset
Summary of 1,211 tumours reviewed at the German Neuropathology Reference Centre for Epilepsy Surgery

WHO Diagnosis	All Cases		Gender Female	Male	Age at onset	Surgery	Duration epilepsy	TEMP	Location FRONT	OTHER
GG	603	49.6%	47.9%	52.1%	12.7	24.5	11.8	84.6%	4.6%	10.8%
DNT	224	18.4%	43.3%	56.7%	15.0	25.8	10.8	71.4%	16.5%	12.1%
O (mixed)*	73	6.0%	45.2%	54.8%	28.8	36.4	7.6	43.8%	30.1%	26.0%
PA	65	5.3%	46.2%	53.8%	14.8	26.2	11.4	69.2%	12.3%	18.5%
Astro*	52	4.3%	48.1%	51.9%	26.0	31.6	5.6	55.8%	25.0%	19.2%
Tumor, NOS	33	2.7%	42.4%	57.6%	17.6	28.5	10.9	78.8%	12.1%	9.1%
AA*	27	2.2%	29.6%	70.4%	34.1	36.6	2.4	48.1%	33.3%	18.5%
PXA*	26	2.1%	65.4%	34.6%	18.8	30.5	11.6	88.5%	0.0%	11.5%
Epithelial Cyst	26	2.1%	53.8%	46.2%	24.0	36.9	13.0	73.1%	15.4%	11.5%
M	24	2.0%	66.7%	33.3%	39.0	48.0	9.0	41.7%	37.5%	20.8%
iA	15	1.2%	33.3%	66.7%	14.6	26.6	12.0	33.3%	13.3%	53.3%
GBM*	12	1.0%	33.3%	66.7%	47.3	50.1	2.8	66.7%	16.7%	16.7%
E*	8	0.7%	37.5%	62.5%	9.6	25.1	15.5	50.0%	12.5%	37.5%
ANET	8	0.7%	37.5%	62.5%	7.0	14.6	7.6	50.0%	~	50.0%
SEGA	7	0.6%	57.1%	42.9%	4.7	13.4	8.7	14.3%	14.3%	71.4%
Neurocytoma	6	0.5%	50.0%	50.0%	12.7	23.7	11.0	100%	~	~
PGNT	2	0.2%	~	100%	31.0	32.5	1.5	100%	~	~
TOTAL	1,211**		46.7%	53.7%	16.6	27.2	10.7	74.1%	11.6%	14.4%

GG: ganglioglioma WHO I/III; DNT: dysembryoplastic neuroepithelial tumour WHO I; O (mixed): oligodendroglioma and mixed oligo-astrocytroma WHO II; PA: pilocytic astrocytoma WHO I; Astro: diffuse astrocytoma WHO II; NOS: not otherwise specified; AA: anaplastic astrocytoma WHO III; PXA: pleomorphic xantoastrocytoma WHO II/III; epithelial cyst: dermoid or epidermoid cysts; M: meningioma WHO I-III; iA: isomorphic astrocytoma variant (analogous to WHO I); GBM: glioblastoma multiforme WHO IV; E: ependymoma WHO II/III; ANET: angiocentric glioma (syn. angiocentric neuroepithelial tumour) WHO I; SEGA: supependymal giant cell astrocytoma WHO I; PGNT: papillary glio-neuronal tumour WHO I; age at operation (mean in years); age at epilepsy onset (mean in years); epilepsy duration until time of surgery; TEMP: temporal lobe; FRONT: frontal lobe; OTHER: comprising all other locations, *i.e.* parietal, occipital, corpus callosum or ventricle.
* Note that common semi-malignant or malignant glial brain tumours represent only 14.5% of cases in this epilepsy surgery cohort.
** 56 patients also suffered from hippocampal sclerosis and were classified as "Dual Pathology" (*see chapter 1, Table I*).

In the following chapters, we will focus on those four tumour entities that occur almost uniquely in patients with early epilepsy onset and which represent 75.3% of our entire case series. These are 1) gangliogliomas (GG); 2) dysembryoplastic neuroepithelial tumours (DNT); 3) angiocentric gliomas (syn. angiocentric neuroepithelial tumours, ANET); and 4) a recently described isomorphic astrocytoma (iA), which is not yet included in the WHO classification system of CNS tumours (Blümcke et al., 2004b; Schramm et al., 2004). We further stratify these entities into those with a predominant neuronal-glial phenotype (GG, DNT) or predominant glial (mostly astrocytic) phenotype (ANET, iA), anticipating the notion that variability in their cellular composition and differentiation is huge and may not entirely reflect any description of typical hallmarks determined from routine H&E stainings.

Tumours with predominant neuronal-glial phenotypes

• Ganglioglioma (WHO I°)

Gangliogliomas are the most common tumours in epilepsy surgery case series (*Table I*) and the best studied of the neuronal-glial tumour group; gangliocytomas, by comparison, are less frequently reported and not present in our series at all. By definition, both contain nodular or compact aggregates of dysplastic neurones, though their appearance can largely vary and may also be difficult to recognise without further immunohistochemical studies. Ganglion cell tumours with more diffuse growth patterns have been reported (Ratilal *et al.*, 2007), where the differential diagnosis may include also cortical dysplasia. More recently cases of multinodular and vacuolating neuronal tumours were reported (Huse *et al.*, 2013; Bodi *et al.*, 2014; Fukushima *et al.*, 2014). An example of this new tumour entity is presented in chapter 7. Although arising in any location, gangliogliomas strongly favour the temporal lobe with a slight male predominance (Yang *et al.*, 2011). The majority of gangliogliomas are WHO I° neoplasms with a favourable prognosis and over 90% of patients have recurrence-free, long-term survivals (Luyken *et al.*, 2004).

Gangliogliomas present with a broad spectrum of histopathological alterations. The recognition of dysplastic neurones is obligatory but often challenging. We recommend the following diagnostic criteria: clusters of neurones with irregular orientation, that cannot be anatomically explained otherwise as pre-existing neurones overrun by glial tumour cells (*Figure 1C*), and/or bi- or multi-nucleated neurones. The glial cell population is considered as the neoplastically transformed component of ganglioglioma (Becker *et al.*, 2001), and most commonly shows features of astrocytic differentiation, but oligodendroglial-like cells can also be recognized. The composition of neuronal and glial cells varies to a considerable extent, with tumours presenting a predominantly neuronal phenotype (in these cases, the differential diagnosis of a gangliocytoma may be considered) or predominantly glial phenotype (the differential diagnosis of a diffusely infiltrating glioma need consideration). Additional histopathological features which can be observed in gangliogliomas are calcification, lymphocytic infiltrates, Rosenthal fibres or eosinophilic granular bodies as well as microcysts (often as white matter rarefaction). Tumours also may present with increased vasculature, mimicking cavernomas. Subarachnoidal spread of the tumour can be detected and confirm autonomous growth. Additional variants with papillary architecture or rosetted neuropil islands have been identified (Komori *et al.*, 1998; Broholm *et al.*, 2002; Dim *et al.*, 2006) and were listed as distinct neuronal-glial tumour entities in the WHO classification of brain tumours.

Immunohistochemical reactions are recommended to confirm the diagnosis of gangliogliomas. Almost 80% of tumours are labelled with antibodies against the class II stem cell epitope CD34 (Blümcke *et al.*, 1999b), which is not expressed in the adult mammalian central nervous system or any neuroimmunological or neurodegenerative disease. In gangliogliomas, CD34 immunolabelling presents three distinguishable patterns (*Figure 1D*): 1) dense CD34 immunoreactivity in the tumour mass; 2) clusters of CD34-positive tumour cells (often resemble oligodendroglia-like cells in H&E stain); 3) tumour cells infiltrating diffusely into remote cortical areas. These may not be detectable by H&E, and often cause misinterpretation as FCD Type IIIb (Blümcke *et al.*, 2011). Such satellites can be immunohistochemically recognized even if only small or fragmented surgical specimens are available for histopathological review. However, described patterns for CD34 immunoreactivity may not be simultaneously present in each tumour specimen. Some tumours will reveal all three patterns, which usually require an anatomically well preserved surgical specimen to recognise. On the other hand, gangliogliomas may only show type 1 or 2 patterns, in particular if fragmented specimens are available. However, their presence is sufficient to classify them as remnant of a neuronal-glial tumour as normal brain cells were never shown to express this class II CD34 epitope. Its differential diagnosis in tumour diagnosis should always include pleomorphic xanthroastrocytomas (Reifenberger et al., 2003) and haemangiopericytomas (Perry et al., 1997), solitary fibrous tumours (Katenkamp et al., 1996) and has been reported in giant cell variants of GBM (Galloway, 2010) or the sarcomatous portion of gliosarcomas (Wharton et al., 2001; Rodriguez et al., 2007). CD34 positive cells more often co-express neuronal markers such as NeuN (Blümcke et al., 1999b) and nestin (Thom et al., 2011) than astrocytic markers.

Dysplastic neurones may also accumulate neurofilament proteins or harbour a perisomatic rim of synatophysin ("corona"). The glial tumour population often expresses GFAP whereas glial MAP2-staining is absent (Blümcke et al., 2004a). The proliferative index is low (1-2% of cells are labelled with the Ki67 epitope). Higher proliferation activities may result from CD68-positive microglia cell infiltration and should be further investigated. If the glial cell component contributes to higher proliferation activity, atypical or anaplastic variants of gangliogliomas will need consideration. Whereas atypical gangliogliomas of WHO II° were not recognized by the WHO grading scale, malignant variants (WHO III) should reveal frank signs of anaplasia, i.e. necrosis, microvascular proliferation and increased mitotic figures in the glial cell component. The latter criterion also is not well defined in the WHO blue book, but should exceed more than 4 mitosis in 10 high power fields. Cellular pleomorphisms should not be mistaken with histopathological criteria for atypia or anaplasia!

It is important to consider the diagnosis of ganglioglioma in the differential diagnosis of any low grade tumour in a young patient with temporal lobe epilepsy and not to overlook a minor ganglion cell component. However, over-diagnosis of a pleomorphically composed "benign" ganglioglioma as malignant glioma or misinterpretation of a diffuse glioma overrunning and distorting (often enlarging)

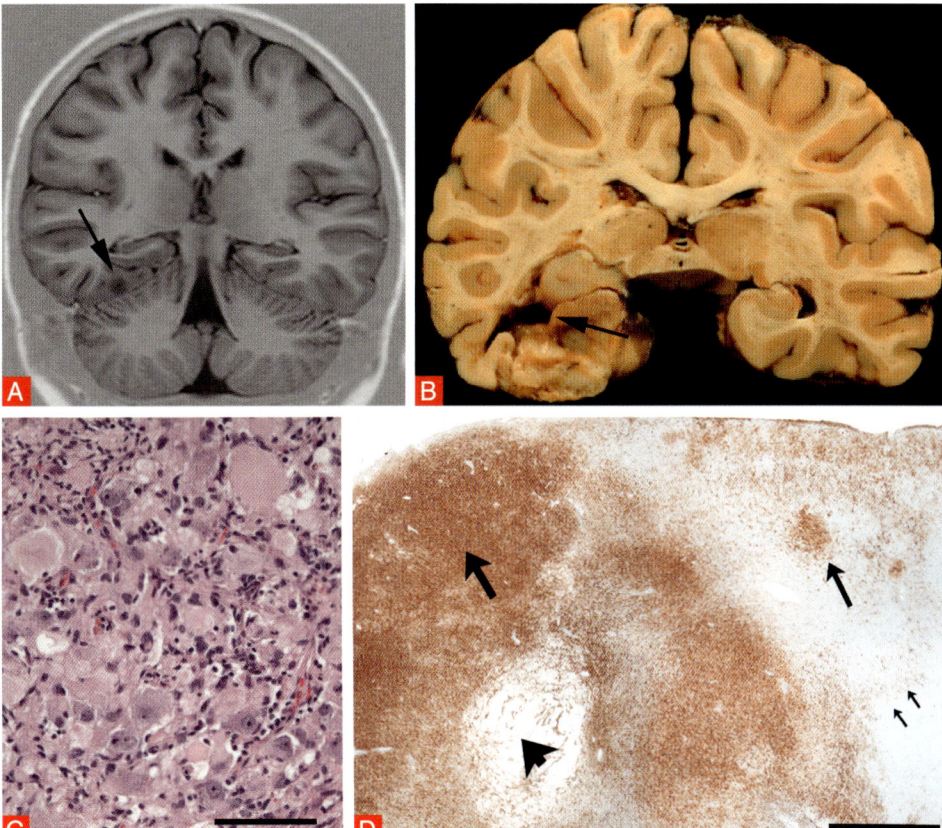

Figure 1
Ganglioglioma (WHO I)

A. Magnetic resonance imaging in a patient with intractable seizures and a small multi-nodular lesion within the right mesial temporal lobe (arrow). Courtesy of Prof. H. Urbach, Freiburg, Germany. B. Autopsy specimen obtained from an elderly patient with a ganglioglioma located in the left temporal lobe (arrow). Courtesy of Prof. P. Kleihues, Freiburg, Germany (with kind permission). C. High-power magnification of a ganglioglioma (WHO grade I). Note the clusters of irregular oriented, dysplastic neurones with large nuclei and prominent nucleoli and neoplastic glia cells. H&E-staining. D. Gangliogliomas frequently are labelled with antibodies directed against the class II oncofoetal epitope CD34 (labelled in brownish colour). Three distinct labelling patterns can be recognised: 1: tumour mass (thick arrow); 2: clusters or nodules of CD34+ tumour cells (smaller arrow); 3. Diffusely infiltrating CD34+ cells into remote cortical areas (thin arrows). Microcysts (or white matter rarefication) are frequently encountered in gangliogliomas (arrowhead). Scale bars in C = 50 µm, in D = 2 mm.

cortical neurones is clinically more demanding, as it immediately calls for adjunct chemo- and/or radiation therapy. On the other hand, poor inter-observer reliability in the diagnosis of ganglio-gliomas has been reported also between experienced pathologists, when differentiating infiltrative gliomas from classical gangliogliomas on H&E-stained sections, with agreement rates of only 55% (Horbinski et al., 2011). NeuN immunohistochemistry as well as CD34 and MAP2 is advocated as superior to H&E as it help to clarify a pre-existing cortical lamination overrun by tumour. Only a small proportion of gangliogliomas display a more aggressive biology with recurrence and progression (Majores et al., 2008). Anaplastic gangliogliomas (WHO III°) represent about 1% of all gangliogliomas (Luyken et al., 2004). They less frequently involve the temporal lobe than their WHO I counterparts, and are more common in young males at the time of presentation (Majores et al., 2008; Selvanathan et al., 2011) but seizures are still the most frequent clinical symptom (Karremann et al., 2009). Predicting those gangliogliomas that are more likely to progress is imperative and should be classified as atypical ganglioglioma (analogue WHO II°). However, this definition has not been included into the 2007 WHO classification system of brain tumours. Clinico-pathological risk factors include age over 40, a non-temporal lobe tumour, incomplete resection and histologically glial cell atypia (increased cell densities and Ki67 labelling indices, nuclear TP53 expression). We have good evidence for improved seizure control following early surgical intervention in patients with gangliogliomas (Yang et al., 2011). Gross total resection is recommended (Luyken et al., 2003; Luyken et al., 2004) and a review of 402 patients supported also a role for radiotherapy when only partial resection was possible, even for low grade ganglioglioma (Rades et al., 2010). However, other studies could not confirm a benefit of radiotherapy on overall survival in anaplastic ganglioglioma (Selvanathan et al., 2011) with good outcome following gross tumour resection alone (Karremann et al., 2009).

Distinct molecular-genetic signatures may play an important role in future diagnostic work-up protocols of tumours associated with early epilepsy onset. Poor interobserver agreement still hampers interpretation of published tumour series and reliable molecular signatures in these tumour entities. As a prominent example, *BRAF* mutations have been identified in up to 50% of gangliogliomas (Dougherty et al., 2010; Schindler et al., 2011) linking ganglioglioma also with PXA (Reifenberger et al., 2003) and pilocytic astrocytomas. Recent reports of oligodendrogliomas that harbour foci of ganglion cell differentiation have been described (Perry et al., 2010; Yamashita et al., 2011). In order to distinguish these from gangliogliomas with oligodendroglial-like cell differentiation, analysis of tumoural CD34 expression and 1p/19q status may be helpful. Gangliogliomas have been reported in patients with neurofibromatosis type 1 (Rodriguez et al., 2008). Histological similarities to cortical tubers called for molecular analysis of *TSC1 and TSC2* genes, with detection of loss of heterozygosity at the TSC1 and TSC2 loci in 30% of patients (Parry et al., 2000), a splice site associated polymorphism in TSC2 (Platten et al., 1997) and a TSC2 mutation in the glial cell component following laser-microdissection (Becker et al., 2001). Enhanced Pi3K-mTOR signalling pathway activation was also shown to play a role in gangliogliomas, rather than in DNT (Boer et al., 2010). *IDH*1 R132H mutations were observed in 8% of a cohort of 98 gangliogliomas and associated with advanced age, increased atypia or anaplasia and worse outcome (Horbinski et al., 2011). It remains possible that IDH1 mutant-positive cases actually represent conventional gliomas misdiagnozed as gangliogliomas. Nevertheless, these studies highlight molecular screening as a useful adjunct and important prognostic information for patient management (Capper et al., 2010; Hartmann et al., 2010; Capper et al., 2011; Reuss et al., 2015).

• Dysembryoplastic neuroepithelial tumour (DNT; WHO I)

DNTs virtually always present with seizures (Daumas-Duport et al., 1988) and comprise the second largest group of tumours in our epilepsy surgery series (*Table I*). The term "dysembryoplastic neuroepithelial tumour, DNT" was coined in recognition of their early presentation with mean age at seizure onset of 15 years and slow progression in a quasi-hamartomatous fashion. These tumours share a characteristic intracortical, nodular growth pattern with a predilection for the temporal lobe (70%, *Figure 2*). The 2007 WHO classification system for brain tumours specifies two subtypes, simple and complex DNTs, which both belong into the category of WHO I° brain tumours (Louis et al., 2007a). Both subtypes failed to demonstrate predictive value in clinical practise (Thom *et al.*, 2011; Thom *et al.*, 2012; Blümcke *et al.*, 2014). The histopathological hallmark of a DNT is the "specific glio-neuronal element", characterized by oligodendroglial-like cells (OLC) and floating neurones embedded into a mucoid matrix, typically with cortical involvement (*Figure 2*). The proteinaceous mucoid fluid usually is contained within fields of multiple micro-cysts of variable size. These characteristic cellular arrangements can show a nodular appearance with or without a diffuse growth pattern. Some DNTs display histopathological features of composite tumours with neoplastic differentiation patterns of DNTs and pilocytic astrocytomas or gangliogliomas. These variants should be classified as complex DNT (Prayson and Napekoski, 2012; Blümcke *et al.*, 2014). Various publications are in favour of two additional variants, i.e. "diffuse" or "non-specific" DNTs (Honavar *et al.*, 1999; Thom *et al.*, 2011; Bodi *et al.*, 2012; Chassoux and Daumas-Duport, 2013; Chassoux *et al.*, 2013). These diffuse and non-specific forms were, however, not officially approved by the WHO panel, failed to demonstrate predictive value in clinical practice (Thom *et al.*, 2011; Thom *et al.*, 2012; Blümcke *et al.*, 2014), and these terms will not further be used herein.

Confirmation of the "specific glio-neuronal element" and multinodular occurrence should be decisive for the diagnosis of DNT. However, a prominent clear cell phenotype warrants the differential diagnosis of oligodendrogliomas. In fact, the DNT was recognized more than 20 years ago from a cohort of epilepsy-associated oligodendrogliomas with benign prognosis (Daumas-Duport *et al.*, 1988). Routine histopathology and immunohistochemistry should be used to confirm the diagnosis. Floating neurones are usually mature, lack dysmorphisms (characteristic for gangliogliomas, *i.e.* excessive clustering or bi-nucleated neurones), can be immunohistochemically characterized by NeuN, MAP2 or synaptophysin (Wolf *et al.*, 1997; Blümcke *et al.*, 2004a), and tend to express markers appropriate to corresponding cortical layers (Hadjivassiliou *et al.*, 2010). The glial component of this tumour usually does not react for GFAP, but expresses S-100β and partially also MAP2 (Wolf *et al.*, 1997; Blümcke *et al.*, 2004a). In our experience, CD34 immunoreactivity is absent in DNTs (Blümcke *et al.*, 2004a). Those reports describing CD34 immunoreactivity in a DNT may not have applied strict WHO criteria as used herein (Deb *et al.*, 2006; Sung *et al.*, 2011), and such tumours may share features also common in GG. Proliferative Ki67-positive nuclei are rare in DNTs (below 1%), supporting the concept of a dysembryoplastic or developmental origin of this tumour entity.

Differences in diagnostic criteria for DNTs are overt and largely due to recognition of simple, complex, non-specific or diffuse variants, which help to explain controversial results in published series for surgical outcome, molecular signatures and their relative incidence in epilepsy surgery centres. As prominent example, the frequency of DNTs vary from 7-80% in a meta-analysis of 8 series reporting on 2,055 tumours in patients with epilepsy (Thom *et al.*, 2012). Molecular-diagnostic signatures will be most helpful to better classify DNT in the future and their distinction from other brain tumours with/without clear cell composition (Fujisawa *et al.*, 2002; Thom *et al.*, 2011; Chappe *et al.*, 2013), such as gangliogliomas (GG), oligodendrogliomas, neurocytomas, or pleomorphic xanthoastrocytomas (PXA). Compared to oligodendrogliomas, loss of heterozygosity testing has not revealed alterations at chromosome 1p and 19q, nor have TP53 mutations been identified in a DNT (Fujisawa *et al.*, 2002; Thom *et al.*, 2011; Padovani *et al.*, 2012). IDH1 mutations are absent in DNTs, compared to their frequent occurrence in oligodendrogliomas, but this may partially reflect their occurrence in the young population of patients (Capper *et al.*, 2011; Padovani *et al.*, 2012). On the other hand, DNT may share similar B-RAF mutations with PXA and GG (Chappe *et al.*, 2013; Prabowo *et al.*, 2014). Although the molecular pathogenesis of DNTs remains unknown, one report described familial occurrence at same age and cortical location (Hasselblatt *et al.*, 2004). Thus, genetic analysis of affected family members may provide clues to its pathogenesis in the future.

The vast majority of DNT behave in a benign fashion as slowly growing WHO I tumours. However, tumours with more accelerated growth rates have been recognized (Nakatsuka *et al.*, 2000). Considering the diagnostic difficulties mentioned above, published reports describing tumour relapse following surgical removal (more often when initial tumours are partially resected but also in a few cases following gross total resection) may need a careful review using strict histopathological criteria (Fernandez *et al.*, 2003; Maher *et al.*, 2008; Minkin *et al.*, 2008; Ray *et al.*, 2009). Of interest, recurrence of DNT has been reported more often with

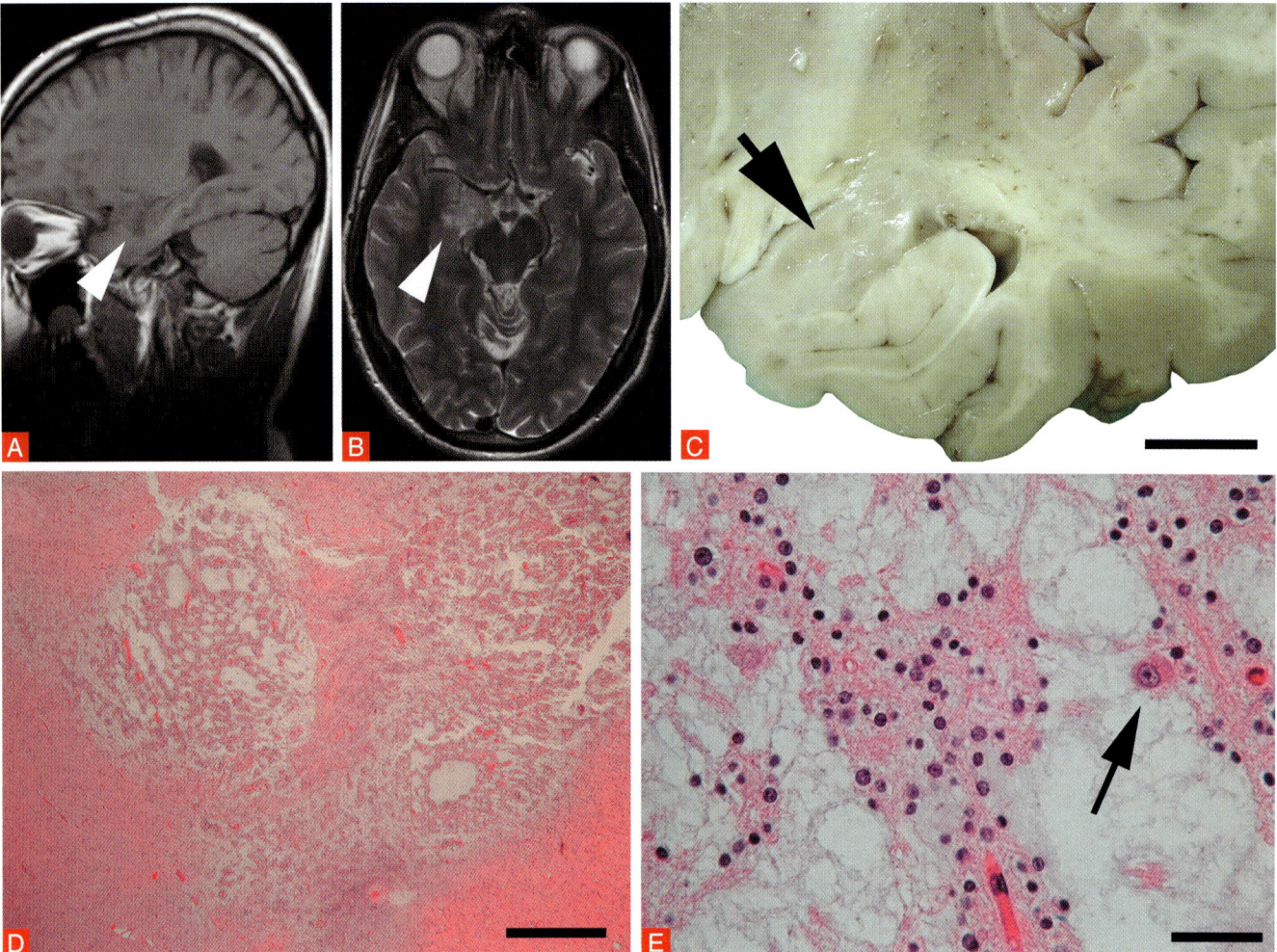

Figure 2

Dysembryoplastic neuroepithelial tumour (WHO I)

53-year old patient with temporal lobe epilepsy. Consecutive MRI scans did not reveal tumour growth (arrow in A: T1 parasagittal, in B: T2 axial) **C.** Post-mortem specimen of same patient shown in A/B with multinodular, intracortical growth into right mesial temporal lobe (arrow). **D.** microscopic image with characteristic multinodular growth (H&E staining). **E.** specific neuronal-glial element at higher magnification with arrow pointing to a "floating neurone". Scale bar in C = 1.5 cm; D = 1 mm; E = 40 μm. Courtesy of Dr. Macaulay, Halifax, Canada.

extra-temporal tumours. Overall the chance of malignant transformation of a DNT is likely to be less than 1%. Transformation was associated with post-operative adjuvant treatment in two cases following the initial resection (Rushing et al., 2003; Ray et al., 2009) and in another case with late initial surgical resection and focally elevated Ki67 index in the initial tumour (Thom et al., 2011). Extended follow-up periods in the post-operative periods are therefore probably justified, particularly following partial tumour resection, in extra-temporal DNTs and specimens with increased Ki67-labelling indices (> 5%).

Reported seizure-free outcomes following surgery vary from 62 to 100% (Honavar et al., 1999; Takahashi et al., 2005). There are reports of late seizure recurrences, even in the absence of tumour regrowth (Campos et al., 2009). In a study with longer follow-up periods of 10 years, 42% of patients had remained seizure-free (de Tisi et al., 2011). Partial resections have been associated with continuation of seizures (Nolan et al., 2004; Chang et al., 2010) often necessitating second surgeries. In terms of histological predictors of a seizure-free outcome there is no evidence that described DNT variants (simple, complex, diffuse, non-specific) influences outcome (Thom et al., 2011). Comparison between paediatric and adult series do not disclose obvious outcome differences, although single reports suggest older age and longer duration of epilepsy is associated with poorer outcome (Nolan *et al.*, 2004). Associated cortical dysplasia was reported in 0-83% of surgical samples (Takahashi *et al.*, 2005; Burneo *et al.*, 2008; Chang *et al.*, 2010), which may also determine and/or predict postsurgical seizure control (Sakuta *et al.*, 2005; Lee *et al.*, 2009). Significant inconsistencies in these published series are, again, mostly influenced by differences in histopathological criteria (2 *vs.* 4 DNT variants), but extra-temporal DNT tend to be associated with greater risk of continued seizures (Luyken *et al.*, 2003; Chang *et al.*, 2010). Another challenging issue herein is the classification of any abnormal (dysplastic) neurone or cortical dyslamination in the vicinity of a DNT, which should be regarded as component of its dysontogenic origin (such as FCD Type IIIb) rather than as "double pathology", a term used to describe lesions with independent aetiology and molecular pathogenesis (Blümcke *et al.*, 2011). Using a strict definition of the ILAE classification of FCD and as exemplified above in the GG chapter, FCD IIIb should be diagnosed only in areas of adjacent or remote neocortex not infiltrated by any tumour cells (Blümcke *et al.*, 2011).

Tumours with predominant glial (astrocytic) phenotype

• Angiocentric glioma (ANET; WHO I°)

Angiocentric glioma (syn. angiocentric neuroepithelial tumour, ANET) represent rare and slowly growing cerebral tumour classified by the WHO as grade I (Louis *et al.*, 2007a). ANETs occur in children and adults with chronic epilepsy (Lellouch-Tubiana *et al.*, 2005; Wang *et al.*, 2005; Louis *et al.*, 2007a; Majores *et al.*, 2007; Preusser *et al.*, 2007; Urbach *et al.*, 2007; Fulton *et al.*, 2009; Shakur *et al.*, 2009; Prayson, 2010; Prayson *et al.*, 2010; Marburger and Prayson, 2011; Miyata *et al.*, 2012) and present at any location (preferentially temporal and frontal lobes; *Table I*). Characteristic of ANET is the intrinsically high signal on T1-weighted MRI, as well as a stalk-like extension to the ventricle (Lellouch-Tubiana *et al.*, 2005; Wang *et al.*, 2005; Majores *et al.*, 2007; Preusser *et al.*, 2007; Urbach *et al.*, 2007; Ma *et al.*, 2010). Macroscopically, ANET may produce expansion of the involved region with blurring of anatomical structures. Histopathologically, ANETs consist of monomorphic, bipolar spindle cells with elongated nuclei and with a characteristic angiocentric arrangement around blood vessels, similar to perivascular pseudorosettes in ependymomas (Louis *et al.*, 2007a). However, variable histopathological features have been reported (Arsene *et al.*, 2008; Miyata *et al.*, 2012), and we also identify tumour components with neuronal differentiation in our series of 12 cases. We would prefer, therefore, the term "angiocentric neuroepithelial tumour, ANET" rather than angiocentric glioma, which is suggestive of pure glial differentiation. Mitoses, necrosis, microvascular proliferation are usually absent. The MIB-1 (Ki-67) labelling index ranges from 1% to less than 5% (Louis *et al.*, 2007a). A case with anaplastic recurrence and increased Ki67-labelling index of 10% has been reported (Wang *et al.*, 2005). This contrasts another series reporting three ANETs with elevated proliferation indices of 10% as well as increased mitotic activity, but benign behaviour with recurrence-free survival after 6 years of follow-up (Li *et al.*, 2012). Immunohistochemistry is positive for GFAP, S-100β protein and vimentin, whereas neuronal markers (such as MAP2, synaptophysin, chromogranin and NeuN) are reported mostly negative. In our experience, neuronal components can be also present in ANET. However, expression of epithelial membrane antigen (EMA) with a "dot-like" cytoplasmic labelling is frequently detected in these tumours (particularly in cells forming pseudorosettes) and recommended as most significant marker to confirm the diagnosis.

The histogenesis of ANET is a matter of ongoing debate (Miyata *et al.*, 2012). Morphological, immunohistochemical and ultrastructural features support a hypothesis that ANET could arise from an ependymal precursor cell (Lehman, 2008), but cortical location of these tumours argues against an origin from native ependymocytes or tanycytes. Another hypothesis suggests, therefore, that ANET develop from bipolar radial glia during early stages of corticogenesis (Lellouch-Tubiana *et al.*, 2005; Mott *et al.*, 2010). Accordingly, the reported association with cortical dysplasia and the benign clinical course supports a developmental origin of these tumours, possibly from multipotential neuroectodermal precursor cells (Prayson, 2010). Molecular genetic studies were not helpful thus far to clarify the nature of this tumour. As a prominent example, cytogenetic analysis revealed loss at chromosomal bands 6q24-25 in 1 of 8 cases and a copy number gain at 11p11.2 containing the protein-tyrosine phosphatase receptor type gene in 1 of 3 cases (Preusser et al., 2007). Losses at 1p/19q were never reported so far (Prayson et al., 2010), nor were IDH1, IDH2 and B-RAFV600E mutations detectable in ANET (Buccoliero et al., 2013). However, a deletion-truncation breakpoint v-myb avian myeloblastosis viral oncogene (MYB) was reported in ANET, similar to those observed in a series of pediatric low-grade gliomas (PLGG), suggesting molecular subclasses of diffuse PLGGs (Ramkissoon et al., 2013). Surgery represent the treatment of choice and ANET have a favourable prognosis with respect to long-term survival and post-operative seizure control (Majores et al., 2007; Preusser et al., 2007; Ma et al., 2010; Mott et al., 2010; Prayson, 2010).

• Isomorphic astrocytoma (iA; analogue WHO I°)

We have identified an isomorphic subtype of diffuse astrocytomas in a series of 24 patients with long-term epilepsy associated gliomas (Blümcke et al., 2004b; Schramm et al., 2004). Seven of these tumours were microscopically characterized by highly differentiated astroglial cell elements with small, rounded nuclei and regular chromatin structure. Fine arborizations of cellular processes built a homogenous fibrillary tumour matrix. Consistent with this observation, ubiquitous GFAP immunoreactivity was detected in all of the reported tumour specimens. The cellularity of isomorphic astrocytoma is always lower compared to "classical" variants of diffuse astrocytomas (WHO II). The mass tumour lesion is localized either in white matter or neocortex of preferably temporal and fronto-parietal lobes, but always presents with an ill-defined demarcation and infiltration into surrounding brain parenchyma, e.g. hippocampus. Exophytic growth into the subarachnoidal space was observed in one of the reported specimen (Schramm et al., 2004). All tumour samples reveal a non-proliferative capillary network with smooth endothelia. Necrosis, calcification nor lymphocytic infiltrates never occur in isomorphic astrocytoma.

Residual neuronal elements can be recognized in many tumour specimens, making it difficult to distinguish isomorphic astrocytoma from neuronal-glial tumours, i.e. gangliogliomas or glioneuronal hamartomas. As some neuronal profiles may show an atypical orientation and organization, antibodies directed against MAP2, synaptophysin and neurofilament protein were useful in clarifying the nature of these neurones. Differentiated neurones with a pyramidal cell shape can be identified using cytoskeletal markers such as MAP2 and neurofilaments, whereas preexisting neuropil shows a characteristic and densely distributed immunoreactivity for synaptophysin with a more or less sharp border towards white matter. These observations led us to conclude that such elements represent pre-existing neurones with degenerative changes that were overrun by glial tumour cells, but do not constitute a distinct component of iA (Blümcke et al., 2004b). No mitotic figures were found within any of our 14 tumour specimens (Table I), and low proliferation activities were confirmed by Ki67 immunohistochemistry (< 1%). In addition, nuclear p53 accumulation or IDH1 staining was never observed. In contrast to gangliogliomas, CD34 immunoreactivity is consistently absent in iA. In some specimens it will be difficult to discriminate an isomorphic astrocytoma from reactive astrogliosis, which is often seen in surgical specimens obtained from patients with long-term focal epilepsies (in particular after invasive EEG recordings). MRI should, therefore, always be requested to prove a mass lesion.

So far, long-term follow-up studies were reported only for 7 patients and clinical histories were also compared with epilepsy-associated diffuse astrocytomas (WHO II°) (Schramm et al., 2004). None of the reported patients with isomorphic astrocytoma died after a total follow-up period of up to 13 years, and only 1 patient of this series had to undergo a second tumour resection after 3 years due to local recurrence of residual tumour. Patients presenting with diffuse astrocytomas and epilepsy had later onset and shorter duration of their epilepsy. Temporal tumour location occurred more frequently in isomorphic astrocytoma. Seizure activity was well controlled in all patients following extensive presurgical evaluation of the seizure focus and tailored surgical procedures. Although the WHO has not yet introduced this tumour variant into their classification scheme, we suggest to provisionally describe its biological nature and behaviour analogous to WHO I°.

Associated pathologies including cortical dysplasia

The main types of pathology co-existing with tumours associated with early epilepsy onset include hippocampal sclerosis and focal cortical dysplasia (FCD) (Blümcke *et al.*, 2011; Blümcke *et al.*, 2013). The presence of hippocampal sclerosis in association with a tumour should be considered as dual pathology, but is extremely rare in our large series of 5,603 cases. When hippocampal sclerosis was present, atypical patterns predominated over classical hippocampal sclerosis. In contrast, diffuse or nodular tumour cell invasion into hippocampal structures is common, which also can mimic segmental hippocampal cell loss. But this condition should not be confused with proper hippocampal sclerosis. Cytoarchitectural abnormalities in the cortex adjacent to low grade glial and neuronal-glial tumours have long been recognized, albeit variably reported (Daumas-Duport, 1993; Sakuta *et al.*, 2005; Marburger and Prayson, 2011; Chassoux and Daumas-Duport, 2013). Previously classified either as FCD Palmini Type I or II (Palmini *et al.*, 2004), the ILAE classification of FCD has grouped them together as FCD Type IIIb (Blümcke *et al.*, 2011). The ILAE classification of cortical dysplasias now recognizes that acquired "re-organizational" cortical changes can occur in the maturing post-natal brain, simulating a developmental dysplasia. It seems more likely that peri-tumoural FCD-like changes develop in synchrony with or secondary to a slowly growing tumour rather than follows an independent aetiopathogenesis. Common cytoarchitectural changes reported in the adjacent cortex are layer I hypercellularity, cortical (and white matter) satellites of small immature cells (can be highlighted with CD34 and may not be recognizable on H&E) and a paucicellular cortex with less distinct lamination. In addition, white matter rarefaction may be present, reminiscent of developmental hypomyelination observed in FCD IIb (Campos *et al.*, 2009). The interpretation of these histological features, either as tumour precursor lesion or secondary to tumour growth, remains speculative and further harmonization of diagnostic criteria for FCD IIIb is required. This is exemplified by marked variation in published series. For example, FCD was reported in 47% of DNT (Daumas-Duport *et al.*, 1988) but varied between 0% (Burneo *et al.*, 2008) and 83% of cases (Takahashi *et al.*, 2005) in subsequent series. It most likely relates to variable diagnostic criteria (Chamberlain *et al.*, 2009), as mentioned above. Using NeuN as a recommended immunohistochemical marker in the evaluation of cyto-architecture will likely improve our accuracy to distinguish FCD from tumour infiltration zones (Blümcke *et al.*, 2011). The contribution of perilesional dysplastic cortex to epileptogenesis is of fundamental importance and pertinent to surgical planning (Barba *et al.*, 2011). To answer the question whether tumour cell infiltration into adjacent cortex or FCD contributes to the epileptogenic zone and how large peritumoural resections should be planned will require prospective clinical trials based on reliable pathological and electrophysiological correlation, rather than anecdotal case reports. Availability of surgical tumour specimens also should open the possibility of better characterizing the molecular signature of each tumour variant along with their molecular pathogenesis and epileptogenic potential. Notwithstanding, such studies will require use of reliable terminology and histopathological classification that can be reproduced in any other laboratory.

Mechanisms of epileptogenesis

The association between epilepsy and brain tumours has been observed for over a century. In 1882, Hughlings Jackson made the important observation that epilepsy often represents the initial and only clinical manifestation of glial tumours. In addition, Jackson was the first to recognize the relationship between tumour epileptogenicity and involvement of cortical grey matter in patients with brain tumours (Jackson, 1882; York and Steinberg, 2011). Jackson's ideas of brain tumour epileptogenicity have subsequently been reinforced by clinical studies emphasizing that pharmacologically intractable epilepsy critically affects quality of life in patients with brain tumours, even if the tumour is otherwise under control (van Breemen *et al.*, 2007; Rajneesh and Binder, 2009; de Groot *et al.*, 2012). The incidence of brain tumours in patients with epilepsy is about 4% and the frequency of epilepsy in patients with brain tumours is 30% or more depending on the type of the tumour (van Breemen *et al.*, 2007). In principle, any tumour or hamartomatous lesion (extra-axial, intra-axial, benign or malignant, common or uncommon) can cause seizures, *i.e.* hypothalamus (Cascino *et al.*, 1993; Fenoglio *et al.*, 2007) or cerebellum (Chae *et al.*, 2001; Delande *et al.*, 2001). However, patients with supratentorial low-grade glial and neuronal-glial tumours are more likely to develop epilepsy (van Breemen *et al.*, 2007; de Groot *et al.*, 2012). In particular, those entities discussed above are associated with long histories of pharmacologically intractable seizures, which represent the first, and in some cases, the only clinical manifestation of the tumour (Blümcke and Wiestler, 2002; Luyken *et al.*, 2004; van Breemen *et al.*, 2007). Understanding the mechanisms that underlie epileptogenesis in these tumours is essential to identify new treatment targets and to develop effective therapy. A number of hypotheses have been put forward during the past decades that could explain increased excitability in patients with brain tumours. It is likely that multiple mechanisms are involved, including both tumour related factors (tumour size, tumour location, molecular pathways affecting electrical properties), as well as peri-tumoural architectural or cytological changes (van Breemen *et al.*, 2007; Rajneesh and Binder, 2009; de Groot *et al.*, 2012).

References

Arsene D, Ardeleanu C, Ogrezeanu I, Danaila L. Angiocentric glioma: presentation of two cases with dissimilar histology. *Clin Neuropathol* 2008; 27: 391-5.

Balss J, Meyer J, Mueller W, Korshunov A, Hartmann C, von Deimling A. Analysis of the IDH1 codon 132 mutation in brain tumors. *Acta Neuropathol* 2008; 116: 597-602.

Barba C, Coras R, Giordano F, *et al*. Intrinsic epileptogenicity of gangliogliomas may be independent from co-occurring focal cortical dysplasia. *Epilepsy Res* 2011; 97: 208-13.

Becker AJ, Lobach M, Klein H, *et al*. Mutational analysis of TSC1 and TSC2 genes in gangliogliomas. *Neuropathol Appl Neurobiol* 2001; 27: 105-14.

Blümcke I, Wiestler OD. Gangliogliomas: an intriguing tumor entity associated with focal epilepsies. *J Neuropathol Exp Neurol* 2002; 61: 575-84.

Blümcke I, Löbach M, Wolf HK, Wiestler OD. Evidence for developmental precursor lesions in epilepsy-associated glioneuronal tumors. *Microsc Res Tech* 1999a; 46: 53-8.

Blümcke I, Müller S, Buslei R, Riederer BM, Wiestler OD. Microtubule-associated protein-2 immunoreactivity: a useful tool in the differential diagnosis of low-grade neuroepithelial tumors. *Acta Neuropathol* (Berl) 2004a; 108: 89-96.

Blümcke I, Luyken C, Urbach H, Schramm J, Wiestler OD. An isomorphic subtype of long-term epilepsy-associated astrocytomas associated with benign prognosis. *Acta Neuropathol* 2004b; 107: 381-8.

Blümcke I, Aronica E, Urbach H, Alexopoulos A, Gonzalez-Martinez JA. A neuropathology-based approach to epilepsy surgery in brain tumors and proposal for a new terminology use for long-term epilepsy-associated brain tumors. *Acta Neuropathol* 2014; 128: 39-54.

Blümcke I, Giencke K, Wardelmann E, *et al*. The CD34 epitope is expressed in neoplastic and malformative lesions associated with chronic, focal epilepsies. *Acta Neuropathol* 1999b; 97: 481-90.

Blümcke I, *et al*. International consensus classification of hippocampal sclerosis in temporal lobe epilepsy: a Task Force report from the ILAE Commission on Diagnostic Methods. *Epilepsia* 2013; 54: 1315-29.

Blümcke I, *et al*. The clinico-pathological spectrum of Focal Cortical Dysplasias: a consensus classification proposed by an ad hoc Task Force of the ILAE Diagnostic Methods Commission. *Epilepsia* 2011; 52: 158-74.

Bodi I, Selway R, Bannister P, *et al*. Diffuse form of dysembryoplastic neuroepithelial tumour: the histological and immunohistochemical features of a distinct entity showing transition to dysembryoplastic neuroepithelial tumour and ganglioglioma. *Neuropathol Appl Neurobiol* 2012; 38: 411-25.

Bodi I, Curran O, Selway R, *et al*. Two cases of multinodular and vacuolating neuronal tumour. *Acta Neuropathol Comm* 2014; 2: 7.

Boer K, Troost D, Timmermans W, van Rijen PC, Spliet WG, Aronica E. Pi3K-mTOR signaling and AMOG expression in epilepsy-associated glioneuronal tumors. *Brain Pathol* 2010; 20: 234-44.

Broholm H, Madsen FF, Wagner AA, Laursen H. Papillary glioneuronal tumor – a new tumor entity. *Clin Neuropathol* 2002; 21: 1-4.

Buccoliero AM, Castiglione F, Degl'Innocenti DR, *et al*. Angiocentric glioma: clinical, morphological, immunohistochemical and molecular features in three pediatric cases. *Clin Neuropathol* 2013; 32: 107-13.

Burneo JG, Tellez-Zenteno J, Steven DA, *et al*. Adult-onset epilepsy associated with dysembryoplastic neuroepithelial tumors. *Seizure* 2008; 17: 498-504.

Campos AR, Clusmann H, von Lehe M, *et al*. Simple and complex dysembryoplastic neuroepithelial tumors (DNT) variants: clinical profile, MRI, and histopathology. *Neuroradiology* 2009; 51: 433-43.

Capper D, Reuss D, Schittenhelm J, *et al*. Mutation-specific IDH1 antibody differentiates oligodendrogliomas and oligoastrocytomas from other brain tumors with oligodendroglioma-like morphology. *Acta Neuropathol* 2011; 121: 241-52.

Capper D, Weissert S, Balss J, *et al*. Characterization of R132H mutation-specific IDH1 antibody binding in brain tumors. *Brain Pathol* 2010; 20: 245-54.

Cascino GD, Andermann F, Berkovic SF, *et al*. Gelastic seizures and hypothalamic hamartomas: evaluation of patients undergoing chronic intracranial EEG monitoring and outcome of surgical treatment. *Neurology* 1993; 43: 747-50.

Chae JH, Kim SK, Wang KC, Kim KJ, Hwang YS, Cho BK. Hemifacial seizure of cerebellar ganglioglioma origin: seizure control by tumor resection. *Epilepsia* 2001; 42: 1204-7.

Chamberlain WA, Cohen ML, Gyure KA, *et al*. Interobserver and intraobserver reproducibility in focal cortical dysplasia (malformations of cortical development). *Epilepsia* 2009; 50: 2593-8.

Chang EF, Christie C, Sullivan JE, *et al*. Seizure control outcomes after resection of dysembryoplastic neuroepithelial tumor in 50 patients. *J Neurosurg Pediatr* 2010; 5: 123-30.

Chappe C, Padovani L, Scavarda D, *et al*. Dysembryoplastic Neuroepithelial Tumors Share with Pleomorphic Xanthoastrocytomas and Gangliogliomas BRAF Mutation and Expression. *Brain Pathol* 2013; 23: 574-83.

Chassoux F, Daumas-Duport C. Dysembryoplastic neuroepithelial tumors: where are we now? *Epilepsia* 2013; 54 (Suppl 9): 129-34.

Chassoux F, Landre E, Mellerio C, Laschet J, Devaux B, Daumas-Duport C. Dysembryoplastic neuroepithelial tumors: epileptogenicity related to histologic subtypes. *Clin Neurophysiol* 2013; 124: 1068-78.

Daumas-Duport C. Dysembryoplastic neuroepithelial tumours. *Brain Pathol* 1993; 3: 283-95.

Daumas-Duport C, Scheithauer BW, Chodkiewicz JP, Laws ER, Jr., Vedrenne C. Dysembryoplastic neuroepithelial tumor: a surgically curable tumor of young patients with intractable partial seizures. Report of thirty-nine cases. *Neurosurgery* 1988; 23: 545-56.

de Groot M, Reijneveld JC, Aronica E, Heimans JJ. Epilepsy in patients with a brain tumour: focal epilepsy requires focused treatment. *Brain* 2012; 135: 1002-16.

de Tisi J, Bell GS, Peacock JL, et al. The long-term outcome of adult epilepsy surgery, patterns of seizure remission, and relapse: a cohort study. *Lancet* 2011; 378: 1388-95.

Deb P, Sharma MC, Tripathi M, et al. Expression of CD34 as a novel marker for glioneuronal lesions associated with chronic intractable epilepsy. *Neuropathol Appl Neurobiol* 2006; 32: 461-8.

Delande O, Rodriguez D, Chiron C, Fohlen M. Successful surgical relief of seizures associated with hamartoma of the floor of the fourth ventricle in children: report of two cases. *Neurosurgery* 2001; 49: 726-30; discussion: 730-1.

Dim DC, Lingamfelter DC, Taboada EM, Fiorella RM. Papillary glioneuronal tumor: a case report and review of the literature. *Hum Pathol* 2006; 37: 914-8.

Dougherty MJ, Santi M, Brose MS *et al*. Activating mutations in BRAF characterize a spectrum of pediatric low-grade gliomas. *Neuro-oncology* 2010; 12: 621-30.

Duncan JS, de Tisi J. MRI in the diagnosis and management of epileptomas. *Epilepsia* 2013; 54 (Suppl 9): 40-3.

Fenoglio KA, Wu J, Kim do Y, et al. Hypothalamic hamartoma: basic mechanisms of intrinsic epileptogenesis. *Semin Pediatr Neurol* 2007; 14: 51-9.

Fernandez C, Girard N, Paz Paredes A, Bouvier-Labit C, Lena G, Figarella-Branger D. The usefulness of MR imaging in the diagnosis of dysembryoplastic neuroepithelial tumor in children: a study of 14 cases. *AJNR Am J Neuroradiol* 2003; 24: 829-34.

Fujisawa H, Marukawa K, Hasegawa M, et al. Genetic differences between neurocytoma and dysembryoplastic neuroepithelial tumor and oligodendroglial tumors. *J Neurosurg* 2002; 97: 1350-5.

Fukushima S, Yoshida A, Narita Y, et al. Multinodular and vacuolating neuronal tumor of the cerebrum. *Brain Tumor Pathol* 2015; 32: 131-6.

Fulton SP, Clarke DF, Wheless JW, Ellison DW, Ogg R, Boop FA. Angiocentric glioma-induced seizures in a 2-year-old child. *J Child Neurol* 2009; 24: 852-6.

Galloway M. CD34 expression in glioblastoma and giant cell glioblastoma. *Clin Neuropathol* 2010; 29: 89-93.

Hadjivassiliou G, Martinian L, Squier W, et al. The application of cortical layer markers in the evaluation of cortical dysplasias in epilepsy. *Acta Neuropathol* 2010; 120: 517-28.

Hamer HM, Hong SB. Is an epilepsy presurgical evaluation necessary for midgrade and high-grade brain tumors presenting with seizures? *Epilepsia* 2013; 54 (Suppl 9): 56-60.

Hartmann C, Hentschel B, Wick W, et al. Patients with IDH1 wild type anaplastic astrocytomas exhibit worse prognosis than IDH1-mutated glioblastomas, and IDH1 mutation status accounts for the unfavorable prognostic effect of higher age: implications for classification of gliomas. *Acta Neuropathol* 2010; 120: 707-18.

Harvey AS, Cross JH, Shinnar S, Mathern GW. Defining the spectrum of international practice in pediatric epilepsy surgery patients. *Epilepsia* 2008; 49: 146-55.

Hasselblatt M, Kurlemann G, Rickert CH, et al. Familial occurrence of dysembryoplastic neuroepithelial tumor. *Neurology* 2004; 62: 1020-1.

Hoischen A, Ehrler M, Fassunke J, et al. Comprehensive characterization of genomic aberrations in gangliogliomas by CGH, array-based CGH and interphase FISH. *Brain Pathol* 2008; 18: 326-37.

Honavar M, Janota I, Polkey CE. Histological heterogeneity of dysembryoplastic neuroepithelial tumour: identification and differential diagnosis in a series of 74 cases. *Histopathology* 1999; 34: 342-56.

Horbinski C, Kofler J, Yeaney G, et al. Isocitrate dehydrogenase 1 analysis differentiates gangliogliomas from infiltrative gliomas. *Brain Pathol* 2011; 21: 564-74.

Huse JT, Edgar M, Halliday J, Mikolaenko I, Lavi E, Rosenblum MK. Multinodular and vacuolating neuronal tumors of the cerebrum: 10 cases of a distinctive seizure-associated lesion. *Brain Pathol* 2013; 23: 515-24.

Jackson JH. Localized convulsions from tumor of the brain. *Brain* 1882; 5: 364-74.

Japp A, Gielen GH, Becker AJ. Recent aspects of classification and epidemiology of epilepsy-associated tumors. *Epilepsia* 2013; 54 (Suppl 9): 5-11.

Karremann M, Pietsch T, Janssen G, Kramm CM, Wolff JE. Anaplastic ganglioglioma in children. *J Neuro Oncol* 2009; 92: 157-63.

Katenkamp D, Mentzel T, Kosmehl H. CD34 detection-an immunohistochemical contribution to differential diagnosis of soft tissue tumors. *Der Pathologe* 1996; 17: 195-201.

Kennedy J, Schuele SU. Long-term monitoring of brain tumors: when is it necessary? *Epilepsia* 2013; 54 (Suppl 9): 50-5.

Koelsche C, Wohrer A, Jeibmann A, et al. Mutant BRAF V600E protein in ganglioglioma is predominantly expressed by neuronal tumor cells. *Acta Neuropathol* 2013; 125: 891-900.

Koelsche C, Sahm F, Paulus W, et al. BRAF V600E expression and distribution in desmoplastic infantile astrocytoma/ganglioglioma. *Neuropathol Appl Neurobiol* 2014; 40: 337-44.

Komori T, Scheithauer BW, Anthony DC, et al. Papillary glioneuronal tumor: a new variant of mixed neuronal-glial neoplasm. *Am J Surg Pathol* 1998; 22: 1171-83.

Lee J, Lee BL, Joo EY, et al. Dysembryoplastic neuroepithelial tumors in pediatric patients. *Brain Dev* 2009; 31: 671-81.

Lehman NL. Central nervous system tumors with ependymal features: a broadened spectrum of primarily ependymal differentiation? *J Neuropathol Exp Neurol* 2008; 67: 177-88.

Lellouch-Tubiana A, Boddaert N, Bourgeois M, et al. Angiocentric neuroepithelial tumor (ANET): a new epilepsy-related clinicopathological entity with distinctive MRI. *Brain Pathol* 2005; 15: 281-6.

Li JY, Langford LA, Adesina A, Bodhireddy SR, Wang M, Fuller GN. The high mitotic count detected by phospho-histone H3 immunostain does not alter the benign behavior of angiocentric glioma. *Brain Tumor Pathol* 2012; 29: 68-72.

Louis DN, Ohgaki H, Wiestler OD, Cavenee WK. WHO Classification of Tumours of the Central Nervous System. In: *World Health Organization Classification of Tumours*. Lyon: IARC, 2007a.

Louis DN, Ohgaki H, Wiestler OD, et al. The 2007 WHO classification of tumours of the central nervous system. *Acta Neuropathol* 2007b; 114: 97-109.

Luyken C, Blümcke I, Fimmers R, Urbach H, Wiestler OD, Schramm J. Supratentorial gangliogliomas: histopathologic grading and tumor recurrence in 184 patients with a median follow-up of 8 years. *Cancer* 2004; 101: 146-55.

Luyken C, Blümcke I, Fimmers R, et al. The spectrum of long-term epilepsy-associated tumors: long-term seizure and tumor outcome and neurosurgical aspects. *Epilepsia* 2003; 44: 822-30.

Ma X, Ge J, Wang L, et al. A 25-year-old woman with a mass in the hippocampus. *Brain Pathology* 2010; 20: 503-6.

Maher CO, White JB, Scheithauer BW, Raffel C. Recurrence of dysembryoplastic neuroepithelial tumor following resection. *Pediatr Neurosurg* 2008; 44: 333-6.

Majores M, Niehusmann P, von Lehe M, Blümcke I, Urbach H. Angiocentric neuroepithelial tumor mimicking Ammon's horn sclerosis – case report. *Clin Neuropathol* 2007; 26: 311-6.

Majores M, von Lehe M, Fassunke J, Schramm J, Becker AJ, Simon M. Tumor recurrence and malignant progression of gangliogliomas. *Cancer* 2008; 113: 3355-63.

Marburger T, Prayson R. Angiocentric glioma: a clinicopathologic review of 5 tumors with identification of associated cortical dysplasia. *Arch Pathol Lab Med* 2011; 135: 1037-41.

Minkin K, Klein O, Mancini J, Lena G. Surgical strategies and seizure control in pediatric patients with dysembryoplastic neuroepithelial tumors: a single-institution experience. *J Neurosurg Pediatr* 2008; 1: 206-10.

Miyata H, Ryufuku M, Kubota Y, Ochiai T, Niimura K, Hori T. Adult-onset angiocentric glioma of epithelioid cell-predominant type of the mesial temporal lobe suggestive of a rare but distinct clinicopathological subset within a spectrum of angiocentric cortical ependymal tumors. *Neuropathology* 2012; 32: 479-91.

Mott RT, Ellis TL, Geisinger KR. Angiocentric glioma: a case report and review of the literature. *Diagn Cytopathol* 2010; 38: 452-6.

Nakatsuka M, Mizuno S, Kimura T, Hara K. A case of an unclassified tumor closely resembling dysembryoplastic neuroepithelial tumor with rapid growth. *Brain Tumor Pathol* 2000; 17: 41-5.

Nolan MA, Sakuta R, Chuang N, et al. Dysembryoplastic neuroepithelial tumors in childhood: long-term outcome and prognostic features. *Neurology* 2004; 62: 2270-6.

Ostrom Q, Cohen ML, Ondracek A, Sloan A, Barnholtz-Sloan J. Gene markers in brain tumors: what the epileptologist should know. *Epilepsia* 2013; 54 (Suppl 9): 25-9.

Padovani L, Colin C, Fernandez C, et al. Search for distinctive markers in DNT and cortical grade II glioma in children: same clinicopathological and molecular entities? *Curr Topics Med Chem* 2012; 12: 1683-92.

Palmini A, Paglioli E, Silva VD. Developmental tumors and adjacent cortical dysplasia: single or dual pathology? *Epilepsia* 2013; 54 (Suppl 9): 18-24.

Palmini A, Najm I, Avanzini G, et al. Terminology and classification of the cortical dysplasias. *Neurology* 2004; 62: S2-8.

Parry L, Maynard JH, Patel A, et al. Molecular analysis of the TSC1 and TSC2 tumour suppressor genes in sporadic glial and glioneuronal tumours. *Hum Genet* 2000; 107: 350-6.

Parsons DW, et al. An integrated genomic analysis of human glioblastoma multiforme. *Science* 2008; 321: 1807-12.

Perry A, Scheithauer BW, Nascimento AG. The immunophenotypic spectrum of meningeal hemangiopericytoma: a comparison with fibrous meningioma and solitary fibrous tumor of meninges. *Am J Surg Pathol* 1997; 21: 1354-60.

Perry A, Burton SS, Fuller GN, et al. Oligodendroglial neoplasms with ganglioglioma-like maturation: a diagnostic pitfall. *Acta Neuropathol* 2010; 120: 237-52.

Piao YS, Lu DH, Chen L, et al. Neuropathological findings in intractable epilepsy: 435 Chinese cases. *Brain Pathol* 2010; 20: 902-8.

Platten M, Meyer Puttlitz B, Blümcke I, et al. A novel splice site associated polymorphism in the tuberous sclerosis 2 (TSC2) gene may predispose to the development of sporadic gangliogliomas. *J Neuropathol Exp Neurol* 1997; 56: 806-10.

Prabowo AS, Iyer AM, Veersema TJ, et al. BRAF V600E mutation is associated with mTOR signaling activation in glioneuronal tumors. *Brain Pathol* 2014; 24: 52-66.

Prayson RA. Tumours arising in the setting of paediatric chronic epilepsy. *Pathology* 2010; 42: 426-31.

Prayson RA. Brain tumors in adults with medically intractable epilepsy. *Am J Clin Pathol* 2011; 136: 557-63.

Prayson RA, Napekoski KM. Composite ganglioglioma/dysembryoplastic neuroepithelial tumor: a clinicopathologic study of 8 cases. *Hum Pathol* 2012; 43: 1113-8.

Prayson RA, Fong J, Najm I. Coexistent pathology in chronic epilepsy patients with neoplasms. *Mod Pathol* 2010; 23: 1097-103.

Preusser M, Hoischen A, Novak K, et al. Angiocentric glioma: report of clinicopathologic and genetic findings in 8 cases. *Am J Surg Pathol* 2007; 31: 1709-18.

Rades D, Zwick L, Leppert J, et al. The role of postoperative radiotherapy for the treatment of gangliogliomas. *Cancer* 2010; 116: 432-42.

Rajneesh KF, Binder DK. Tumor-associated epilepsy. *Neurosurg Focus* 2009; 27: E4.

Ramkissoon LA, et al. Genomic analysis of diffuse pediatric low-grade gliomas identifies recurrent oncogenic truncating rearrangements in the transcription factor MYBL1. *Proc Natl Acad Sci USA* 2013; 110: 8188-93.

Ratilal B, McEvoy A, Sisodiya S, Thom M, Toma A. Diffuse cerebral gangliocytoma in an adult with late-onset refractory epilepsy. *Neuropathol App Neurobiol* 2007; 33: 706-9.

Ray WZ, Blackburn SL, Casavilca-Zambrano S, et al. Clinicopathologic features of recurrent dysembryoplastic neuroepithelial tumor and rare malignant transformation: a report of 5 cases and review of the literature. *J Neuro Oncol* 2009; 94: 283-92.

Reifenberger G, Kaulich K, Wiestler OD, Blümcke I. Expression of the CD34 antigen in pleomorphic xanthoastrocytomas. *Acta Neuropathol* 2003; 105: 358-64.

Reuss DE, Sahm F, Schrimpf D, et al. ATRX and IDH1-R132H immunohistochemistry with subsequent copy number analysis and IDH sequencing as a basis for an "integrated" diagnostic approach for adult astrocytoma, oligodendroglioma and glioblastoma. *Acta Neuropathol* 2015; 129: 133-46.

Rodriguez FJ, Perry A, Gutmann DH, et al. Gliomas in neurofibromatosis type 1: a clinicopathologic study of 100 patients. *J Neuropathol Exp Neurol* 2008; 67: 240-9.

Rodriguez FJ, Scheithauer BW, Jenkins R, et al. Gliosarcoma arising in oligodendroglial tumors ("oligosarcoma"): a clinicopathologic study. *Am J Surg Pathol* 2007; 31: 351-62.

Rosenow F, Menzler K. Invasive EEG studies in tumor-related epilepsy: when are they indicated and with what kind of electrodes? *Epilepsia* 2013; 54 (Suppl 9): 61-5.

Rushing EJ, Thompson LD, Mena H. Malignant transformation of a dysembryoplastic neuroepithelial tumor after radiation and chemotherapy. *Ann Diagn Pathol* 2003; 7: 240-4.

Sakuta R, Otsubo H, Nolan MA, et al. Recurrent intractable seizures in children with cortical dysplasia adjacent to dysembryoplastic neuroepithelial tumor. *J Child Neurol* 2005; 20: 377-84.

Schindler G, Capper D, Meyer J, et al. Analysis of BRAF V600E mutation in 1,320 nervous system tumors reveals high mutation frequencies in pleomorphic xanthoastrocytoma, ganglioglioma and extra-cerebellar pilocytic astrocytoma. *Acta Neuropathol* 2011; 121: 397-405.

Schramm J, Luyken C, Urbach H, Fimmers R, Blümcke I. Evidence for a clinically distinct new subtype of grade II astrocytomas in patients with long-term epilepsy. *Neurosurgery* 2004; 55: 340-7; discussion: 347-8.

Selvanathan SK, Hammouche S, Salminen HJ, Jenkinson MD. Outcome and prognostic features in anaplastic ganglioglioma: analysis of cases from the SEER database. *J Neuro Oncol* 2011; 105: 539-45.

Shakur SF, McGirt MJ, Johnson MW, et al. Angiocentric glioma: a case series. *J Neurosurg Pediatr* 2009; 3: 197-202.

Sung CO, Suh YL, Hong SC. CD34 and microtubule-associated protein 2 expression in dysembryoplastic neuroepithelial tumours with an emphasis on dual expression in non-specific types. *Histopathology* 2011; 59: 308-17.

Takahashi A, Hong SC, Seo DW, Hong SB, Lee M, Suh YL. Frequent association of cortical dysplasia in dysembryoplastic neuroepithelial tumor treated by epilepsy surgery. *Surg Neurol* 2005; 64: 419-27.

Thom M, Blümcke I, Aronica E. Long-term epilepsy-associated tumors. *Brain Pathol* 2012; 22: 350-79.

Thom M, Toma A, An S, et al. One hundred and one dysembryoplastic neuroepithelial tumors: an adult epilepsy series with immunohistochemical, molecular genetic, and clinical correlations and a review of the literature. *J Neuropathol Exp Neurol* 2011; 70: 859-78.

Urbach H, Binder D, von Lehe M, et al. Correlation of MRI and histopathology in epileptogenic parietal and occipital lobe lesions. *Seizure* 2007; 16: 608-14.

van Breemen MS, Wilms EB, Vecht CJ. Epilepsy in patients with brain tumours: epidemiology, mechanisms, and management. *Lancet Neurology* 2007; 6: 421-30.

Wang M, Tihan T, Rojiani AM, et al. Monomorphous angiocentric glioma: a distinctive epileptogenic neoplasm with features of infiltrating astrocytoma and ependymoma. *J Neuropathol Exp Neurol* 2005; 64: 875-81.

Wharton SB, Whittle IR, Collie DA, Bell HS, Ironside JW. Gliosarcoma with areas of primitive neuroepithelial differentiation and extracranial metastasis. *Clin Neuropathol* 2001; 20: 212-8.

Wolf HK, Wiestler OD. Surgical pathology of chronic epileptic seizure disorders. *Brain Pathol* 1993; 3: 371-80.

Wolf HK, Buslei R, Blümcke I, Wiestler OD, Pietsch T. Neural antigens in oligodendrogliomas and dysembryoplastic neuroepithelial tumors. *Acta Neuropathol* 1997; 94: 436-43.

Yamashita S, Yokogami K, Niibo T, et al. Oligodendroglial ganglioglioma. *Brain Tumor Pathol* 2011; 28: 311-6.

Yan H, Parsons DW, Jin G, et al. IDH1 and IDH2 mutations in gliomas. *N Engl J Med* 2009; 360: 765-73.

Yang I, Chang EF, Han SJ et al. Early surgical intervention in adult patients with ganglioglioma is associated with improved clinical seizure outcomes. *J Clin Neurosci* 2011; 18: 29-33.

York GK, 3rd, Steinberg DA. Hughlings Jackson's neurological ideas. *Brain* 2011; 134: 3106-13.

5. Encephalitis

Ingmar Blümcke

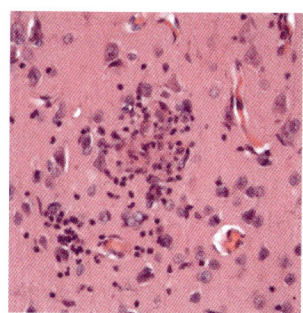

Seizures are a prominent clinical feature in encephalitis (Bauer *et al.*, 2012). Encephalitis-associated epilepsies account for 1.7% of patients collected at the German Neuropathological Reference Centre for Epilepsy Surgery (see chapter 1, *Table I*), with seizure onset at a mean age of 11.3 years. Previous studies suggest the adaptive as well as innate immune system (see below) to be directly involved in pathomechanisms of epileptogenesis (Bauer *et al.*, 2012; Bien *et al.*, 2012). Cytotoxic T-lymphocytes and antibody-mediated complement activation are major components of the adaptive immune system. They can provoke neuroepithelial cellular loss and epileptic encephalitis (Bien *et al.*, 2002b). The innate immune system operates via interleukin-1 and Toll-like-receptor-associated mechanisms, and shown to also play a direct role in epileptogenesis (Maroso *et al.*, 2010; Vezzani *et al.*, 2011). Neuropathological investigations have made important contributions to determine cellular components and molecular mechanisms of neurotoxicity and epileptogenesis provoked by the immune system (Varadkar *et al.*, 2014). These studies helped to also discover encephalitis subtypes associated with antibodies against voltage-gated-potassium-channel-complex (VGKC), N-methyl-D-aspartate-receptor (NMDAR) or glutamic-acid-decarboxylase (GAD) (Vincent *et al.*, 2011; Bauer *et al.*, 2012). Knowledge of the role of the innate immunity can be translated already into clinical treatment strategies and can help discover specific drug targets for this challenging group of epileptic disorders (Bien *et al.*, 2004; Bien *et al.*, 2013; Bittner *et al.*, 2013).

Rasmussen encephalitis (RE)

Theodore Rasmussen published his series of three paediatric patients under the title "Focal seizures due to chronic localized encephalitis" in 1958 (Rasmussen *et al.*, 1958). Most researchers and clinicians nowadays use the term Rasmussen encephalitis (RE) for drug-resistant epilepsy with progressive hemiplegia, cognitive decline and unilateral hemispheric atrophy (Piatt *et al.*, 1988; Andermann, 1991; Bien *et al.*, 2005; Bauer *et al.*, 2012; Varadkar *et al.*, 2014). Its incidence in Germany is estimated to affect 2-4 patients per 10 million people per year aged 18 and younger (Bien *et al.*, 2013). Unilateral myoclonic twitching of the distal extremities or the face, *i.e.* epilepsia partialis continua (EPC) is observed in approximately half of the patients (Thomas *et al.*, 1977; Bien *et al.*, 2005). Loss of neurological function follows progressive brain damage in the affected hemisphere and typically advances into hemiparesis, hemianopia, cognitive deterioration and aphasia, if the dominant hemisphere is affected (Bauer *et al.*, 2012). Seizure frequency can remain high also in the residual stage of the disease but is in general lower when compared to "acute stages" (Oguni *et al.*, 1991; Bien *et al.*, 2002a; Granata, 2003). Changes in seizure semiology most likely reflect disease progression with involvement of newly affected regions of the brain.

Neuropathological hallmarks of RE are lymphocytic T-cell infiltration (mostly CD8-positive cytotoxic T-cells), microglial activation and nodules, astrogliosis and in later stages prominent neuronal and astroglial loss confined to one hemisphere (Bien *et al.*, 2005; Varadkar *et al.*, 2014). Immunohistochemical reactivities are helpful to selectively highlight and confirm cellular damage, *i.e.* using CD4 and CD8 to differentiate helping from cytotoxic T-lymphocytes (pathognomic when more than 10 T-cells per high power microscopic field can be identified in brain parenchyma outside blood vessels), CD68 to detect microglial nodules, GFAP to detect astrogliosis (which follows progression of cortical damage up to glial scarring) and NeuN to characterize abnormalities in neocortical architecture (*i.e.* FCD ILAE Type IIId) or cellular loss. These histopathological hallmarks can be detected in same brain regions but usually help to classify disease spread and progression, *i.e.* stage 1 (early: T-cell infiltration and microglial nodules) – stage 2 (intermediate: + reactive gliosis) – stage 3 (late: ++ neuronal cell loss) – stage 4 (residual or end-stage: +++ glial scarring) (Robitaille, 1991; Farrell *et al.*, 1995; Pardo *et al.*, 2004; Wang *et al.*, 2013). It may be difficult microscopically to identify these histopathological features in a given neurosurgical specimen when sampled outside affected brain areas, and *en bloc* resected surgical specimens are recommended for diagnostic purpose to identify anatomical landmarks and to correlate them with clinical findings. Associated pathology has been reported such as hippocampal sclerosis and focal cortical dysplasia ILAE Type IIId, but also vascular abnormalities, tuberous sclerosis or FCD ILAE Type IIb (Hart *et al.*, 1998; Palmer *et al.*, 1999; Takei *et al.*, 2010; Wang *et al.*, 2013). It remains controversial whether these lesions trigger the encephalitic pathomechanism or develop secondary to brain inflammation, *i.e.* HS and FCD IIId.

Involvement of the adaptive immune system for inducing seizures and progressive neuroepithelial cell loss are subject of scientific studies. A first report described pathogenic antibodies against the glutamate receptor 3 (GluR3) in serum of RE patients (Rogers *et al.*, 1994). These antibodies were thought to kill neurones by antibody or complement mediated attacks (Whitney *et al.*, 1999). Plasmapheresis in RE patients seemed to diminish progression, but recovery was limited to a short period of time (Andrews *et al.*, 1996). Consecutive studies could not confirm anti-GluR3 antibodies in RE patients (Wiendl *et al.*, 2001) and some patients failed to clinically improve after plasmapheresis (Granata *et al.*, 2003). By contrast, neuropathological studies have nicely proven cytotoxic T-lymphocytes in close apposition to neurones as well as to astrocytes (Bien *et al.*, 2002b). These T-cells contain granzyme-B immunoreactive granules and accumulate at the contact zone with neuronal or astrocytic membranes, suggesting a direct cytotoxic effect (Bien *et al.*, 2002b). Inflammation may also contribute to epileptogenic pathomechanisms as it can precede the occurrence of seizures (Korn-Lubetzki *et al.*, 2004; Bien *et al.*, 2007; Vezzani *et al.*, 2011). In addition, MRI studies detected inflammatory disease activity outside the epileptic network in RE, suggesting that inflammation occurs independently from seizures (Hauf *et al.*, 2009). Further evidence arguing against a direct effect of infiltrating immune cells on seizure induction comes from therapeutic studies using tacrolimus to suppress inflammation. In RE patients, tacrolimus had a positive effect on conservation of motor and cognitive function and on brain tissue, but had no effect on seizure frequency (Bien *et al.*, 2004).

Antibody-associated encephalitis

The second group of patients with encephalitis and epilepsy is now recognized as antibody-associated encephalitis, either classified as paraneoplastic (PE) or non-paraneoplastic limbic encephalitis (Bien and Elger, 2007; Bauer *et al.*, 2012). Paraneoplastic neurological disorders can harm any part of the central nervous system, such as brainstem, the limbic system or just single cell types, i.e. Purkinje cells in paraneoplastic cerebellar degeneration. Although multiple areas of the CNS can be involved, PE most often affect the limbic system and termed already in 1968 as limbic encephalitis by J.A.N. Corsellis (Corsellis *et al.*, 1968). Antibodies can react with both, the nervous system and the underlying cancer, but some evidence suggests a correlation between neurological deficits and antibody targets rather than with an underlying specific tumour (Bauer *et al.*, 2012). These studies have supported the concept of non-paraneoplastic antibody-mediated encephalitis (NPE), in which encephalitic patients present with similar neurological deficits, including epilepsy, but extensive diagnostic tests and follow-up failed to detect cancer.

At present, antibody-mediated encephalitis can be classified according to serum antibodies and their specific targets: 1. Antibodies directed against intracellular antigens (such as GAD65); 2. Intranuclear antigens (such as Hu, Yo and Ma2) as prototypic onco-neural antigens (Graus *et al.*, 1990; Posner, 1991; Jean *et al.*, 1994; Verschuuren *et al.*, 1996; Giometto *et al.*, 1997;

Dalmau et al., 1999); 3. Antibodies directed against neuronal membrane antigens such as the VGKC complex, various glutamate receptors (NMDA or AMPA receptors or metabotropic glutamate receptor subunits) or the GABA-B receptor.

Table I
Spectrum of antibody-associated epileptic encephalitis
Most of these antibody-associated encephalitis can occur with or without an underlying neoplasm

Antibody – target	Epitopes	Clinics	Neuropathology
Intracellular	GAD65, AMP	VAR. (NPE)	CD8 positive T-cells and neuronal cell loss preferentially in hippocampus
Intranuclear	Hu, Yo, Ma2	PE	CD8 positive T-cells attacking neurones
Voltage-gated potassium channel complex (VGKC)	LGI1 Caspr2	NPE (PE)	CD8 positive T-cells attacking neurones, severe cell loss preferentially in hippocampus
Glutamate receptors	NMDA R1	NPE (PE)	few T-cells, only mild neuronal cell loss

GAD: glutamic acid decarboxylase; AMP: amphiphysin; VAR: variable; NPE: non-paraneoplastic encephalitis; PE: paraneoplastic encephalitis; LGI1: leucine-rich glia-inactivated 1; Caspr2: contactin-associated protein-like 2; NMDA: N-methyl-D-aspartate.

Detection of these antibodies is clinically relevant and should be confirmed in specialized laboratories using a patient's serum. However, their pathogenic role is still matter of ongoing investigations. Generally it is assumed that antibodies against intracellular antigens are less or not pathogenic (Graus et al., 2008) because antibodies hardly reach intracellularly located neural antigens in normal brain. Exceptions may be antibodies against GAD65 (Manto et al., 2007) or amphiphysin (Geis et al., 2010). In neuropathological studies of PE with anti-Hu, anti-Yo, or anti-Ma antibodies CD8 positive T-cells dominate inflammatory infiltrates (Graus et al., 1990; Posner, 1991; Jean et al., 1994; Verschuuren et al., 1996; Giometto et al., 1997; Dalmau et al., 1999), which possess cytotoxic granules and are in close apposition to neurones suggesting that cytotoxic T-lymphocytes play a role in neuronal cell death (Tanaka et al., 1999; Bernal et al., 2002; Blumenthal et al., 2006).

VGKC complex encephalitis

Antibodies against VGKC complex were detected first in PE (Buckley et al., 2001) but more patients present with non-paraneoplastic ("idiopathic") limbic encephalitis (Pozo-Rosich et al., 2003). Antibodies are directed to potassium channel complex proteins, such as contactin-associated protein-like 2 (Caspr2)(Lancaster et al., 2011) and leucine-rich, glioma-inactivated 1 (LGI1) (Irani et al., 2010a; Lai et al., 2010). Antibodies against LGI1 are more often found than antibodies against Caspr2 (Irani et al., 2010a). Clinically, these patients present with memory loss, confusion, behavioural changes and seizures (Vincent et al., 2004; Chan et al., 2007). In addition, patients with LGi1 antibodies present with facio-brachial dystonic seizures preceding limbic encephalitis (Irani et al., 2011). Histopathologically, surgical specimens obtained from patients with anti-VGKC complex reveal neuronal cell loss in the presence of infiltrating T cells and perivascular B cells (Vincent et al., 2004; Dunstan and Winer, 2006; Park et al., 2007; Khan et al., 2009). Patients with antibodies specific for LGI1 or caspr2 show inflammation and severe degeneration in the hippocampus. Importantly, antibody lowering treatments like plasma exchange have been found to improve neurological deficits in these patients, suggesting that antibodies directed against the VGKC complex are responsible for clinical symptoms (Vincent et al., 2004; Wong et al., 2010).

NMDAR encephalitis

Histopathology findings in patients with antibodies directed against the NMDA receptor differs from most other antibody-associated encephalitis. Although the disease is defined as "encephalitis", brain parenchyma of PE patients reveals relatively few inflammatory cells (Tüzün et al., 2009; Camdessanche et al., 2011), and T-cells, B-cells and plasma cells remain in the perivascular space of blood vessels (Martinez-Hernandez et al., 2011). It is important to note that neuronal loss is remarkably mild in these patients. Neuronal loss was confirmed in only one of four hippocampal samples studied by Dalmau et al. (Dalmau et al., 2007). In some reports this syndrome therefore is referred to as "encephalopathy" rather than encephalitis, thereby underlining the functional character of damage in contrast to only mild structural signatures in this disease (Irani et al., 2010b).

The clinical presentation of patients with NMDA receptor associated encephalitis is remarkable. It occurs mainly in young females with a peak of age at onset between 19 and 24 years (Dalmau et al., 2011). Clinically, a prodromal stage with symptoms such as fever, nausea, vomiting or diarrhoea may be found in retrospect (Iizuka et al., 2007). After few weeks, patients develop seizures, (partial) status epilepticus, short-term memory loss and, in addition, psychiatric symptoms such as anxiety, insomnia, fear, mania and paranoia. This phase is followed by the initiation of abnormal movements of limb and trunk and oro-lingual-facial dyskinesias, a sudden spontaneous fall in consciousness and autonomic manifestations such as tachy- or bradycardia, hyperventilation and central hypoventilation (Dalmau et al., 2007; Dalmau et al., 2011). At this stage, patients need to be managed in intensive care units. However, most patients recover completely (Dalmau et al., 2011), and follow-up MRI studies do not detect permanent brain atrophy (Iizuka et al., 2010).

The clinical syndrome of NMDAR encephalitis was first reported in 2005 in patients with paraneoplastic encephalitis resulting from ovarian teratomas harbouring antibodies to hippocampal neuropil (Ances et al., 2005). Soon after, it was discovered that this particular syndrome was associated with antibodies against the NR1 subunit of the NMDAR (Dalmau et al., 2008). Anti-NMDAR encephalitis was also found in the absence of tumour in a large number of patients (Dalmau et al., 2008; Irani et al., 2010b). Anti-NMDAR antibodies do not activate complement (Tüzün et al., 2009; Martinez-Hernandez et al., 2011), but decrease the NMDA receptor density by cross-linking and subsequent internalization, leading to a state of reversible NMDAR hypofunction (Hughes et al., 2010). Further studies with CSF from patients with anti-NMDAR antibody encephalitis suppressed induction of long-term potentiation (LTP) in mouse hippocampal slices (Zhang et al., 2012), suggesting that these antibodies can act as an NMDAR antagonist and thus may be involved in amnesia. However, there is yet no evidence for complement mediated or cytotoxic T-cell mediated neuronal cell death in this disease (Bauer et al., 2012).

GAD65 encephalitis

GAD antibodies are associated with a broad spectrum of diseases, i.e. patients with neurological disorders or diabetes mellitus type 1 (Solimena et al., 1988; Striano et al., 2006). Neurological diseases are associated with very high GAD antibody concentrations being two to three log ranks higher than in the diabetic population (Meinck et al., 2001). The spectrum of neurological conditions associated with GAD antibodies ranges is broad (Saiz et al., 2008), including stiff-man syndrome (Meinck and Thompson, 2002), cerebellar ataxia (Saiz et al., 1997; Honnorat et al., 2001), limbic encephalitis (Malter et al., 2010) and pharmaco-resistant temporal lobe epilepsy (Liimatainen et al., 2010), which is probably the chronic form of GAD antibody associated limbic encephalitis (Vincent et al., 2011). Some experimental conditions have provided evidence that these antibodies might contribute to a loss of GABAergic inhibition (GAD being the rate limiting enzyme in the biosynthesis of GABA) (Manto et al., 2007; Manto et al., 2011). Histopathological studies have shown neuronal loss and axonal dystrophy in the hippocampi of these patients, whereas Ig and complement deposition was absent from these brains. Since the antigen is intracellular, a T-cell mediated pathology would be a likely mechanism (Graus et al., 2010).

The innate immune system can induce seizures

Microglia and astroglia are the brain's principle cells of the innate immune system. Upon activation, these cells can produce a variety of soluble mediators of inflammation, including cytokines (i.e. interleukin IL1β), chemokines, prostaglandins and complement factors (Vezzani et al., 2011). In addition, glia and neurones can overexpress receptors for proinflammatory cytokines, i.e. IL-1β, IL-6 or tumour-necrosis-factor-α, as well as toll-like-receptors (Rivest, 2009). The innate immune response is different, therefore, from the adaptive immune system representing T-cell, antibody and complement-mediated cytotoxicity and degeneration of neuroepithelial tissue, as discussed above. Experimental evidence suggests, however, that the innate immune system, in particular interleukin IL1β, contributes directly to seizures. This was initially suggested from administration of convulsant drugs such as kainic acid, which increase mRNA and protein levels of inflammatory molecules. Rapid effects of cytokines or prostaglandins on neuronal excitability have been then reported as post-translational change in receptor coupled- or voltage-dependent ion channels and increased glutamatergic neurotransmission (Viviani et al., 2007). Proinflammatory cytokines also decrease glutamate re-uptake by astrocytes. Long-term effects of inflammatory mediators involve gene transcription of proinflammatory genes perpetuating brain inflammation and challenging blood-brain barrier's permeability (BBB). A compromised BBB lowers in turn seizure thresholds due to imbalance of ionic homeostasis in the extracellular milieu, as well as astrocytes and microglia dysfunction. The persistence of transcript and protein up-regulation is likely determined by severity and frequency of seizure activity, as well as by the underlying neuropathology (Minami et al., 1990; Minami et al., 1991; Nishiyori et al., 1997; Eriksson et al., 1999; De Simoni et al., 2000). As an example, the cytokine IL-1β is up-regulated in glial cells of normal brain following central or peripheral administration of bacterial lipopolysaccharides that mimicks infectious processes, and mediates endotoxin-induced response such as fever, sleep and anorexia (Busbridge et al., 1989; Van Dam et al., 1995). In the absence of infection, IL1β can be also induced in brain by various epileptogenic injuries, such as trauma, stroke, or seizures (Vezzani et al., 2011). In human temporal lobe epilepsy or malformations of cortical development, IL-1β and its receptor IL-1R1 are up-regulated, suggesting activation of IL-1 β signalling (Ravizza et al., 2006; Ravizza et al., 2008). Neuropathologic analysis revealed up-regulation of IL-1β in balloon cells, dysmorphic neurones as well as in activated microglia and astrocytes, in focal cortical dysplasia (FCD) Type II but only to a minor extent in glia in FCD Type I (Iyer et al., 2010). Interestingly, patients with FCD Type II have infiltration of cytotoxic T-cells suggesting different immune mechanisms in FCD Type I compared to FCD Type II.

References

Ances BM, Vitaliani R, Taylor RA, et al. Treatment-responsive limbic encephalitis identified by neuropil antibodies: MRI and PET correlates. *Brain* 2005; 128: 1764-77.

Andermann F. *Chronic Encephalitis and Epilepsy. Rasmussen's Syndrome.* Boston: Butterworth-Heinemann, 1991.

Andrews PI, Dichter MA, Berkovic SF, Newton MR, McNamara JO. Plasmapheresis in Rasmussen's encephalitis. *Neurology* 1996; 46: 242-6.

Bauer J, Vezzani A, Bien CG. Epileptic encephalitis: the role of the innate and adaptive immune system. *Brain Pathol* 2012; 22: 412-21.

Bernal F, Graus F, Pifarre A, Saiz A, Benyahia B, Ribalta T. Immunohistochemical analysis of anti-Hu-associated paraneoplastic encephalomyelitis. *Acta Neuropathol* 2002; 103: 509-15.

Bien CG, Elger CE. Limbic encephalitis: a cause of temporal lobe epilepsy with onset in adult life. *Epilepsy Behav* 2007; 10: 529-38.

Bien CG, Gleissner U, Sassen R, Widman G, Urbach H, Elger CE. An open study of tacrolimus therapy in Rasmussen encephalitis. *Neurology* 2004; 62: 2106-9.

Bien CG, Widman G, Urbach H, et al. The natural history of Rasmussen's encephalitis. *Brain* 2002a; 125: 1751-9.

Bien CG, Elger CE, Leitner Y, et al. Slowly progressive hemiparesis in childhood as a consequence of Rasmussen encephalitis without or with delayed-onset seizures. *Eur J Neurol* 2007; 14: 387-90.

Bien CG, Bauer J, Deckwerth TL, et al. Destruction of neurons by cytotoxic T cells: a new pathogenic mechanism in Rasmussen's encephalitis. *Ann Neurol* 2002b; 51: 311-8.

Bien CG, Granata T, Antozzi C, et al. Pathogenesis, diagnosis and treatment of Rasmussen encephalitis: a European consensus statement. *Brain* 2005; 128: 454-71.

Bien CG, Vincent A, Barnett MH, et al. Immunopathology of autoantibody-associated encephalitides: clues for pathogenesis. *Brain* 2012; 135: 1622-38.

Bien CG, Tiemeier H, Sassen R, et al. Rasmussen encephalitis: incidence and course under randomized therapy with tacrolimus or intravenous immunoglobulins. *Epilepsia* 2013; 54: 543-50.

Bittner S, Simon OJ, Gobel K, Bien CG, Meuth SG, Wiendl H. Rasmussen encephalitis treated with natalizumab. *Neurology* 2013; 81: 395-7.

Blumenthal DT, Salzman KL, Digre KB, Jensen RL, Dunson WA, Dalmau J. Early pathologic findings and long-term improvement in anti-Ma2-associated encephalitis. *Neurology* 2006; 67: 146-9.

Buckley C, Oger J, Clover L, et al. Potassium channel antibodies in two patients with reversible limbic encephalitis. *Ann Neurol* 2001; 50: 73-8.

Busbridge NJ, Dascombe MJ, Tilders FJ, van Oers JW, Linton EA, Rothwell NJ. Central activation of thermogenesis and fever by interleukin-1 beta and interleukin-1 alpha involves different mechanisms. *Biochem Biophys Res Commun* 1989; 162: 591-6.

Camdessanche JP, Streichenberger N, Cavillon G, et al. Brain immunohistopathological study in a patient with anti-NMDAR encephalitis. *Eur J Neurol* 2011; 18: 929-31.

Chan D, Henley SM, Rossor MN, Warrington EK. Extensive and temporally ungraded retrograde amnesia in encephalitis associated with antibodies to voltage-gated potassium channels. *Arch Neurol* 2007; 64: 404-10.

Corsellis JA, Goldberg GJ, Norton AR. "Limbic encephalitis" and its association with carcinoma. *Brain* 1968; 91: 481-96.

Dalmau J, Lancaster E, Martinez-Hernandez E, Rosenfeld MR, Balice-Gordon R. Clinical experience and laboratory investigations in patients with anti-NMDAR encephalitis. *Lancet Neurol* 2011; 10: 63-74.

Dalmau J, Gleichman AJ, Hughes EG, et al. Anti-NMDA-receptor encephalitis: case series and analysis of the effects of antibodies. *Lancet Neurol* 2008; 7: 1091-8.

Dalmau J, Gultekin SH, Voltz R, et al. Ma1, a novel neuron- and testis-specific protein, is recognized by the serum of patients with paraneoplastic neurological disorders. *Brain* 1999; 122: 27-39.

Dalmau J, Tüzün E, Wu HY, et al. Paraneoplastic anti-N-methyl-D-aspartate receptor encephalitis associated with ovarian teratoma. *Ann Neurol* 2007; 61: 25-36.

De Simoni MG, Perego C, Ravizza T, et al. Inflammatory cytokines and related genes are induced in the rat hippocampus by limbic status epilepticus. *EurJ Neurosci* 2000; 12: 2623-33.

Dunstan EJ, Winer JB. Autoimmune limbic encephalitis causing fits, rapidly progressive confusion and hyponatraemia. *Age Ageing* 2006; 35: 536-7.

Eriksson C, Van Dam AM, Lucassen PJ, Bol JG, Winblad B, Schultzberg M. Immunohistochemical localization of interleukin-1beta, interleukin-1 receptor antagonist and interleukin-1beta converting enzyme/caspase-1 in the rat brain after peripheral administration of kainic acid. *Neuroscience* 1999; 93: 915-30.

Farrell MA, Droogan O, Secor DL, Poukens V, Quinn B, Vinters HV. Chronic encephalitis associated with epilepsy: immunohistochemical and ultrastructural studies. *Acta Neuropathol* 1995; 89: 313-21.

Geis C, Weishaupt A, Hallermann S, et al. Stiff person syndrome-associated autoantibodies to amphiphysin mediate reduced GABAergic inhibition. *Brain* 2010; 133: 3166-80.

Giometto B, Marchiori GC, Nicolao P, Scaravilli T, Lion A, Bardin PG, Tavolato B. Sub-acute cerebellar degeneration with anti-Yo autoantibodies: immuno-histochemical analysis of the immune reaction in the central nervous system. *NeuropatholAppl Neurobiol* 1997; 23: 468-74.

Granata T. Rasmussen's syndrome. *Neurol Sci* 2003; 24 (Suppl 4): S239-43.

Granata T, Fusco L, Gobbi G, et al. Experience with immunomodulatory treatments in Rasmussen's encephalitis. *Neurology* 2003; 61: 1807-10.

Graus F, Saiz A, Dalmau J. Antibodies and neuronal autoimmune disorders of the CNS. *J Neurol* 2010; 257: 509-17.

Graus F, Ribalta T, Campo E, Monforte R, Urbano A, Rozman C. Immunohistochemical analysis of the immune reaction in the nervous system in paraneoplastic encephalomyelitis. *Neurology* 1990; 40: 219-22.

Graus F, Saiz A, Lai M, et al. Neuronal surface antigen antibodies in limbic encephalitis: clinical-immunologic associations. *Neurology* 2008; 71: 930-6.

Hart YM, Andermann F, Robitaille Y, Laxer KD, Rasmussen T, Davis R. Double pathology in Rasmussen's syndrome: a window on the etiology? *Neurology* 1998; 50: 731-5.

Hauf M, Wiest R, Nirkko A, Strozzi S, Federspiel A. Dissociation of epileptic and inflammatory activity in Rasmussen Encephalitis. *Epilepsy Res* 2009; 83 (2-3): 265-8.

Honnorat J, Saiz A, Giometto B, et al. Cerebellar ataxia with anti-glutamic acid decarboxylase antibodies: study of 14 patients. *ArchNeurol* 2001; 58: 225-30.

Hughes EG, Peng X, Gleichman AJ, et al. Cellular and synaptic mechanisms of anti-NMDA receptor encephalitis. *J Neurosci* 2010; 30: 5866-75.

Iizuka T, Yoshii S, Kan S, et al. Reversible brain atrophy in anti-NMDA receptor encephalitis: a long-term observational study. *J Neurol* 2010; 257: 1686-91.

Iizuka T, Sakai F, Ide T, et al. Anti-NMDA receptor encephalitis in Japan. Long-term outcome without tumor removal. *Neurology* 2007; 70: 504-11.

Irani SR, Alexander S, Waters P, et al. Antibodies to Kv1 potassium channel-complex proteins leucine-rich, glioma inactivated 1 protein and contactin-associated protein-2 in limbic encephalitis, Morvan's syndrome and acquired neuromyotonia. *Brain* 2010a; 133: 2734-48.

Irani SR, Bera K, Waters P, et al. N-methyl-D-aspartate antibody encephalitis: temporal progression of clinical and paraclinical observations in a predominantly non-paraneoplastic disorder of both sexes. *Brain* 2010b; 133: 1655-67.

Irani SR, Michell AW, Lang B, et al. Faciobrachial dystonic seizures precede Lgi1 antibody limbic encephalitis. *Ann Neurol* 2011; 69: 892-900.

Iyer A, Zurolo E, Spliet WG, et al. Evaluation of the innate and adaptive immunity in type I and type II focal cortical dysplasias. *Epilepsia* 2010; 51: 1763-73.

Jean WC, Dalmau J, Ho A, Posner JB. Analysis of the IgG subclass distribution and inflammatory infiltrates in patients with anti-Hu-associated paraneoplastic encephalomyelitis. *Neurology* 1994; 44: 140-7.

Khan NL, Jeffree MA, Good C, Macleod W, Al-Sarraj S. Histopathology of VGKC antibody-associated limbic encephalitis. *Neurology* 2009; 72: 1703-5.

Korn-Lubetzki I, Bien CG, Bauer J, et al. Rasmussen encephalitis with active inflammation and delayed seizures onset. *Neurology* 2004; 62: 984-6.

Lai M, Huijbers MG, Lancaster E, et al. Investigation of LGI1 as the antigen in limbic encephalitis previously attributed to potassium channels: a case series. *Lancet Neurol* 2010; 9: 776-85.

Lancaster E, Huijbers MG, Bar V, et al. Investigations of caspr2, an autoantigen of encephalitis and neuromyotonia. *Ann Neurol* 2011; 69: 303-11.

Liimatainen S, Peltola M, Sabater L, et al. Clinical significance of glutamic acid decarboxylase antibodies in patients with epilepsy. *Epilepsia* 2010; 51: 760-7.

Malter MP, Helmstaedter C, Urbach H, Vincent A, Bien CG. Antibodies to glutamic acid decarboxylase define a form of limbic encephalitis. *Ann Neurol* 2010; 67: 470-8.

Manto M, Dalmau J, Didelot A, Rogemond V, Honnorat J. Afferent facilitation of corticomotor responses is increased by IgGs of patients with NMDA-receptor antibodies. *J Neurol* 2011; 258: 27-33.

Manto MU, Laute MA, Aguera M, Rogemond V, Pandolfo M, Honnorat J. Effects of anti-glutamic acid decarboxylase antibodies associated with neurological diseases. *Ann Neurol* 2007; 61: 544-51.

Maroso M, Balosso S, Ravizza T, et al. Toll-like receptor 4 and high-mobility group box-1 are involved in ictogenesis and can be targeted to reduce seizures. *Nat Med* 2010; 16: 413-9.

Martinez-Hernandez E, Horvath J, Shiloh-Malawsky Y, Sangha N, Martinez-Lage M, Dalmau J. Analysis of complement and plasma cells in the brain of patients with anti-NMDAR encephalitis. *Neurology* 2011; 77: 589-93.

Meinck HM, Thompson PD. Stiff man syndrome and related conditions. *Mov Disord* 2002; 17: 853-66.

Meinck HM, Faber L, Morgenthaler N, et al. Antibodies against glutamic acid decarboxylase: prevalence in neurological diseases. *J Neurol Neurosurg Psychiatry* 2001; 71: 100-3.

Minami M, Kuraishi Y, Satoh M. Effects of kainic acid on messenger RNA levels of IL-1 beta, IL-6, TNF alpha and LIF in the rat brain. *Biochem Biophys Res Commun* 1991; 176: 593-8.

Minami M, Kuraishi Y, Yamaguchi T, Nakai S, Hirai Y, Satoh M. Convulsants induce interleukin-1 beta messenger RNA in rat brain. *Biochem Biophys Res Commun* 1990; 171: 832-7.

Nishiyori A, Minami M, Takami S, Satoh M. Type 2 interleukin-1 receptor mRNA is induced by kainic acid in the rat brain. *Brain Res Mol Brain Res* 1997; 50: 237-45.

Oguni H, Olivier A, Andermann F, Comair J. Anterior callosotomy in the treatment of medically intractable epilepsies: a study of 43 patients with a mean follow-up of 39 months. *Ann Neurol* 1991; 30: 357-64.

Palmer CA, Geyer JD, Keating JM, et al. Rasmussen's encephalitis with concomitant cortical dysplasia: the role of GluR3. *Epilepsia* 1999; 40: 242-7.

Pardo CA, Vining EP, Guo L, Skolasky RL, Carson BS, Freeman JM. The pathology of Rasmussen syndrome: stages of cortical involvement and neuropathological studies in 45 hemispherectomies. *Epilepsia* 2004; 45: 516-26.

Park DC, Murman DL, Perry KD, Bruch LA. An autopsy case of limbic encephalitis with voltage-gated potassium channel antibodies. *Eur J Neurol* 2007; 14: e5-6.

Piatt JH, Jr., Hwang PA, Armstrong DC, Becker LE, Hoffman HJ. Chronic focal encephalitis (Rasmussen syndrome): six cases. *Epilepsia* 1988; 29: 268-79.

Posner JB. Paraneoplastic syndromes. *NeurolClin* 1991; 9: 919-36.

Pozo-Rosich P, Clover L, Saiz A, Vincent A, Graus F. Voltage-gated potassium channel antibodies in limbic encephalitis. *Ann Neurol* 2003; 54: 530-3.

Rasmussen T, Olszewski J, Lloyd-Smith D. Focal seizures due to chronic localized encephalitis. *Neurology* 1958; 8: 435-45.

Ravizza T, Gagliardi B, Noe F, Boer K, Aronica E, Vezzani A. Innate and adaptive immunity during epileptogenesis and spontaneous seizures: evidence from experimental models and human temporal lobe epilepsy. *Neurobiol Dis* 2008; 29: 142-60.

Ravizza T, Boer K, Redeker S, et al. The IL-1beta system in epilepsy-associated malformations of cortical development. *Neurobiol Dis* 2006; 24: 128-43.

Rivest S. Regulation of innate immune responses in the brain. *Nat Rev Immunol* 2009; 9: 429-39.

Robitaille Y. Neuropathologic aspects of chronic encephalitis. In: Andermann F, ed. *Chronic Encephalitis and Epilepsy. Rasmussen's Syndrome*, pp. 79-110. Boston: Butterworth-Heinemann, 1991.

Rogers SW, Andrews PI, Gahring LC, et al. Autoantibodies to glutamate receptor GluR3 in Rasmussen's encephalitis. *Science* 1994; 265: 648-51.

Saiz A, Arpa J, Sagasta A, Casamitjana R, Zarranz JJ, Tolosa E, Graus F. Autoantibodies to glutamic acid decarboxylase in three patients with cerebellar ataxia, late-onset insulin-dependent diabetes mellitus, and polyendocrine autoimmunity. *Neurology* 1997; 49: 1026-30.

Saiz A, Blanco Y, Sabater L, et al. Spectrum of neurological syndromes associated with glutamic acid decarboxylase antibodies: diagnostic clues for this association. *Brain* 2008; 131 (Pt 10): 2553-63.

Solimena M, Folli F, Denis Donini S, et al. Autoantibodies to glutamic acid decarboxylase in a patient with stiff-man syndrome, epilepsy, and type I diabetes mellitus. *N Eng l J Med* 1988; 318: 1012-20.

Striano P, Perruolo G, Errichiello L, Formisano P, Beguinot F, Zara F, Striano S. Glutamic acid decarboxylase antibodies in idiopathic generalized epilepsy and type 1 diabetes. *Ann Neurol* 2006; 63: 127-8.

Takei H, Wilfong A, Malphrus A, et al. Dual pathology in Rasmussen's encephalitis: a study of seven cases and review of the literature. *Neuropathology* 2010; 30: 381-91.

Tanaka K, Tanaka M, Inuzuka T, Nakano R, Tsuji S. Cytotoxic T lymphocyte-mediated cell death in paraneoplastic sensory neuronopathy with anti-Hu antibody. *J Neurol Sci* 1999; 163: 159-62.

Thomas JE, Reagan TJ, Klass DW. Epilepsia partialis continua. A review of 32 cases. *Arch Neurol* 1977; 34: 266-75.

Tüzün E, Zhou L, Baehring JM, Bannykh S, Rosenfeld MR, Dalmau J. Evidence for antibody-mediated pathogenesis in anti-NMDAR encephalitis associated with ovarian teratoma. *Acta Neuropathol* 2009; 118: 737-43.

Van Dam AM, Bauer J, Tilders FJ, Berkenbosch F. Endotoxin-induced appearance of immunoreactive interleukin-1 beta in ramified microglia in rat brain: a light and electron microscopic study. *Neuroscience* 1995; 65: 815-26.

Varadkar S, Bien CG, Kruse CA, et al. Rasmussen's encephalitis: clinical features, pathobiology, and treatment advances. *Lancet Neurol* 2014; 13: 195-205.

Verschuuren J, Chuang L, Rosenblum MK, et al. Inflammatory infiltrates and complete absence of Purkinje cells in anti-Yo-associated paraneoplastic cerebellar degeneration. *Acta Neuropathol* 1996; 91: 519-25.

Vezzani A, French J, Bartfai T, Baram TZ. The role of inflammation in epilepsy. *Nature Rev Neurol* 2011; 7: 31-40.

Vincent A, Bien CG, Irani SR, Waters P. Autoantibodies associated with diseases of the CNS: new developments and future challenges. *Lancet Neurol* 2011; 10: 759-72.

Vincent A, Buckley C, Schott JM, et al. Potassium channel antibody-associated encephalopathy: a potentially immunotherapy-responsive form of limbic encephalitis. *Brain* 2004; 127: 701-12.

Viviani B, Gardoni F, Marinovich M. Cytokines and neuronal ion channels in health and disease. *Int Rev Neurobiol* 2007; 82: 247-63.

Wang D, Blümcke I, Gui Q, Zhou W, Zuo H, Lin J, Luo Y. Clinico-pathological investigations of Rasmussen encephalitis suggest multifocal disease progression and associated focal cortical dysplasia. *Epileptic Disord* 2013; 15: 32-43.

Whitney KD, Andrews JM, McNamara JO. Immunoglobulin G and complement immunoreactivity in the cerebral cortex of patients with Rasmussen's encephalitis. *Neurology* 1999; 53: 699-708.

Wiendl H, Bien CG, Bernasconi P, et al. GluR3 antibodies: Prevalence in focal epilepsy but no specificity for Rasmussen's encephalitis. *Neurology* 2001; 57: 1511-4.

Wong SH, Saunders MD, Larner AJ, Das K, Hart IK. An effective immunotherapy regimen for VGKC antibody-positive limbic encephalitis. *J Neurol Neurosurg Psychiatry* 2010; 81: 1167-9.

Zhang Q, Tanaka K, Sun P, et al. Suppression of synaptic plasticity by cerebrospinal fluid from anti-NMDA receptor encephalitis patients. *Neurobiol Dis* 2012; 45: 610-5.

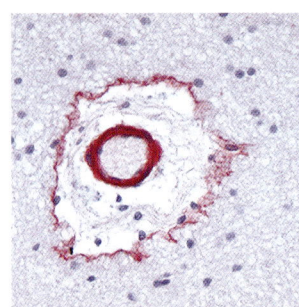

6. Vascular lesions associated with focal epilepsies

Ingmar Blümcke, Harvey B. Sarnat

The differential diagnosis of vascular lesions in histopathological specimens obtained from epilepsy surgery covers primarily the spectrum of vascular malformations with cavernous haemangioma, capillary telangiectasia, arterio-venous malformations, and Sturge-Weber syndrome (*i.e.* encephalo-facial angiomatosis) as most significant examples. Vascular malformations represent congenital lesions with compromised mesodermal differentiation occurring between the third to eighth weeks of gestation (Rammos *et al.*, 2009). These vascular malformations are histopathologically classified by different architectural abnormalities of vessel walls, continuity with normal cerebral vasculature and the amount of intervening brain parenchyma. However, epilepsy surgery specimens often reveal also angiopathic alterations in white matter with abnormal enlargement of their perivascular space. These features were frequently observed in children and adults, although its origin remains hitherto unknown. In our opinion, a secondary pathogenesis related to repetitive seizure-related blood-brain-barrier (BBB) breakdown is more likely and would provisionally classify as white matter angiopathy in epilepsy (Hildebrandt *et al.*, 2008).

White matter angiopathy in focal epilepsies

An intriguing pattern of white matter angiopathy can be frequently observed in surgical brain tissue obtained from patients with drug-resistant focal epilepsy, either in adults or children (Hildebrandt *et al.*, 2008). Neuropathology hallmarks include splitting of the basal membrane into endothelial and parenchymal leaves (*Figure 1C*), which results in an extensively enlarged perivascular space (*Figure 1B*). These cavities also contain activated microglial cells and macrophages, T-lymphocytes or cell detritus (*Figure 1D*). Additional findings include swelling and vacuolation of endothelial cells, invasion of astrocytic end-feet, degeneration of pericytes as well as newly build capillaries (*Figure 1D*). Angiopathic changes occur independently of and also distant to specific epilepsy-associated lesions, *i.e.* dysplasia, neoplasia or hippocampal sclerosis, and were encountered more frequently in temporal *vs.* extratemporal localization (Hildebrandt *et al.*, 2008). Only half the white matter vessels reveal such prominent perivascular spaces, more frequently around arterioles (74.7%) than around capillaries (44.8%). There is no difference in overall white matter vessel density when comparing epilepsy surgery tissue with age- and location-matched autopsy specimens. Moreover, this histopathological pattern is distinct from vascular changes in chronic hypertensive angiopathy, which is typically associated with thickening of the tunica media of affected blood vessels, i.e. arteriolosclerosis or small vessel disease (Graham and Lantos, 2002).

During development, all parenchymal arterioles branch exactly three times before feeding into the capillary network. The smooth muscular walls of these arterioles are not acquired until the mid-3rd trimester. This late maturation explains why premature infants of less than 37 weeks lack the auto-regulation of cerebral blood flow that term neonates possess: even if the autonomic neural mechanism is present, the end-organ vessel cannot respond by vasoconstriction. In some neonatal angiitis cases, such as those associated with congenital infections, this may be an additional factor in the neurological morbidity of survivors. Neonatal seizures are common in such infants. The perivascular space represents an abnormally enlarged Virchow-Robin compartment, which is built normally early during brain development. The

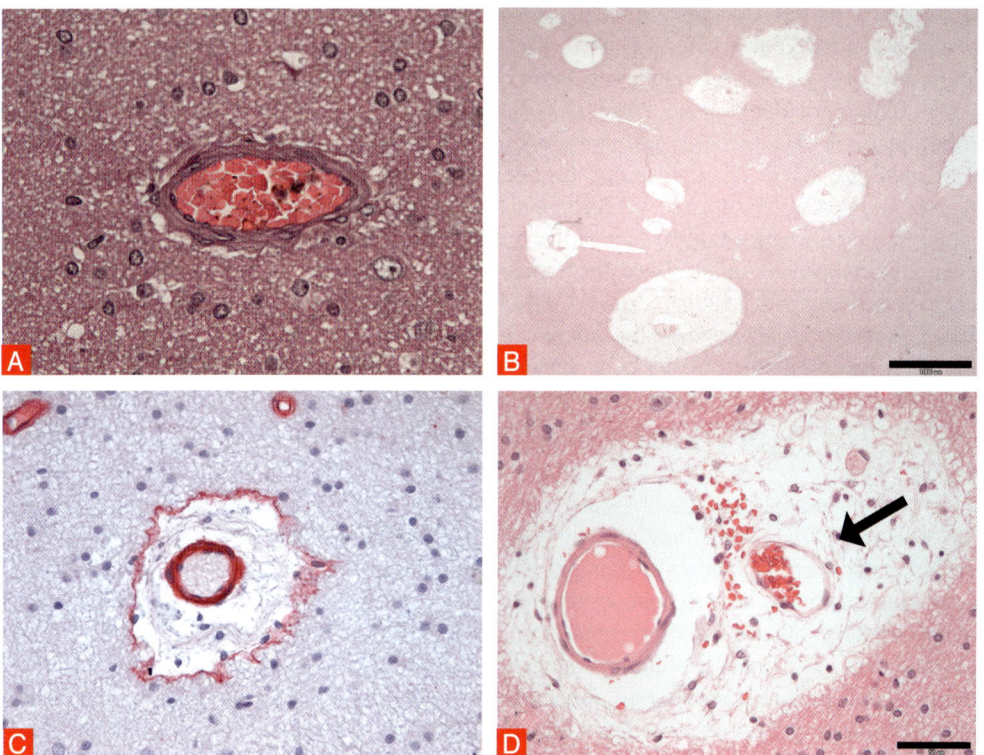

Figure 1

White matter angiopathy in epilepsy tissue.

A: Small arteriole in white matter without any perivascular space detectable. Technical procedures for tissue dehydration prior to paraffin embedding were same in A to D (see appendix). **B:** Significantly enlarged perivascular spaces can be seen in white matter of this young patient with drug-resistant epilepsy. **C:** splitting of the basal lamina into endothelial and parenchymal leaves visualized by collagen-immunohistochemistry (red colour with blue haematoxylin counterstaining). **D:** enlarged perivascular space often contains macrophages, T-lymphocytes or cell detritus. Newly built capillaries (arrow) also were encountered in this example.

brain's vascular system derives from pial vessels perforating the cortex towards the subependymal zone (Marin-Padilla, 2011). Perforating vessels are surrounded and accompanied throughout their entire length by a Virchow-Robin compartment (V-RC), keeping the perforating vessels extrinsic to the nervous system. V-RC remains open and likely function as a pre-lymphatic drainage system, in both physiological and pathological conditions (Marin-Padilla, 2011). There are no lymphatic vessels in the brain, however. The intrinsic micro-vascular system of the neocortex derives from endothelial sprouts communicating between equidistant perforating vessels (Marin-Padilla, 2011). These early anastomotic capillary plexus is devoid of the V-RC and surrounded only by a single basal lamina. Such neocortical vessels rarely show perivascular cavities in epilepsy surgery tissue, another yet unanswered observation within the large spectrum of neuropathological findings in epilepsy surgery.

Virchow-Robin spaces exceeding a critical diameter of 1 mm (VRS) can be readily detected by magnetic resonance imaging (Heier *et al.*, 1989; Song *et al.*, 2000). As an example, VRS can be detected by MRI in the insular cortex and basal ganglia of adults with chronic epilepsy as well as in healthy controls (Song *et al.*, 2000). Its predilection and distribution point to microangiopathic changes of the aging brain. On the other hand, a prospective MRI-study revealed a prevalence of "VRS" in frontal and parietal white matter in 3% of children under the age of 17 years and is associated with neuropsychiatric disorders (Rollins *et al.*, 1993). Their incidence in epilepsy is currently unclear (Song *et al.*, 2000; Lahl *et al.*, 2003). Ample evidence indicates that seizures can harm BBB and cerebral vasculature itself. MRI scans performed early after status epilepticus identify transient brain oedema (Scott *et al.*, 2002; Briellmann *et al.*, 2005); Kim *et al.* 2001) that could also be experimentally induced after kainate injection (Lassmann *et al.*, 1984). In agreement with these findings, seizure activity induces local vasodilatation and enhanced cerebral blood flow. Other pathophysiological consequences of seizure activity include enhanced metabolic activity followed by consumptive hypoxia (Scholz and Jotten, 1951) as well as a transient rise of intracerebral pressure which is rapidly normalized via blood auto-regulation mechanisms. The latter can be impaired by hypercapnia which also results in focal break-down of the BBB and extravasation of protein and liquid into the brain (Faraci *et al.*, 1993). Thus, abundance of substances from blood plasma within perivascular spaces observed in epilepsy surgery tissue supports severe or chronic white matter BBB dysfunction.

Other white matter changes are frequently reported in many epilepsy patients and can be readily recognized during presurgical work-up, such as temporal lobe atrophy with or without blurred white/grey-matter boundaries (Thom *et al.*, 2001; Kasper *et al.*, 2003; Hildebrandt *et al.*, 2005). Temporal polar blurring, however, is caused by degeneration of fibre bundles and redistribution of remaining fibres rather than by focal cortical dysplasia or angiopathic lesions (Garbelli *et al.*, 2012). Whether or not mechanisms of multidrug resistance also relate to white matter angiopathy remains to be further clarified. In our previous study, all patients were reported pharmaco-resistant to first choice antiepileptic drugs (AED) including carbamazepine, phenobarbital or valproic acid and there was no significant difference in AED treatment regimens in patients with compared to patients without VRS prior to surgery (Hildebrandt *et al.*, 2008). Furthermore, neither gender nor side of the operated hemisphere had an influence on the presence of enlarged perivascular spaces along blood vessels of white matter.

Cavernous haemangioma (cavernoma)

Cavernous haemangiomas (cavernomas) occur at any site of the brain as well as in any other tissue (Ferrer *et al.*, 2008). They present usually with a single lesion whereas multiple cavernomas occur more commonly in familial diseases (Moran *et al.*, 1999). Histologically, cavernomas are composed of closely apposed and dilated vascular channels (back-to-back) without mature vessel walls and no intervening brain parenchyma. Elastica-van-Gieson (EvG) staining characterizes vessel walls as fibrous membranes covered by endothelial cells. Calcification or even ossification has been reported. A peripheral rim of haemosiderin (stored in macrophages) is almost always present in surrounding brain parenchyma and can be detected by MRI. However, the concept that cavernomas are static lesions has been revised from longitudinal neuroimaging studies describing growth (Rosenow *et al.*, 2013) and neuropathological studies demonstrated angiogenesis and proliferation using VEGF, endoglin and PCNA immunohistochemistry (Sure *et al.*, 2005). MRI usually reveals a well-circumscribed multi-cystic lesion (resembling mulberry cysts), without or only mild contrast enhancement and no surrounding oedema, unless there has been a recent associated parenchymal haemorrhage. A well-defined rim of haemosiderin also should be identified.

Epileptic seizures are the most frequent symptom in patients with cavernous angiomas, as emphasized and discussed in a Task Force report from the ILAE commission on therapeutic strategies (Rosenow *et al.*, 2013; Rosenow *et al.*, 2014). The prevalence of cavernous angiomas is between 0.02 and 0.5% (Maraire and Awad, 1995; Bertalanffy *et al.*, 2002), whereas 4-6% of pharmaco-resistant epilepsies are caused by cerebral cavernomas. Indeed, they represent 3.9% of all cases collected at the German Neuropathology Reference Centre for Epilepsy Surgery (see *chapter 1, Table I*), with epilepsy onset occurring at a mean age of 27.2 years in our series of 218 patients (see *Appendix, Table I*). The 5-year risk of a first seizure in adult patients with a cavernoma and intracerebral haemorrhage or focal neurological deficit is 6% compared to 4% in patients with incidentally detected cavernomas (Josephson *et al.*, 2011). The risk of recurrence after a first unprovoked seizure is 94% (Josephson *et al.*, 2011) so that the diagnosis of epilepsy should be made and antiepileptic treatment is justified when a first cavernoma related seizure occurs (Fisher *et al.*, 2005; Fisher *et al.*, 2014).

The epileptogenic mechanisms in cavernomas remain an issue of ongoing debate (Kraemer and Awad, 1994; Willmore *et al.*, 1978). Repeated micro-haemorrhage and haemosiderin deposits in surrounding cortical tissue are believed to cause hyperexcitability by iron ions, providing free radicals and lipid peroxides. Furthermore, reactive glial proliferation and their innate immune system's response is epileptogenic (see above, *chapter 5, section "The innate immune system can induce seizures"*). Dual pathology with hippocampal sclerosis has also been described (Stefan and Hammen, 2004). However, major risk factors for epilepsy in patients with cavernomas have been specified by the Task Force report to include: 1) supratentorial localization; 2) cortical involvement *vs.* exclusively subcortical localization; 3) archicortical/mesio-temporal involvement *vs.* exclusively neocortical localization (Rosenow *et al.*, 2013). Surgical resection achieves postoperative seizure control in about 75% of patients with cavernoma related epilepsy (Englot *et al.*, 2011). Surgical failures may result from insufficient efforts to adequately define and resect the epileptogenic zone (Schwartz, 2010), in particular when the dominant hemisphere is affected, and long duration of epilepsy (> 5 years) contributes usually as another risk factor for unfavourable postsurgical seizure control (Simasathien *et al.*, 2013).

Reported families with cerebral cavernous malformations (CCM) showed autosomal dominant inheritance, and three genes have been identified, *i.e. CCM1* (Laberge-le Couteulx *et al.*, 1999), *CCM2* (Liquori *et al.*, 2003) and *CCM3* (Bergametti *et al.*, 2005). KRIT1 (Krev interaction trapped 1) is likely to represent the disease causing gene in *CCM1* and is located at chromosome 7q11.2-21 (Sahoo *et al.*, 1999). Approximately 40% of families with cerebral cavernous malformations carry KRIT1-mutations (Wang, 2005). Mutations in a phosphortyrosine-binding domain (PTB) at chromosome 7p15-13 occurs in 20% of patients with familial CCM, but its gene function is unknown (Liquori *et al.*, 2003; Denier *et al.*, 2004). Approximately 40% of CCM families are linked to the CCM3 locus, so called PDCD10 (programmed cell death 10). Its role in vascular morphogenesis remains to be investigated (Bergametti *et al.*, 2005). An encephaloclastic cavernous angioma was demonstrated in the opercular region of a mid-gestational foetus, initially mistakenly diagnosed by foetal imaging as schizencephaly (Sarnat *et al.*, 2012); genetic studies of the tissues of this foetus subsequently showed a KRIT1/CCM1 mutation. This is the earliest case of cerebral cavernoma reported to date.

Arteriovenous malformation (AVM)

AVMs occur in all parts of the brain, but most commonly in the territory of the middle cerebral artery. AVMs range in size from grossly invisible to those involving a large portion of the entire hemisphere. They may enlarge over time by recruitment of adjacent blood vessels. MRI shows vascular lesions with abnormal vessels and arteriovenous shunts following angiography. Histological examination discovers vessels of irregular size, shape and abnormalities in the organization of vessel walls. Arteries with intact media and a lamina elastica interna can be observed adjacent to veins. Arteriovenous shunt vessels are pathognomic for the histopathological diagnosis. Using EvG-staining, shunt vessels are defined by transition from arteries into venous calibres without intervening capillaries. Interposed brain parenchyma is gliotic and may contain haemosiderin storing macrophages after recurrent bleeding. Remnants of preoperative AVM embolization may be detected in vascular lumen. AVMs arise during embryogenesis and account for 70% of all cerebral vascular malformations in children. Immature veins and arteries contact with each other before development of capillaries. Lack of the capillary bed results in arteriovenous shunt vessels with consecutive dilatation of the receptive venous system. AVMs become symptomatic at any age but most commonly present in the second to forth decade with recurrent subarachnoidal bleeding. AVMs account for 0.6% of surgical brain samples collected at the German Neuropathology Reference Centre for Epilepsy Surgery (see *Chapter 8, Table I*) with a mean age at epilepsy onset at 20.7 years and late surgery at 37.3 years. Seizures may be related to brain ischemia caused by "steal" of blood from surrounding brain parenchyma into the malformation (Costantino and Vinters, 1986; Scaravilli, 1998). Similar to cavernomas, iron deposits after bleeding or reactive gliosis are likely to contribute to seizure onset (see above). Most AVMs are sporadic lesions with rare reports of familial inheritance (Amin-Hanjani *et al.*, 1998). However, these rare forms help to decipher candidate genes, likely to be related with angiogenesis. As an example, microarray analysis demonstrated increased mRNA of vascular endothelial growth factor A (VEGF-A) and its protein as well as increased expression of integrin $\alpha v \beta 3$ protein, suggesting a role of integrins in the aetiology of AVMs (Hashimoto *et al.*, 2004). An earlier study reported decreased Tie-2 and also VEGF-R2 expression levels in AVM vessels. Some arteriovenous malformations are associated with hereditary haemorrhagic telangiectasia type 1. Endoglin is the gene mutated in this disorder (see below). Even though endoglin is not involved in the generation of AVMs, the presence of endoglin on fibroblasts in the perivascular stroma suggests an active role for this protein in vascular remodelling as response to increased blood flow (Matsubara *et al.*, 2000).

Capillary telangiectasia

Capillary telangiectasia are often an incidental finding at brain autopsy and cannot be detected by imaging unless lesions are confluent or haemorrhagic. They are composed of dilated blood vessels separated by relatively normal brain parenchyma, which often shows reactive astrogliosis. Capillary telangiectasia have a high prevalence and are usually asymptomatic. Bleeding is rare. If capillary telangiectasia occur in distinct brain regions, e.g. within the hippocampus, or in association with other vascular malformations, seizures may occur. In infant autopsies, occasional brainstem telangiectasia are demonstrated as an incidental finding, usually in the pons; they are not haemorrhagic and have normal neurons and glial cells between the cluster of capillaries. They are asymptomatic during life and are not the cause of death.

However, hereditary haemorrhagic telangiectasia (HHT), an autosomal dominant vascular malformation of skin, mucosa and viscera can also manifest in brain vessels. Three gene loci are known: HHT1 on chromosome 9q34.1, HHT2 on chromosome 12q11-14 and HHT3 on chromosome 5q31.5-32 (Wang, 2005). HHT1 is caused by mutations in endoglin which encodes a TGFβ binding protein expressed predominantly in endothelial cells and plays an important role in vascular remodelling and maintenance of vessel wall integrity (Lebrin et al., 2005). HHT2 results from mutations in the ALK1 gene encoding a type 1 serine-threonine kinase receptor in endothelial cells. Alk1 binds to TGFβ1 and activin-A, and signal through phosphorylation of SMAD1 and SMAD5 (Chen and Massague, 1999). A third genetic locus, HHT3 was identified in a family without linkage to endoglin, ALK1 or SMAD4. However, the specific gene of HHT3 has not been identified yet (Cole et al., 2005). There exists also an association with juvenile polyposis (JP), caused by mutations in the MADH4 gene on chromosome 18q21.1 encoding for SMAD4. SMAD4 is an integral downstream effector on the TGFβ signal transduction pathway.

Sturge-Weber syndrome (SWS)

William A. Sturge reported about a girl with an extensive telangiectatic nevus of the right side of her face and head, and epileptic fits beginning in the left hand (Sturge, 1879). Frederik Parkes Weber demonstrated cortical calcifications in this group of patients and suggested the possibility of brain atrophy as a consequence of steal phenomena from the angiodysplastic cortex surrounding the vascular malformation (Weber, 1922). Nowadays, Sturge-Weber syndrome (SWS) is classified as neurocutaneous phacomatosis presenting with 1) unilateral (less frequently bilateral) facial nevus, typically located with a port-wine patch appearance in V1 or V2 regions of trigeminal nerve innervation; 2) dural and leptomeningeal angiomatosis affecting more often unilateral occipital and posterior parietal lobes; 3) haemangiomas of the choroid; 4) congenital glaucoma. The clinical SWS phenotype is most diverse with partial or incomplete manifestation of these lesions (Roach, 1992; Wang et al., 2015).

Microscopically, large tortuous and abnormal venous angioma in thickened leptomeninges can be defined as leptomeningeal angiomatosis. The underlying brain tissue is atrophic and displays neuronal loss, reactive astrogliosis and calcification. Laminar cortical necrosis may occur, suggesting ischemic damage secondary to venous stasis in leptomeninges and cerebral vessels. However, intraoperative electro-corticographic recordings also documented epileptogenic areas beyond angiomatous patches (Rasmussen et al., 1972). Few reports highlighted the coexistence of SWS with cortical malformations such as FCD and polymicrogyria (Simonati et al., 1994; Pal et al., 2002; Comi, 2003; Maton et al., 2010; Murakami et al., 2012). These studies revealed FCD IA or FCD IIA using Palmini's classification scheme (Palmini et al., 2004). In contrast, the ILAE classification of FCDs would classify architectural abnormalities with or without hypertrophic neurons outside layer 5 of the neocortex in association with any other principal lesion as FCD Type III (Blümcke et al., 2011), i.e. FCD Type IIIc in SWS with extensive capillary-venous malformations (Wang et al., 2015).

Difficult-to-treat focal epilepsies are frequent clinical symptoms and observed in almost 80% of patients with SWS (Kossoff et al., 2005). Decrease of cerebral blood flow within affected cortical areas by leptomeningeal angiomatosis as well as decreased venous return, focal ischemia, and decreased neuronal metabolism are considered as the main pathogenetic mechanisms. Imaging and gross examination reveal widespread, usually unilateral leptomeningeal angiomatosis, cortical calcifications in a "railroad track" pattern and less frequently atrophy of the underlying neocortex. White matter abnormalities are common and may be linked to chronic ischemia and reactive gliosis. Angiography demonstrates an overall lack of superficial cortical veins, non-filling of the dural sinuses and tortuous course of veins towards the vein of Galen (Thomas-Sohl et al., 2004). Functional brain imaging has demonstrated decreased glucose metabolism and hypoperfusion of the affected neocortex (Lee et al., 2001).

Early onset seizures in patients with SWS typically respond less well to medical treatment and are associated with greater neurological and cognitive impairments than late-onset seizures (Bourgeois et al., 2007). Complete resection of the epileptogenic zone is a prognostic factor determining outcome of epilepsy surgery (Morioka et al., 1999). It is important to also consider invasive recording modalities, anatomic and functional neuroimaging including FDG-PET and SPECT to localize and characterize the epileptogenic network in patients with SWS (Wang et al., 2015). Different strategies were proposed for surgical treatment of SWS, including cortical excisions, lobectomy, or hemispherectomy owing to the unilateral and focal character of the condition in a majority of cases (Di Rocco and Tamburrini, 2006). In a large meta-analysis including 16 anatomic hemispherectomies, 14 functional hemispherectomies, and two hemidecortications in children with SWS, hemispherectomies were reported most successful (82%) (Kossoff et al., 2002). As for cortical excisions, most resection procedures achieved a reduction of epileptic activity but followed later on by seizure relapse. It was already T. Rasmussen in 1972 describing that most active epileptogenic areas involved cortical regions adjacent to the angiomatous patches (Rasmussen et al., 1972). Based on these observations tailored lobectomy was considered.

The underlying cortical vessels are increased in number, typically thin-walled and narrowed by hyalinization and subendothelial proliferation. Repeated stroke-like episodes and thrombosis may result in disease progression and neurological deterioration. SWS occurs sporadically with a frequency of approximately 1/50,000. Inheritance is so far not established. Non-Mendelian genetic hypotheses, including chromosomal instability have been suggested. Spontaneous somatic mutations in a common progenitor cell line of dermal, neuronal and ocular tissue in the first trimester of development may lead to genetic mosaicism of the affected areas (Comi et al., 2005). A case report about one of two monozygotic twins presenting with SWS supports this hypothesis (Pedailles et al., 1993). Another possibility refers to a two-hit model combining hereditary and spontaneous factors. Excessive vascular proliferation of the angioma diverts blood flow from parenchyma and creates an anoxic environment in the surrounding brain, leading to cellular damage. As a result, the underlying cortex becomes atrophied, calcified and eventually dysfunctional (Kotagal and Lüders, 1999), leading to seizures. The endothelial basal lamina contains an extracellular matrix composed of glycoproteins and proteoglycans including laminin, fibronectin and tenascin. Fibronectin has been identified as a key regulator in angiogenesis and vasculogenesis and plays a crucial role in brain tissue response to ischemia and maybe to seizures (Comi et al., 2003). Increased fibronectin gene expression levels were indeed observed in fibroblasts obtained from port-wine haemangiomas compared to normal skin samples. Moreover, there was a trend towards increased fibronectin protein expression in SWS brain samples compared to post-mortem controls. Therefore, fibronectin is supposed to be a likely candidate for SWS. Furthermore, the analysis of families with hereditary port-wine stain identified *RAS1* mutation on chromosome 5q (Eerola et al., 2002). The *RAS1* gene product is p120-RasGAP, a negative regulator of the Ras-mitogen-activated protein kinase signalling pathway. It may also be a candidate for involvement in vascular abnormalities of SWS.

SWS and focal cortical dysplasia

A recent report of six SWS patients with difficult-to-treat epilepsies and large surgical resections showed abnormal neurones with cytological features described also for dysmorphic neurons in FCD Type II or cortical tubers (Wang et al., 2015). These neurones presented with enlarged cell bodies and nuclei, abnormally distributed intracellular Nissl substance, and cytoplasmic accumulation of neurofilament proteins (Blümcke et al., 2011). Notwithstanding, FCD

Type II can occur as double pathology with other principal lesions by two independent pathogenic mechanisms, *i.e.* FCD Type II and cavernomas or tumours. We have proposed, however, that the described histopathology pattern in SWS patients is likely to reflect an associated pathology, *i.e.* FCD ILAE Type IIIc. A major argument is that the overall architecture of the neocortex does not fit into the concept of FCD ILAE Type II, with its severely disturbed architectural layering and many dysmorphic neurones recognizable throughout the cortical thickness as well as in white matter (Muhlebner *et al.*, 2012). Moreover, cell shape is not a defining hallmark of dysmorphic neurones, as these cells can present with pyramidal or interneuronal phenotypes (Blümcke *et al.*, 2011). Hypertrophic pyramidal neurones similar to those described in SWS are reminiscent of those observed in FCD IIa have been reported also in other epileptogenic pathologies, such as hippocampal sclerosis (Kim *et al.*, 2008; Thom *et al.*, 2008; Mirsattari *et al.*, 2009; Miyahara *et al.*, 2011). Long-term plasticity with reorganization or epigenetically driven molecular pathways are likely possibilities to convert the cytological appearance of any pyramidal cells into a cell with dysmorphic-like features (Kobow and Blümcke, 2011, 2012). However, it will need further clarification of the molecular nature and origin of FCD subtypes, as well as deciphering the impact of other pathologies such as ischemia and vascular calcification for aberrant morphogenesis in the developing brain (McCartney and Squier, 2014).

References

Amin-Hanjani S, Robertson R, Arginteanu MS, Scott RM. Familial intracranial arteriovenous malformations. Case report and review of the literature. *Pediatr Neurosurg* 1998; 29: 208-13.

Bergametti F, Denier C, Labauge P, *et al.* Mutations within the programmed cell death 10 gene cause cerebral cavernous malformations. *Am J Hum Genet* 2005; 76: 42-51.

Bertalanffy H, Benes L, Miyazawa T, Alberti O, Siegel AM, Sure U. Cerebral cavernomas in the adult. Review of the literature and analysis of 72 surgically treated patients. *Neurosurg Rev* 2002; 25: 1-53; discussion 54-5.

Blümcke I, *et al.* The clinico-pathological spectrum of Focal Cortical Dysplasias: a consensus classification proposed by an ad hoc Task Force of the ILAE Diagnostic Methods Commission. *Epilepsia* 2011; 52: 158-74.

Bourgeois M, Crimmins DW, de Oliveira RS, *et al.* Surgical treatment of epilepsy in Sturge-Weber syndrome in children. *J Neurosurg* 2007; 106: 20-8.

Briellmann RS, Wellard RM, Jackson GD. Seizure-associated abnormalities in epilepsy: evidence from MR imaging. *Epilepsia* 2005; 46: 760-6.

Chen YG, Massague J. Smad1 recognition and activation by the ALK1 group of transforming growth factor-beta family receptors. *J Biol Chem* 1999; 274: 3672-7.

Cole SG, Begbie ME, Wallace GM, Shovlin CL. A new locus for hereditary haemorrhagic telangiectasia (HHT3) maps to chromosome 5. *J Med Genet* 2005; 42: 577-82.

Comi AM. Pathophysiology of Sturge-Weber syndrome. *J Child Neurol* 2003; 18: 509-16.

Comi AM, Mehta P, Hatfield LA, Dowling MM. Sturge-Weber syndrome associated with other abnormalities: a medical record and literature review. *Arch Neurol* 2005; 62: 1924-7.

Comi AM, Hunt P, Vawter MP, Pardo CA, Becker KG, Pevsner J. Increased fibronectin expression in sturge-weber syndrome fibroblasts and brain tissue. *Pediatr Res* 2003; 53: 762-9.

Costantino A, Vinters HV. A pathologic correlate of the "steal" phenomenon in a patient with cerebral arteriovenous malformation. *Stroke* 1986; 17: 103-6.

Denier C, *et al.* Mutations within the MGC4607 gene cause cerebral cavernous malformations. *Am J Hum Genet* 2004; 74: 326-37.

Di Rocco C, Tamburrini G. Sturge-Weber syndrome. *Child Nerv Syst* 2006; 22: 909-21.

Eerola I, Boon LM, Watanabe S, Grynberg H, Mulliken JB, Vikkula M. Locus for susceptibility for familial capillary malformation ('port-wine stain') maps to 5q. *Eur J Hum Genet* 2002; 10: 375-80.

Faraci FM, Breese KR, Heistad DD. Nitric oxide contributes to dilatation of cerebral arterioles during seizures. *Am J Physiol* 1993; 265: H2209-12.

Ferrer I, Kaste M, Kalimo H. Vascular diseases. In: Love S, Louis DN, Ellison DW, (eds) *Greenfield's Neuropathology*, pp. 121-240. London: Edward Arnold, 2008.

Fisher RS, van Emde Boas W, Blume W, Elger C, Genton P, Lee P, Engel J, Jr. Epileptic seizures and epilepsy: definitions proposed by the International League Against Epilepsy (ILAE) and the International Bureau for Epilepsy (IBE). *Epilepsia* 2005; 46: 470-2.

Fisher RS, Acevedo C, Arzimanoglou A, *et al.* ILAE official report: a practical clinical definition of epilepsy. *Epilepsia* 2014; 55: 475-82.

Garbelli R, Milesi G, Medici V, *et al.* Blurring in patients with temporal lobe epilepsy: clinical, high-field imaging and ultrastructural study. *Brain* 2012; 135: 2337-49.

Graham DI, Lantos PL. *Greenfields' Neuropathology, 7th edition.* London, New York, New Delhi: Arnold, 2002.

Hashimoto T, Lawton MT, Wen G, *et al.* Gene microarray analysis of human brain arteriovenous malformations. *Neurosurgery* 2004; 54: 410-23; discussion 423-5.

Heier LA, Bauer CJ, Schwartz L, Zimmerman RD, Morgello S, Deck MD. Large Virchow-Robin spaces: MR-clinical correlation. *Am J Neuroradiol* 1989; 10: 929-36.

Hildebrandt M, Pieper T, Winkler P, Kolodziejczyk D, Holthausen H, Blümcke I. Neuropathological spectrum of cortical dysplasia in children with severe focal epilepsies. *Acta Neuropathol* 2005; 110: 1-11.

Hildebrandt M, Amann K, Schroder R, *et al.* White matter angiopathy is common in pediatric patients with intractable focal epilepsies. *Epilepsia* 2008; 49: 804-15.

Josephson CB, Leach JP, Duncan R, Roberts RC, Counsell CE, Al-Shahi Salman R. Seizure risk from cavernous or arteriovenous malformations: prospective population-based study. *Neurology* 2011; 76: 1548-54.

Kasper BS, Stefan H, Paulus W. Microdysgenesis in mesial temporal lobe epilepsy: a clinicopathological study. *Ann Neurol* 2003; 54: 501-6.

Kim SH, Cho YJ, Seok Kim H, *et al.* Balloon cells and dysmorphic neurons in the hippocampus associated with epileptic amnesic syndrome: a case report. *Epilepsia* 2008; 49: 905-9.

Kobow K, Blümcke I. The methylation hypothesis: do epigenetic chromatin modifications play a role in epileptogenesis? *Epilepsia* 2011; 52 (Suppl 4): 15-9.

Kobow K, Blümcke I. The emerging role of DNA methylation in epileptogenesis. *Epilepsia* 2012; 53: 11-20.

Kossoff EH, Buck C, Freeman JM. Outcomes of 32 hemispherectomies for Sturge-Weber syndrome worldwide. *Neurology* 2002; 59: 1735-8.

Kossoff EH, Hatfield LA, Ball KL, Comi AM. Comorbidity of epilepsy and headache in patients with Sturge-Weber syndrome. *J Child Neurol* 2005; 20: 678-82.

Kotagal P, Lüders HO. *The Epilepsies*. San Diego, London, Boston, New York, Sydney, Tokyo, Toronto: Academic Press, 1999.

Lahl R, Villagran R, Teixeira W. *Neuropathology of Focal Epilepsies: An Atlas*. Bielefeld: John Libbey and Co. Ltd, 2003.

Lassmann H, Petsche U, Kitz K, Baran H, Sperk G, Seitelberger F, Hornykiewicz O. The role of brain edema in epileptic brain damage induced by systemic kainic acid injection. *Neuroscience* 1984; 13: 691-704.

Lebrin F, Deckers M, Bertolino P, Ten Dijke P. TGF-beta receptor function in the endothelium. *Cardiovasc Res* 2005; 65: 599-608.

Lee JS, Asano E, Muzik O, et al. Sturge-Weber syndrome: correlation between clinical course and FDG PET findings. *Neurology* 2001; 57: 189-95.

Liquori CL, Berg MJ, Siegel, et al. Mutations in a gene encoding a novel protein containing a phosphotyrosine-binding domain cause type 2 cerebral cavernous malformations. *Am J Hum Genet* 2003; 73: 1459-64.

Maraire JN, Awad IA. Intracranial cavernous malformations: lesion behavior and management strategies. *Neurosurgery* 1995; 37: 591-605.

Marin-Padilla M. Human cerebral cortex intrinsic microvascular system: development and cytoarchitecture. In: Marin-Padilla M (ed). *The Human Brain: Prenatal Development and Structure*, pp. 85-99. Berlin Heidelberg: Springer, 2011.

Maton B, Krsek P, Jayakar P, et al. Medically intractable epilepsy in Sturge-Weber syndrome is associated with cortical malformation: implications for surgical therapy. *Epilepsia* 2010; 51: 257-67.

Matsubara S, Bourdeau A, terBrugge KG, Wallace C, Letarte M. Analysis of endoglin expression in normal brain tissue and in cerebral arteriovenous malformations. *Stroke* 2000; 31: 2653-60.

McCartney E, Squier W. Patterns and pathways of calcification in the developing brain. *Dev Med Child Neurol* 2014; 56: 1009-15.

Mirsattari SM, Steven DA, Keith J, Hammond RR. Pathophysiological implications of focal cortical dysplasia of end folium for hippocampal sclerosis. *Epilepsy Res* 2009; 84: 268-72.

Miyahara H, Ryufuku M, Fu YJ, et al. Balloon cells in the dentate gyrus in hippocampal sclerosis associated with non-herpetic acute limbic encephalitis. *Seizure* 2011; 20: 87-9.

Moran NF, Fish DR, Kitchen N, Shorvon S, Kendall BE, Stevens JM. Supratentorial cavernous haemangiomas and epilepsy: a review of the literature and case series. *J Neurol Neurosurg Psychiatry* 1999; 66: 561-8.

Morioka T, Nishio S, Ishibashi H, et al. Intrinsic epileptogenicity of focal cortical dysplasia as revealed by magnetoencephalography and electrocorticography. *Epilepsy Res* 1999; 33: 177-87.

Muhlebner A, Coras R, Kobow K, et al. Neuropathologic measurements in focal cortical dysplasias: validation of the ILAE 2011 classification system and diagnostic implications for MRI. *Acta Neuropathol* 2012; 123: 259-72.

Murakami N, Morioka T, Suzuki SO, et al. Focal cortical dysplasia type IIa underlying epileptogenesis in patients with epilepsy associated with Sturge-Weber syndrome. *Epilepsia* 2012); 53: e184-8.

Pal L, Shankar SK, Santosh V, Yasha TC. Glioneuronal migration and development disorders: histological and immunohistochemical study with a comment on evolution. *Neurology India* 2002; 50: 444-51.

Palmini A, Najm I, Avanzini G, et al. Terminology and classification of the cortical dysplasias. *Neurology* 2004; 62: S2-8.

Pedailles S, Martin N, Launay V, et al. [Sturge-Weber-Krabbe syndrome. A severe form in a monozygote female twin]. *Ann Dermatol Venereol* 1993; 120: 379-82.

Rammos SK, Maina R, Lanzino G. Developmental venous anomalies: current concepts and implications for management. *Neurosurgery* 2009; 65: 20-9; discussion 29-30.

Rasmussen T, Mathieson G, Le Blanc F. Surgical therapy of typical and a forme fruste variety of the Sturge-Weber syndrome. *Schweiz Arch Neurol Neurochir Psychiatr* 1972; 111: 393-409.

Roach ES. Neurocutaneous syndromes. *Pediatr Clin North Am* 1992; 39: 591-620.

Rollins NK, Deline C, Morriss MC. Prevalence and clinical significance of dilated Virchow-Robin spaces in childhood. *Radiology* 1993; 189: 53-7.

Rosenow F, et al. In response to commentary on cavernoma-related epilepsy: review and recommendations for management-report of the surgical task force of the ILAE commission on therapeutic strategies. *Epilepsia* 2014; 55: 466-7.

Rosenow F, et al. Cavernoma-related epilepsy: review and recommendations for management-report of the Surgical Task Force of the ILAE Commission on Therapeutic Strategies. *Epilepsia* 2013; 54: 2025-35.

Sahoo T, Johnson EW, Thomas JW, et al. Mutations in the gene encoding KRIT1, a Krev-1/rap1a binding protein, cause cerebral cavernous malformations (CCM1). *Hum Mol Genet* 1999; 8: 2325-33.

Sarnat HB, Wei XC, Flores-Sarnat L, Trevenen CL, Barlow K. Fetal opercular cavernous angioma causing cerebral cleft: contralateral primitive vascular anomaly and subicular dysgenesis. *J Child Neurol* 2012; 27: 478-84.

Scaravilli F. *Neuropathology of Epilepsy*. Singapore, New Jersey, London, Hong Kong: World ScientificPublishing Co. Pte. Ltd, 1998.

Scholz W, Jotten J. [Disorders of cerebral blood circulation in the cat following a short series of electroshock treatments]. *Arch Psychiatr Nervenkr Z Gesamte Neurol Psychiatr* 1951; 186: 264-79.

Scott RC, Gadian DG, King MD, et al. Magnetic resonance imaging findings within 5 days of status epilepticus in childhood. *Brain* 2002; 125: 1951-9.

Simasathien T, Vadera S, Najm I, Gupta A, Bingaman W, Jehi L. Improved outcomes with earlier surgery for intractable frontal lobe epilepsy. *Ann Neurol* 2013; 73: 646-54.

Simonati A, Colamaria V, Bricolo A, Bernardina BD, Rizzuto N. Microgyria associated with Sturge-Weber angiomatosis. *Child Nerv Sys* 1994; 10: 392-5.

Song CJ, Kim JH, Kier EL, Bronen RA. MR imaging and histologic features of subinsular bright spots on T2-weighted MR images: Virchow-Robin spaces of the extreme capsule and insular cortex. *Radiology* 2000; 214: 671-7.

Stefan H, Hammen T. Cavernous haemangiomas, epilepsy and treatment strategies. *Acta Neurol Scand* 2004; 110: 393-7.

Sturge WA. A case of partial epilepsy, apparently due to a lesion of one of the vasomotor centres of the brain. *Trans Clin Soc Lon* 1879; 12: 162-7.

Sure U, Freman S, Bozinov O, Benes L, Siegel AM, Bertalanffy H. Biological activity of adult cavernous malformations: a study of 56 patients. *J Neurosurg* 2005; 102: 342-7.

Thom M, Sisodiya S, Harkness W, Scaravilli F. Microdysgenesis in temporal lobe epilepsy. A quantitative and immunohistochemical study of white matter neurones. *Brain* 2001; 124: 2299-309.

Thom M, Martinian L, Caboclo LO, McEvoy AW, Sisodiya SM. Balloon cells associated with granule cell dispersion in the dentate gyrus in hippocampal sclerosis. *Acta Neuropathol* 2008; 115: 697-700.

Thomas-Sohl KA, Vaslow DF, Maria BL. Sturge-Weber syndrome: a review. *Pediatr Neurol* 2004; 30: 303-10.

Wang DD, Blümcke I, Coras R, et al. Sturge-Weber syndrome is associated with cortical dysplasia ILAE Type IIIc and excessive hypertrophic pyramidal neurons in brain resections for intractable epilepsy. *Brain Pathol* 2015; 25: 248-55.

Wang QK. Update on the molecular genetics of vascular anomalies. *Lymphat Res Biol* 2005; 3: 226-33.

Weber FP. Right-sided hemi-hypotrophy resulting from right-sided congenital spastic hemiplegia, with a morbid condition of the left side of the brain, revealed by radiograms. *J Neurol Psychopathol* 1922; 3: 134-9.

CHAPTER 7. Atlas of neuropathological lesions in epilepsy surgery

Roland Coras, Ingmar Blümcke

No hippocampal sclerosis (ILAE classification 2013)	83
Hippocampal sclerosis, ILAE Type 1	87
Hippocampal sclerosis, ILAE Type 2 (CA1-predominant neuronal loss)	89
Hippocampal sclerosis, ILAE Type 3 (CA4 predominant neuronal loss)	91
Mild malformation of cortical development (mMCD)	93
Focal cortical dysplasia ILAE Type Ia	95
Focal cortical dysplasia ILAE Type Ib	97
Focal cortical dysplasia ILAE Type Ic	98
Focal cortical dysplasia ILAE Type IIa	100
Focal cortical dysplasia ILAE Type IIb	102
Focal cortical dysplasia ILAE Type IIIa	104
Focal cortical dysplasia ILAE Type IIIb	105
Focal cortical dysplasia ILAE Type IIIc	106
Focal cortical dysplasia ILAE Type IIId	107
Cortical tuber (genetically confirmed TSC)	109
Hemimegalencephaly (HME)	111
Polymicrogyria (PMG) and nodular heterotopia	113
Ganglioglioma (WHO I°)	115
Anaplastic ganglioglioma (WHO III°)	118
Dysembryoplastic neuroepithelial tumour (WHO I°)	119
Dysembryoplastic neuroepithelial tumour (WHO I°)/variant	121
Pilocytic astrocytoma (WHO I°)	123
Isomorphic astrocytoma variant (analogue WHO I°)	125
Angiocentric glioma (WHO I°)	127
Pleomorphic xanthoastrocytoma (WHO II°)	129
Papillary glio-neuronal tumour (WHO I°)	131
Multinodular and vacuolating neuronal tumour (analogue WHO I°)	133
Rasmussen encephalitis	135
Limbic encephalitis	139
Arterio-venous malformation (AVM)	140
Cavernous haemangioma (CAV)	142
Sturge-Weber syndrome (SWS)	144

Abbreviations

AED: antiepileptic drugs
CBZ: carbamazepine
DNT: dysembryoplastic neuroepithelial tumour
EEG: electroencephalography
ESL: eslicarbazepine
FCD: focal cortical dysplasia
LEV: levetiracetam

LTG: lamotrigine
OXC: oxcarbazepine
PHT: phenytoin
TPM: topiramate
TSC: tuberous sclerosis complex
VNS: vagal nerve stimulator
VPA: valproic acid

No hippocampal sclerosis (ILAE classification 2013)

Clinical history

22-year old male patient with Sturge-Weber syndrome. Seizure onset reported at age 9 years. Drug resistant for multiple AED trials, last medication included LEV and LTG. Previous VNS implantation also failed to control his seizures. 1st operation at age 21 years with diagnosis of meningoangiomatosis. Patient was not seizure free and received 2nd operation at age 22 including right mesio-temporal lobe structures. There was no sign for hippocampal atrophy (*Figure 1A*: T2 weighted turbo spin echo MRI) although EEG examination suggested mesial temporal structures to be involved.

Histopathology and immunohistochemistry

We received en bloc resected hippocampal tissue (2.4 × 2 × 1.4 cm; *Figure 1B*). Hippocampal head with its characteristic digitations as well as the midbody could be identified and were dissected perpendicular to the anterior-posterior axis (arrow in

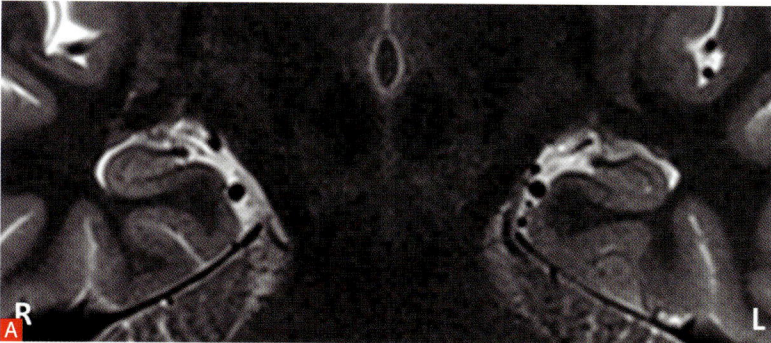
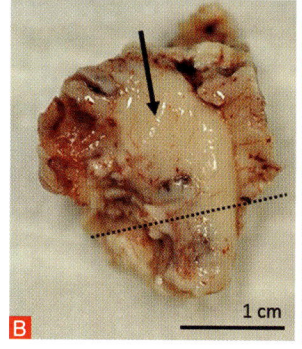
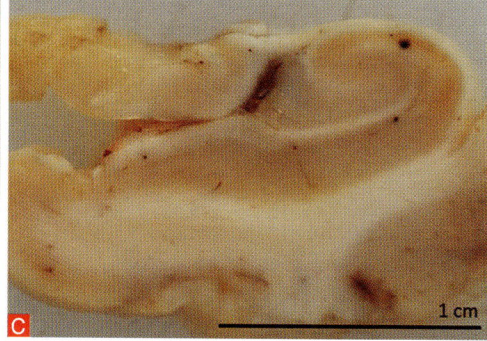

Figure 1

B). Representative samples were fixed in formalin and embedded into paraffin (C: slice through the anterior midbody of the hippocampus as indicated by dotted line in B). One unfixed section was snap frozen in liquid nitrogen for long-term storage at - 80° C.

H&E staining revealed a well preserved hippocampal anatomy with all pyramidal cell layers developed (*Figure 2*). No evidence for segmental neuronal cell loss (see NeuN and GFAP immunohistochemistry). The dentate gyrus also revealed its characteristic densely-packed granule cell layer without signs of cellular loss or dispersion. NeuN immunoreactivity is always recommended to approve lack of segmental cell loss (Wolf *et al.*, 1996). GFAP staining showed reactive "cellular" gliosis only, no dense fibrillary gliosis or "sclerosis".

Comments

Histopathological examination revealed an anatomically well preserved human hippocampus without evidence for segmental neuronal cell loss, tumour or acute/chronic inflammation. Cell density measurements of NeuN immunohistochemistry were consistent with the diagnosis of no-HS (gliosis only), according to the new ILAE classification of HS (Blümcke *et al.*, 2013). No remnants of leptomeningeal angiomatosis were observed.

Microscopic findings in no-HS

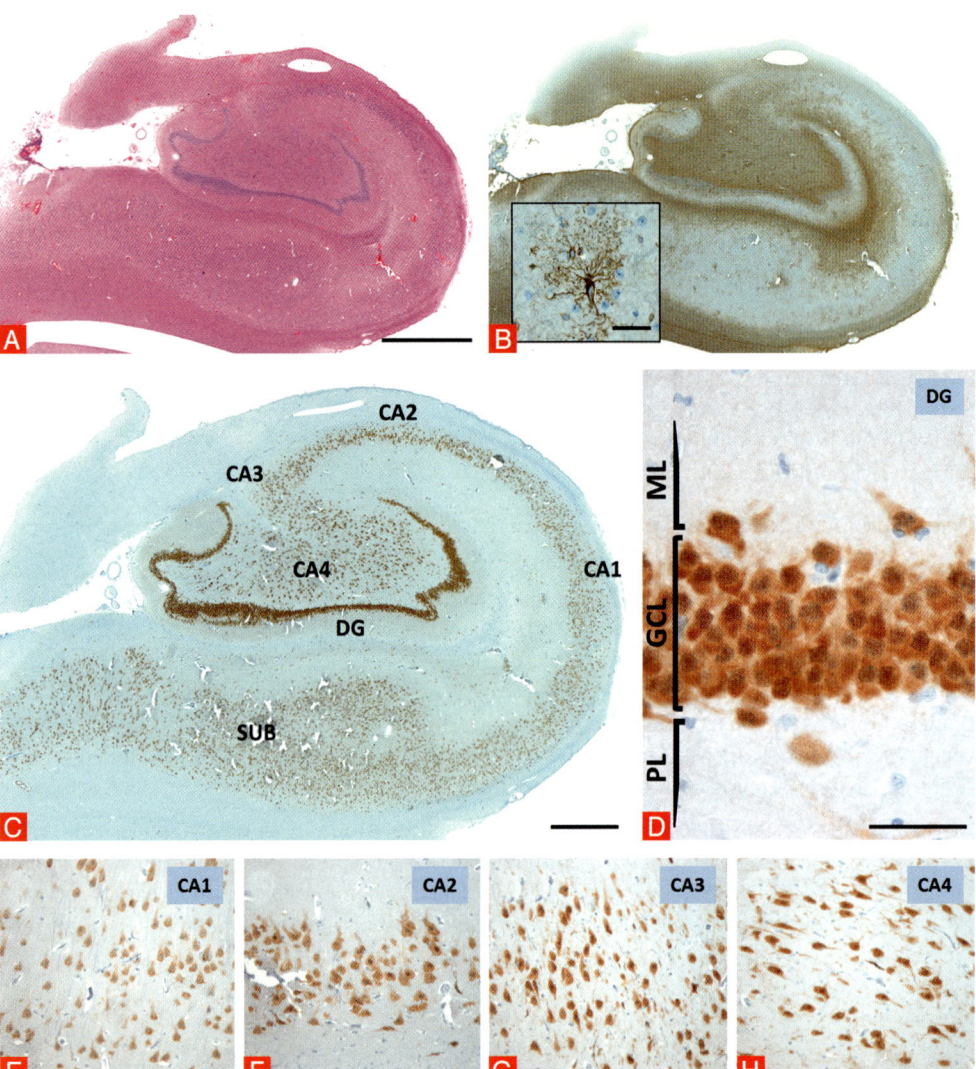

Figure 2

A. H&E staining of the hippocampus. **B.** GFAP immunohistochemistry of the hippocampus. Inset in B: reactive "cellular" gliosis, no sclerosis. **C.** NeuN immunohistochemistry of the hippocampus highlighting the subiculum (SUB), the sectors of the cornu ammonis (CA1-CA4) and the dentate gyrus (DG) without evidence for segmental cell loss. **D.** Higher magnification of the dentate gyrus. Regular package density of the granule cell layer (GCL) without signs of granule cell loss or dispersion. ML: molecular layer of DG. PL: polymorphic layer of DG. **E-H.** Higher magnification of the cornu ammonis sectors with regular pyramidal cell densities. Scale bar in A: 2,000 µm, applies also for B. Scale bar in B (inset): 50 µm. Scale bar in C: 1,000 µm. Scale bar in D: 50 µm. Scale bar in E: 100 µm, applies also for F-H.

Hippocampal anatomy

The anatomy of the human hippocampus has a long and controversial history since its first description by Julius Caesar Arantius in 1587, who was a pupil of the Italian anatomist Andreas Vesalius (Lewis, 1923). Arantius compared the anatomical elevations within the inferior horn of the lateral ventricles with that of a seahorse (Hippocampus), with the animal's head pointing either to the third ventricle or the anterior part of the temporal lobe. De Garengoet compared the mesial view of the hippocampus with the Ammon's horn adopted from the Egyptian god Ammun Kneph (Lewis, 1923; Walther, 2002) and introduced this term in 1742. At present, it is the pyramidal cell layer of the hippocampal subregions that is microscopically recognized as cornu ammonis (CA areas). The anatomical classification of hippocampal subfields is somewhat contradictory with many classification systems available. This may also result from differences between rodent and human hippocampus. The classification introduced by Lorente de Nó in 1933 (Lorente de Nó, 1933) is mostly used designating four hippocampal sectors, namely CA1 to CA4. The transition areas between CA1 and subiculum or between the CA3-CA4 regions remain, however, difficult to clarify using routine staining techniques.

Anatomy of the human hippocampus

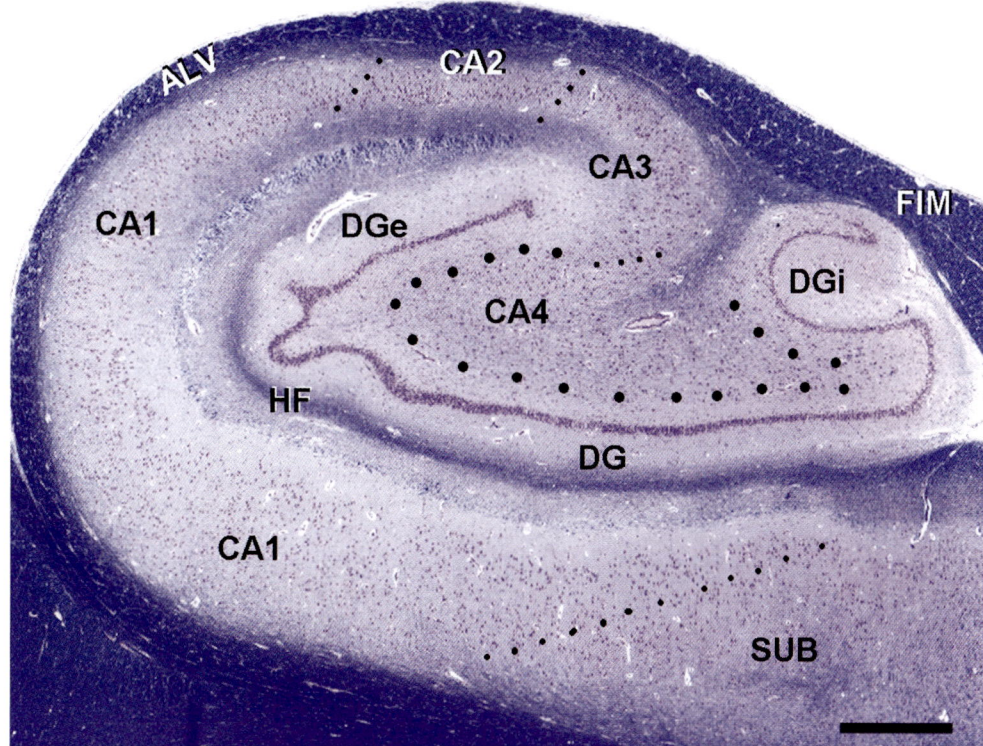

Figure 3

Cresyl violet and luxol fast blue staining of a post-mortem human hippocampus illustrating the ILAE classification use of terminology: SUB: subiculum; CA1-CA4: sectors of the cornu ammonis; DG: dentate gyrus with external (DGe) and internal limbs (DGi); HF: remnant of hippocampal fissure; ALV: alveus; FIM: fimbria. Dotted lines circumscribe anatomical boundaries between CA sectors, and cell quantification should be always performed at the centre of these regions. Scale bar: 1,000 μm.

The hippocampus is a main constituent of the allocortex (Braak, 1980). It is situated in the mesial temporal lobe and occupies the floor of the inferior horn of the lateral ventricle from the level of the corpus amygdaloideum up to the splenium of the corpus callosum. Three major parts can be distinguished: the dentate gyrus (or fascia dentata), the cornu ammonis (Ammon's horn) and the subiculum. The dentate gyrus consists of three laminae: the molecular layer, the granular layer, and an ill-defined plexiform layer. Small nerve cells usually referred to as "granule cells" dominate in the dentate gyrus. The perikarya of granule cells assemble tightly together and form a clear-cut band. The basal tip of the soma shows a distinct axon hillock from which a relatively thick axon is generated which enters the cornu ammonis and forms synaptic contacts with the pyramids of the third and the fourth sector (mossy fibre system). Apical dendrites ramify within the molecular layer and receive topographically restricted efferents from the collateral hippocampus and ipsilateral tractus perforans. The granule cell layer is functionally regarded as "gate keeper" of the hippocampus, as it receives the majority of axonal input. The cornu ammonis displays three laminae on cross-sections: the molecular layer, the pyramidal cell layer and the stratum oriens. The inner surface of the dentate gyrus, within the hilus, is the polymorphic layer that consists of undifferentiated bipolar progenitor cells (i.e. resident "stem cells"), one of two permanent repositories of cells capable of neurogenesis in the mature brain. The other reservoir is the olfactory bulb.

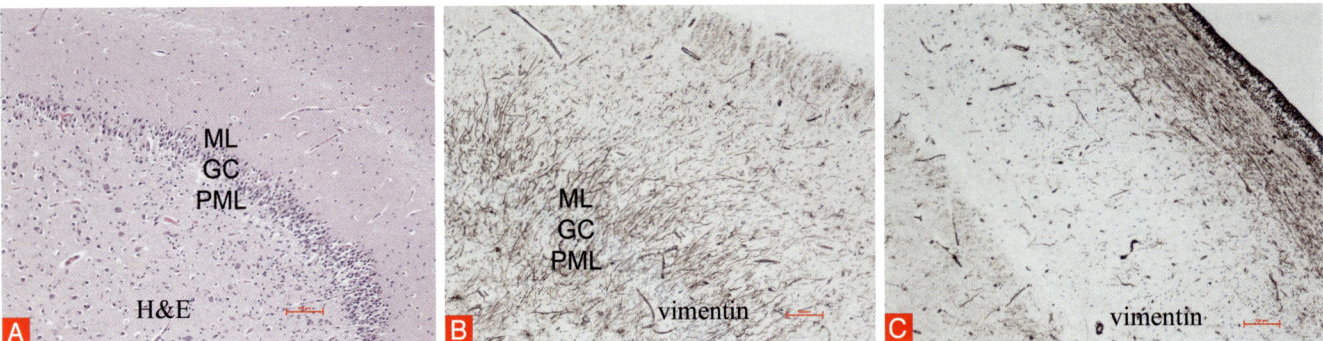

Figure 4

Normal hippocampus of an 8-day-old term male neonate. The polymorphic zone (PML) is a band beneath the inner surface of the dentate gyrus which contains resident progenitor cells that **(A)** are scattered indistinctive small cells and a few scattered large neurones of CA4, as seen with H&E stain, but **(B)** are clearly defined by vimentin immunocytochemistry as bipolar cells with long thin processes extending through the dentate gyrus into its molecular zone. Nestin (not shown) is an alternative immunoreactivity for demonstrating these cells. **(C)** Vimentin-reactive progenitor cells are rare in the cornu ammonis, but long progenitor cell processes are mixed in parallel with axons within the subependymal alveus leading to the fimbria. Vimentin also normally is strongly reactive within endothelial cells at all ages and with ependymocytes, though ependymal reactivity disappears with maturation. The polymorphic layer of progenitor cells appears very similar to this neonate in foetuses as young as 10 weeks, throughout foetal life and childhood, and into late middle-age in adults.

Hippocampal sclerosis, ILAE Type 1

Clinical history
57-year old, left-handed female patient suffering from auto-motor seizures for 35 years. Drug resistant for multiple AED trials, last medication included CBZ, LEV and ESL. MRI revealed left-sided hippocampal atrophy (*Figure 5A*: T2 weighted turbo spin echo MRI; white arrow) with increased signal intensity.

Histopathology and immunohistochemistry
We received en bloc resected hippocampal tissue (2.6 × 1.9 × 1.4 cm). Hippocampal head and mid-body could be identified (*Figure 5B*) and were dissected perpendicular to the anterior-posterior axis. Representative samples (*Figure 5C*) were fixed in formalin and embedded into paraffin. H&E staining revealed well-preserved hippocampal anatomy with severe neuronal loss in sectors CA1, CA3 and CA4 (*Figure 6*). NeuN immunohistochemistry (Wolf *et al.*, 1996) and semi-quantitative cell density measurements detected pyramidal cell loss also in CA2. All areas with severe neuronal loss showed fibrillary gliosis (GFAP). The granule cell layer contained areas of severe granule cell depletion (in both external and internal limbs) and also granule cell dispersion.

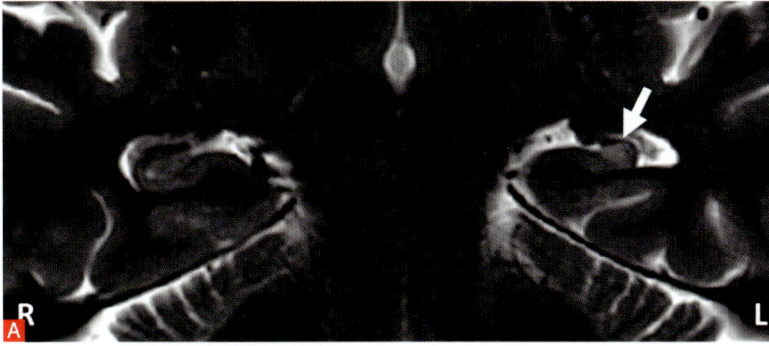
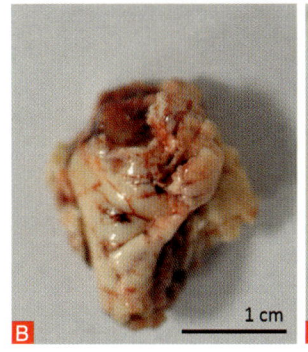
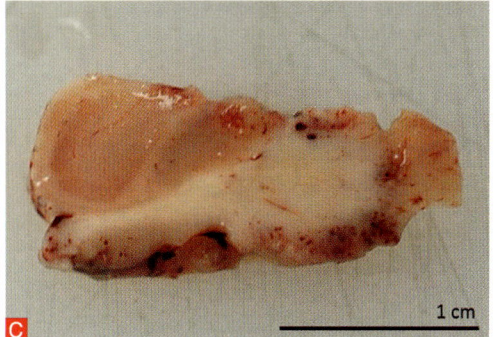

Figure 5

Comments
Neuropathological examination revealed a characteristic pattern of segmental pyramidal cell loss and fibrillary gliosis in the hippocampus consistent with the diagnosis of HS ILAE Type 1 (Blümcke *et al.*, 2013). The dentate gyrus showed severe granule cell depletion and granule cell dispersion. Neither tumour nor acute inflammation was evident.

Microscopic findings in HS ILAE Type 1

Figure 6

A. Severe pyramidal cell loss along the cornu ammonis sectors, already well visible on H&E staining. **B.** GFAP immunohistochemistry highlighting sclerotic sectors CA1-CA4. Inset in B: abundant "fibrillary" gliosis (sclerosis) on higher magnification exemplified from sector CA1. **C.** NeuN immunohistochemistry evidencing neuronal cell loss in sectors CA1-CA4. **D & E.** Higher magnification of the dentate gyrus with areas of severe granule cell depletion (in both external and internal limbs) (D) and focally also of granule cell dispersion (E). **F-I.** Higher magnification of the cornu ammonis sectors with severe pyramidal cell loss in all sectors (CA1, CA3 and CA4 more severe than CA2). Scale bar in A: 1,000 µm, applies also for B. Scale bar in B (inset): 50 µm. Scale bar in C: 1,000 µm. Scale bar in D: 50 µm, applies also for E. Scale bar in F: 100 µm, applies also for G-I.

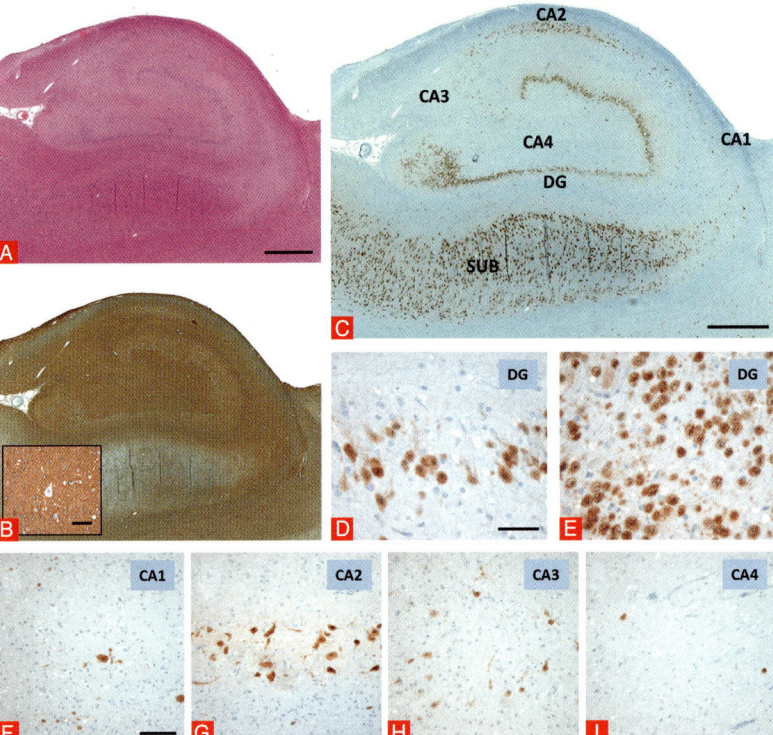

Hippocampal sclerosis, ILAE Type 2 (CA1-predominant neuronal loss)

Clinical history

56-year old female patient with right-sided temporal lobe epilepsy since age 8 years. She suffered from many epigastric auras and auto-motor seizures and also experienced a generalized tonic-clonic seizure. Repeated MRI at 3T revealed no hippocampal abnormality (*Figure 7A*: T2 weighted turbo-spin-echo MRI; white arrow). Neuropsychological examination disclosed no cognitive dysfunction of the right hemisphere. At time of surgery, she was trialed on LEV.

Histopathology and immunohistochemistry

We received en bloc resected hippocampal tissue (3 × 2.2 × 1 cm, *Figure 7B*). The specimen was dissected perpendicular to the anterior-posterior axis into six 5 mm thin sections (*Figure 7C*). All samples were fixed in formalin and embedded into paraffin. H&E staining revealed a well preserved hippocampal anatomy with severe neuronal loss predominately in sector CA1, whereas CA2, CA3 and CA4 remained preserved (*Figure 8*). CA1 showed concomitant fibrillary gliosis (GFAP). The granule cell layer showed a few areas of granule cell dispersion.

Comments

Neuropathological examination revealed a predominant pattern of segmental pyramidal cell loss and fibrillary gliosis in the hippocampal CA1 area consistent with the diagnosis of HS ILAE Type 2 (Blümcke *et al.*, 2013). The dentate gyrus showed no granule cell depletion but foci of granule cell dispersion. No evidence for tumour or acute inflammation was seen.

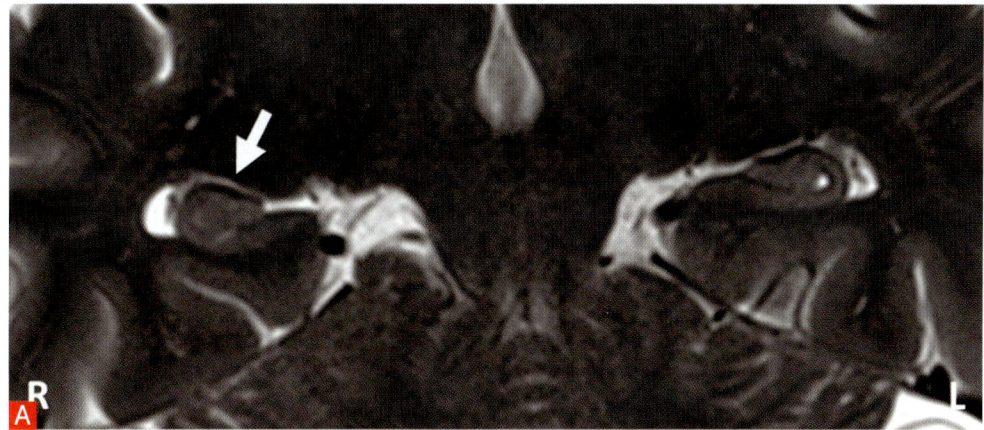
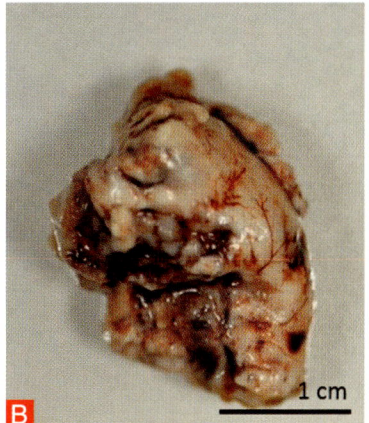
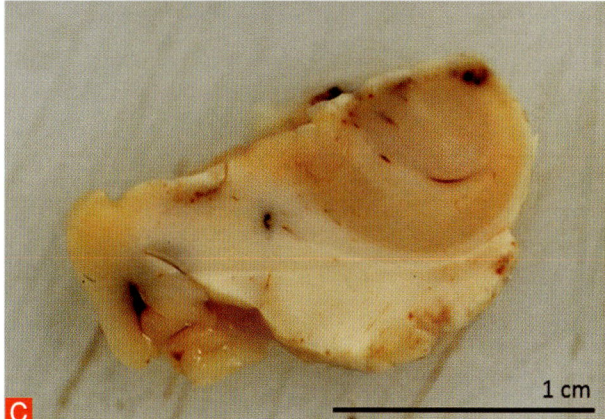

Figure 7

Microscopic findings in HS ILAE Type 2

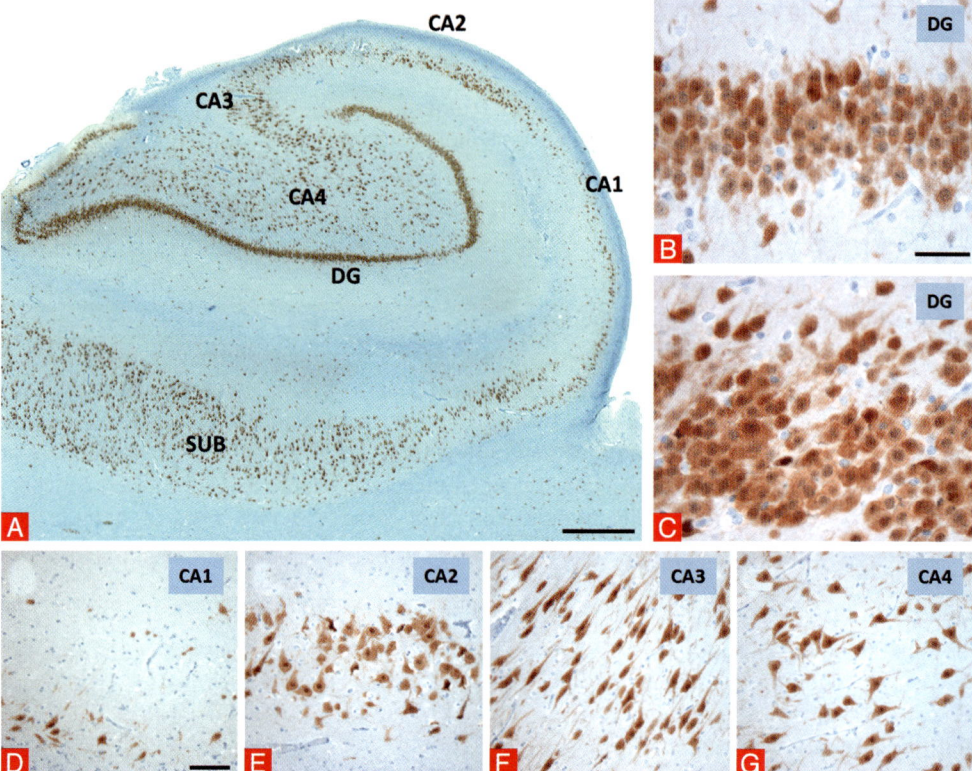

Figure 8

A. Segmental pyramidal cell loss predominantly affecting sector CA1. B & C. The granule cell layer mostly has a normal granule cell density (B), with a few areas of granule cell dispersion (C). D-G. severe neuronal loss predominately in sector CA1, whereas CA2, CA3 and CA4 are preserved. A-G: NeuN immunohistochemistry. Scale bar in A: 1,000 μm. Scale bar in B: 50 μm, applies also for C. Scale bar in D: 100 μm, applies also to E-G.

Hippocampal sclerosis, ILAE Type 3 (CA4 predominant neuronal loss)

Clinical history

10-year old girl with left temporal lobe epilepsy since the age of one year and previous operation of a DNT at another hospital.

Histopathology and immunohistochemistry

We received en bloc resected and formalin fixed hippocampal tissue (1.5 × 1.5 × 0.6 cm). The specimen was dissected at 5 mm thickness along the coronar plane and embedded into paraffin. H&E staining revealed a tumour with moderate cellularity infiltrating the entorhinal cortex and subiculum. The tumour is not displayed here and was predominately composed of glial cells showing small round or ovoid nuclei and eosinophilic cytoplasm with ramifying processes. No mitotic figures were demonstrated. Within the glial tumour matrix, there were dysplastic ganglion cells. Small infiltrating clusters of tumour cells could be identified also in the hippocampus proper. There were decreased pyramidal cell densities in sectors CA1 and CA2, whereas CA3 and CA4 were almost depleted of pyramidal cells (*Figure 9*). Granule cell loss also could be identified in the dentate gyrus, which showed bi-laminated architecture in addition (*Figure 9C*).

NeuN confirmed a slight decrease in neuronal cell density in CA1 and CA2, as well as subtotal pyramidal cell depletion in CA3 and CA4.

Comments

This case presented with dual pathology, *i.e.* hippocampal sclerosis and a CD34 immunoreactive ganglioglioma (WHO I°). The tumour was located outside the hippocampus proper, but showed already infiltrating cell clusters (visible using CD34 immunoreactivity, not shown here). Although pyramidal cell densities were reduced in all segments of the hippocampus, they were most pronounced in CA3 and CA4. We have neither interpreted neuronal cell depletion in CA3 and CA4, nor granule cell dispersion, as result from tumour infiltration, and we classified this atypical pattern of hippocampal sclerosis according to the ILAE system as HS Type 3 (Blümcke *et al.*, 2013). Due to the missmatch of tumour diagnosis, we were asked to review the histopathological specimens obtained from the first operation and could not identify any DNT-specific cellular architecture (*i.e.* specific glio-neuronal element or multinodular growth pattern).

Microscopic findings in HS ILAE Type 3

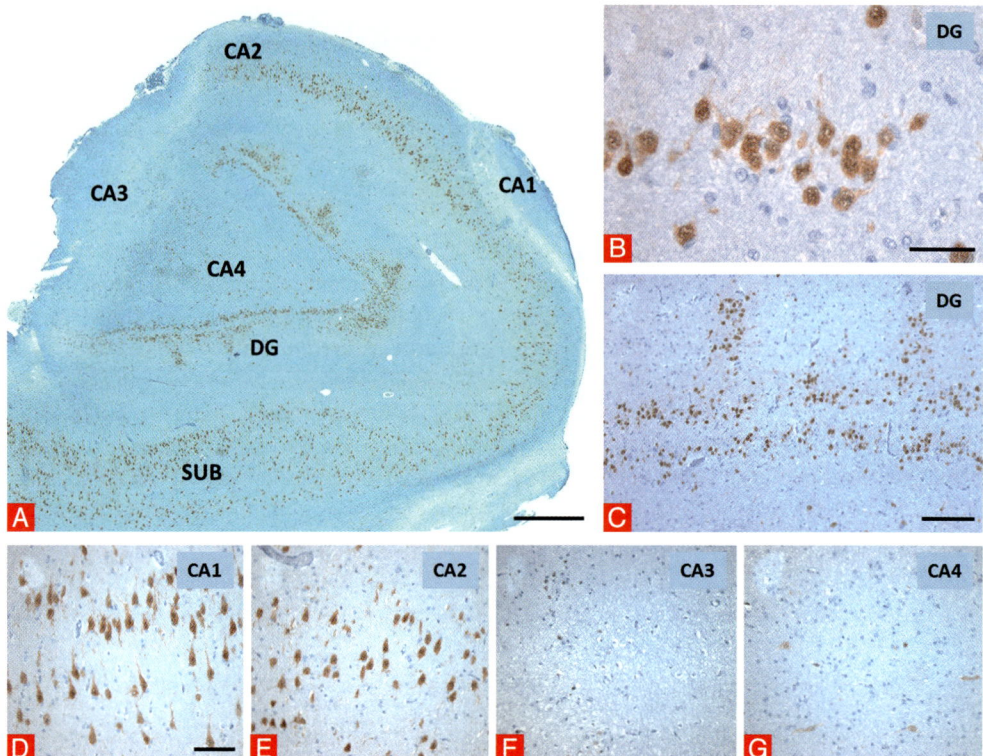

Figure 9

A. Slightly decreased pyramidal cell densities in sectors CA1 and CA2, whereas CA3 and CA4 are almost depleted of pyramidal cells. **B & C.** The granule cell layer with severe cellular loss (B), and also with a bi-laminated architecture and heterotopic clusters in circumscribed areas (C). **D–G.** Slight decrease in neuronal cell density in CA1 and CA2, as well as subtotal pyramidal cell depletion in CA3 and CA4. A–G: NeuN immunohistochemistry. Scale bar in A: 1,000 μm. Scale bar in B: 50 μm. Scale bar in C: 200 μm. Scale bar in D: 100 μm, applies also for E–G.

Mild malformation of cortical development (mMCD)

Clinical history

14-year old female patient with medically refractory temporal lobe epilepsy and clinically suspected temporo-basal/mesial focal cortical dysplasia (FCD).

Histopathology and immunohistochemistry

We received three surgical specimens labelled as temporal lobe (I: 4.8 × 2.8 × 1.5 cm), amygdala (II: 1.8 × 1.2 × 1 cm) and hippocampus (III: 1.7 × 1.5 × 1 cm). On display is fraction I, from which 4 sections were embedded in paraffin. H&E staining revealed neocortex and white matter in normal anatomical configuration. The cortical ribbon presented with its characteristic six-layered architecture and no frank signs for horizontal or vertical dyslamination. There were no dysmorphic neurones or balloon cells visible. Several areas showed prominent blurring of the grey/white matter boundary and increased numbers of heterotopic neurones (*Figure 10*) in subcortical as well as deep areas of white matter (the latter is defined as > 500 µm away from grey/white matter boundary). White matter showed normal myelination on Nissl-LFB stainings. NeuN and MAP2 immunohistochemistry was used to better demonstrate areas with blurring of grey/white matter boundary and abundance of heterotopic neurones in the white matter (more than 20 neurones per high power field). Immunoreactivity for neurofilament protein (SMI32) did not highlight dysmorphic neurones. Immunohistochemistry for GFAP revealed reactive gliosis in both, neocortex and white matter.

Comments

Microscopic inspection revealed cortical grey and subcortical white matter with blurred boundaries and increased numbers of heterotopic neurones in white matter. There were no frank signs for horizontal or vertical cortical dyslamination, *i.e.* **no** FCD Type I. Furthermore, no dysmorphic neurones or balloon cells could be demonstrated by appropriate immunohistochemistry, *i.e.* **no** FCD Type II. This specimen is, therefore, difficult to further classify. Presence of individual hypertrophic neurones may be seen, but should be regarded with caution in an otherwise normal six-layered neocortex. Such finding can often be recognized in chronic epilepsy tissue, as well as normal brain, and do not automatically qualify for the diagnosis of FCD. Areas of blurred grey/white matter boundaries are another frequent finding in epileptic neocortex (Muhlebner *et al.*, 2012). It occurs physiologically at the crowns of gyri and should be determined only at intermediate zones or bottom of sulcus (also see *chapter 3; Figure 6*). In absence of any other pathological findings, we classify this pattern as mild malformation of cortical development (mMCD Type II according to Palmini's and ILAE's FCD classification system; (Blümcke *et al.*, 2011, Palmini *et al.*, 2004). The hippocampus did not show any segmental neuronal cell loss and was classified as ILAE no-HS (not shown here).

Microscopic findings in mMCD Type II

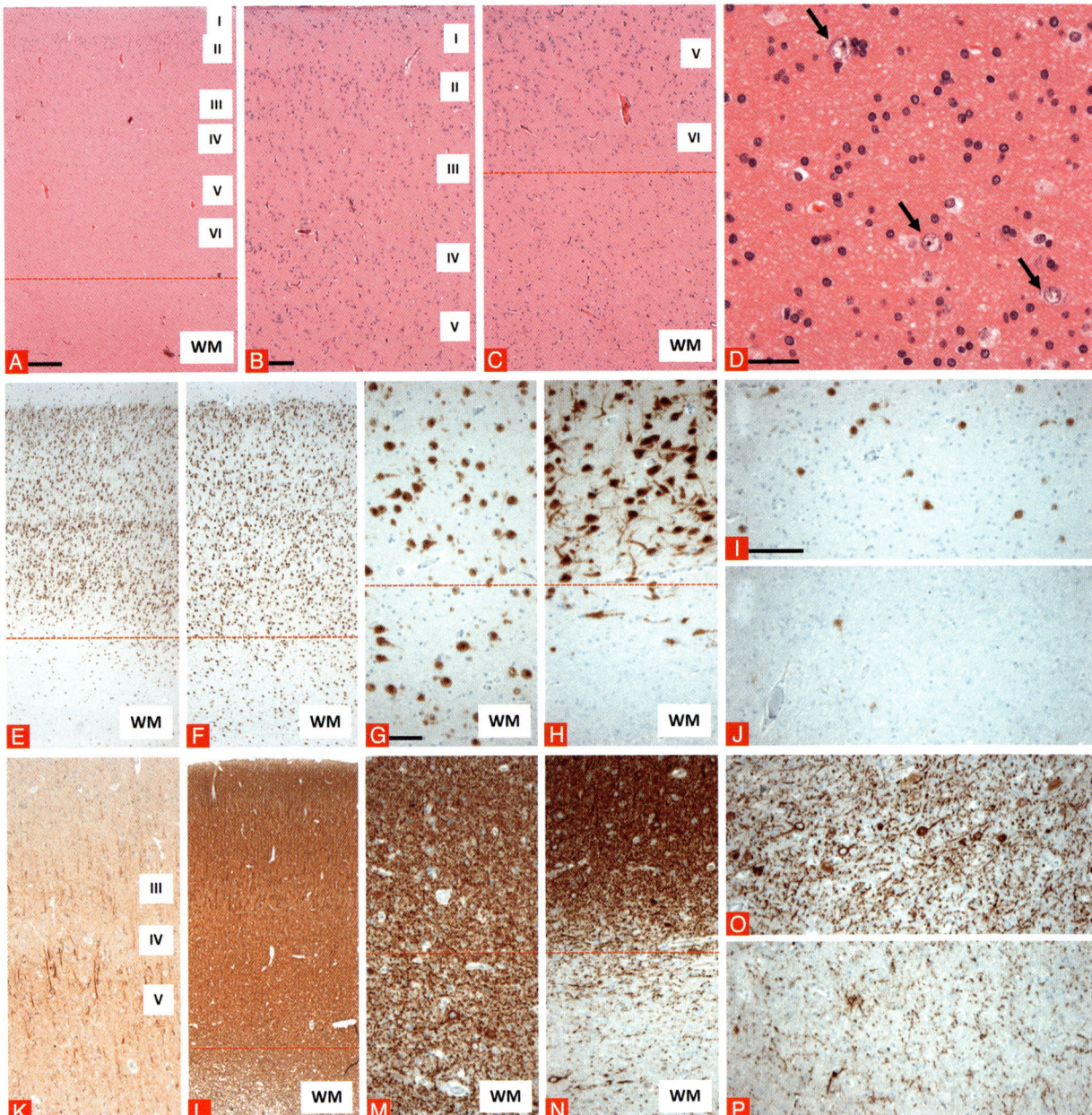

Figure 10

A-B. H&E staining showing a regular architecture of the cortical ribbon, confirmed at higher magnification in B. **C-D.** The grey/white matter boundary is blurred and increased numbers of heterotopic neurones can be detected also in deep white matter areas (D, arrows). **E & K.** NeuN (E) and neurofilament SMI32 (K) immunohistochemistry demonstrates a normal six-layered neocortex with intact grey/white matter boundary (as indicated by dotted red line). Note that SMI32 can also be used as marker for cortical layering. It labels large pyramidal cells in layers III and V when normal order of layers is fully established. **F & L.** In this cortical region, the grey/white matter boundary is severely blurred as visualized by NeuN (F) and MAP2 (L) immunohistochemistry. **G-H & M-N.** blurred grey/white matter boundary at higher objective magnification compared to normal cortex. Dotted red lines always indicate grey/white matter boundary. **G & M.** no frank signs for a boundary between grey and white matter can be demonstrated using either NeuN (G) or MAP2 (M) immunohistochemistry, compared to normal neocortex (H: NeuN; N: MAP2). **I-P.** Increased numbers of heterotopic neurones observed in deep areas or white matter (I: NeuN; O: MAP2), compared to their rare presence in normal brain (J: NeuN; P: MAP2). Scale bar in A: 500 µm, applies also for E, F & L. Scale bar in B: 200 µm, applies also for C & K. Scale bar in D: 50 µm. Scale bar in G: 100 µm, applies also for H, M & N. Scale bar in I: 100 µm, applies also for J, O & P.

Focal cortical dysplasia ILAE Type Ia

Clinical history

3-year old boy with chronic focal epilepsy originating from the left temporo-occipital lobes. Epilepsy onset was at the age of 1 year. Imaging revealed volume reduction (predominantly white matter) of the temporo-occipital lobes without sharp delineation of the grey/white matter boundaries, and subtle increased signals on T2 (*Figure 11A & B*) and FLAIR (*Figure 11C*) images.

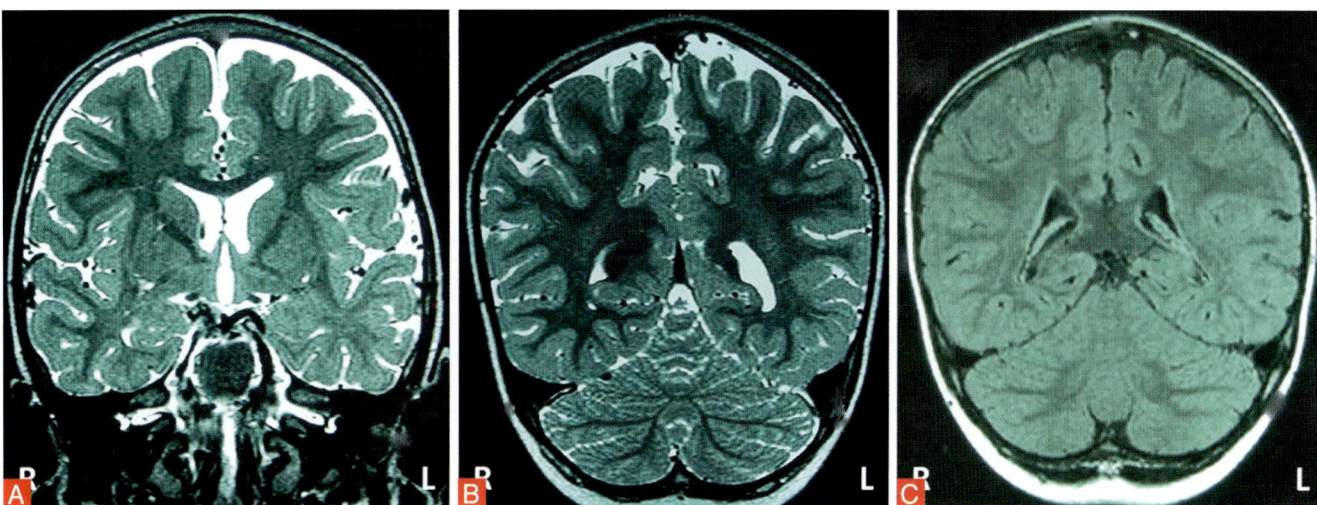

Figure 11

Histopathology and immunohistochemistry

We received three different surgical specimens labelled as temporal lobe (I: 4.5 × 4 × 2 cm), hippocampus (II: 1.5 × 1 × 0.8 cm), occipital lobe (III: 8 × 5.5 × 3.5 cm). On display is specimen III, from which 10 sections were embedded in paraffin. H&E staining revealed neocortex and white matter with architectural dysplasia and abundant vertical organization of pyramidal cells (micro-columns; *Figure 12A-D*). Cortical layers III and IV could not always be identified in affected areas. In addition, neuronal cell clusters could be envisaged. The grey/white matter boundaries were not always well demarcated or were blurred, with abundant heterotopic neurones in white matter (Muhlebner *et al.*, 2012). The latter showed normal myelination with Nissl-LFB staining. Hypertrophic or dysmorphic neurones were not visible. NeuN immunohistochemistry was most helpful in confirming a predominantly micro-columnar arrangement of the neocortex (Hildebrandt *et al.*, 2005). MAP2 demonstrated blurring of grey/white matter boundaries and abundant heterotopic neurones. Immunoreactivity for neurofilament-protein (SMI32) excluded hypertrophic or dysmorphic neurones. Immunohistochemistry for GFAP revealed irregular patterns of reactive gliosis within the neocortex and white matter.

Comments

The most characteristic finding in these large surgical specimens showed a FCD with predominant vertical or radial (micro-columnar) architecture of the neocortex. This pattern is classified as FCD ILAE Type Ia (Blümcke *et al.*, 2011) and was more prominent in parieto-occipital than in temporal lobe (not shown here). The hippocampus did not show any segmental neuronal loss and was classified as "no-HS" (not shown here).

Microscopic findings in FCD ILAE Type Ia

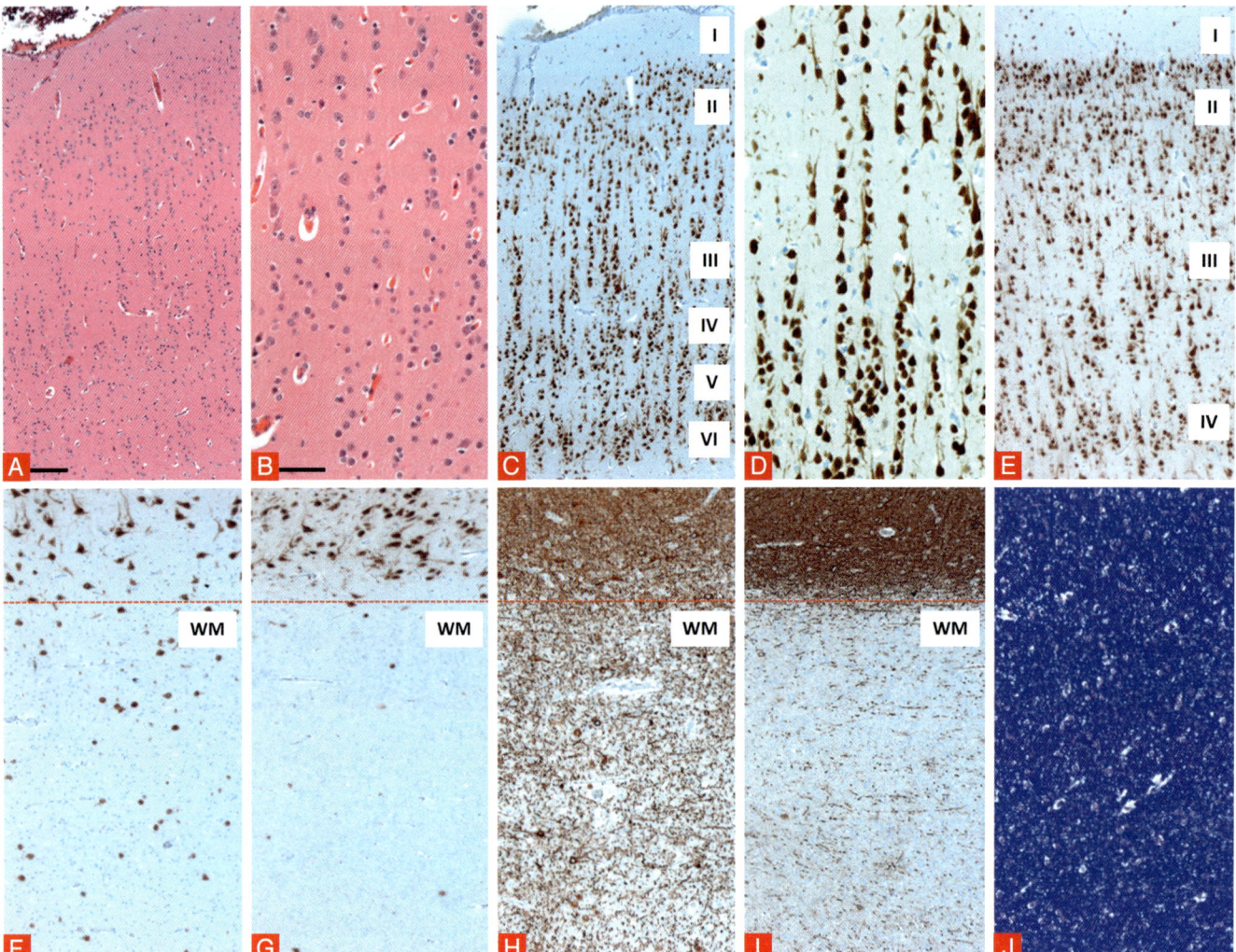

Figure 12

A & B. H&E staining with a prominent radial organization of pyramidal cells. **C–E.** NeuN immunohistochemistry showing abundant micro-columnar arrangement of the neocortex (higher magnification in D) and overall thinning of the cortical ribbon (C) compared with regular cortical architecture (E). **F & I.** Blurring of grey/white matter boundaries with abundant heterotopic neurones within deeper white matter regions (F: NeuN immunohistochemistry; H: MAP2 immunohistochemistry) compared to regular grey/white matter junctions in corresponding immunohistochemical stainings in G (NeuN) and I (MAP2). **J.** No hypo- or dys-myelination in deep cortical areas (Nissl–LFB staining). Dotted red line in F–I: grey/white matter boundaries. I–IV: cortical layers. WM: white matter. Scale bar in A: 200 μm, applies also for C and E. Scale bar in B: 100 μm, applies also for D and F–G.

Focal cortical dysplasia ILAE Type Ib

Clinical history

23-year old male patient with clinically and radiologically suspected mesial temporal sclerosis.

Histopathology and immunohistochemistry

We received formalin-fixed fragments of white to light-brownish tissue with a total size of 7 × 5 × 1.5 cm. Representative material was embedded into 10 paraffin blocks.

1-5: Temporal neocortex: Microscopic inspection revealed central nervous tissue. Large neocortical areas showed a six-layered architecture. There were foci of tangential cortical dyslamination with a thinned cortical ribbon (*Figure 13*). Here, neuronal loss with a maximum of four visible layers. The grey/white matter boundaries were almost sharp. No dysmorphic or hypertrophic neurones were visible.

6-10: Hippocampus (not on display). Microscopic inspection revealed well preserved hippocampal tissue. The pyramidal cell layer showed no segmental neuronal loss. There was a regular configuration of the granule cell layer without granule cell loss or granule cell dispersion.

NeuN and MAP2- immunoreactivities highlighted the focally thinned cortical ribbon with neuronal cell reduction. There were numerous reactive astrocytes within the cortex (GFAP). No hypertrophic or dysmorphic neurones with intra-cytoplasmatic neurofilament-protein accumulation (SMI32). NeuN immunoreactivity showed no segmental cell loss within the hippocampal formation (not on display).

Comments

Microscopic inspection revealed central nervous tissue originating from the temporal cortex and the hippocampal formation. The temporal neocortex has foci of tangential cortical dyslamination and a thinned cortical ribbon. Here, neuronal cell loss with a maximum of four visible layers. The grey/white matter boundaries were sharp. No dysmorphic or hypertrophic neurones visible. In summary, these changes are consistent with a FCD Type Ib (ILAE classification 2011; Blümcke et al., 2011). Microscopic inspection of the hippocampal tissue revealed a regular configuration of the pyramidal and granule cell layer without significant segmental cell loss. Focally, there was gliosis within CA4 but no clues for hippocampal sclerosis. No signs of an inflammatory process or tumour.

Microscopic findings in FCD ILAE Type Ib

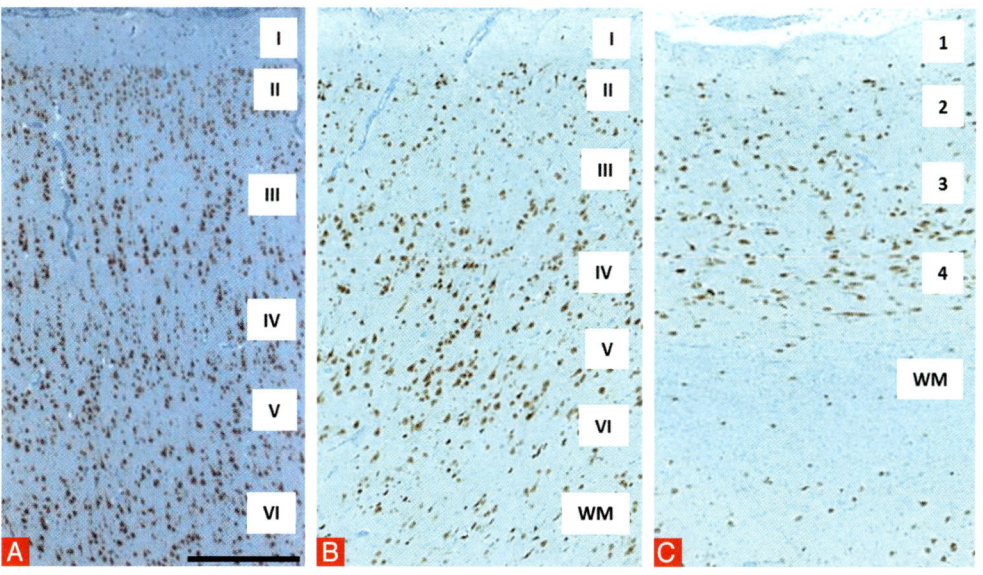

Figure 13

A. Regular six-layered cortical ribbon for comparison with findings in FCD ILAE Type Ib (B and C). Of note A-C are of same magnification. B. Six-layered cortex with patchy neuronal cell loss within the supra- and infra-granular layers as well as blurred grey/white matter boundaries. C. Area with severely thinned cortical ribbon with only four visible layers (1-4). A-C: NeuN immunohistochemistry. I-IV: cortical layers. WM: white matter. Scale bar in A: 500 μm, applies also to B and C.

Focal cortical dysplasia ILAE Type Ic

Clinical history

24-year old woman with focal refractory epilepsy. Epilepsy onset was at the age of 8 years with daily complex partial seizures and monthly generalized tonic-clonic seizures that have evolved over the last years. MRI did not reveal any lesions. PET showed extensive hypo-metabolism over the right temporal lobe and the right occipito-temporal junction. A right temporal lobectomy, including temporo-occipital areas was performed.

Histopathology and immunohistochemistry

We received two different surgical specimens labelled as temporal lobe (I: 7.5 × 5 × 2 cm) and temporo-occipital lobe (II: 4 × 1.7 × 1.5 cm). Specimen II is illustrated, from which three sections were embedded in paraffin.

H&E staining revealed cortical grey and subcortical white matter with alterations of the cortical ribbon. On the one hand, there were areas with a vertical dyslamination and micro-columnar arrangement of neurones (*Figure 14C & D*). Other areas were characterized by horizontal abnormalities of the cortical ribbon and patchy neuronal loss, both in supra- as well in infra-granular layers, focally also with thinning of the neocortex (*Figure 14B*). In addition, blurring of grey/white-matter boundaries with increased numbers of heterotopic neurones within the white matter were demonstrated. NeuN and MAP2 immunohistochemistry were most helpful to confirm the horizontal and vertical dyslamination of the cortical ribbon. Hypertrophic or dysmorphic neurones with intra-cytoplasmatic accumulation of neurofilament-protein were not present (SMI32). GFAP immunohistochemistry showed alternating degrees of reactive gliosis in neocortical and subcortical areas.

Comments

Microscopic inspection revealed in both fractions central nervous tissue with a prominent cortical dyslamination. There were areas with vertical dyslamination as well as regions with a horizontal disturbance of cortical architecture with blurring of the grey/white-matter boundaries and heterotopic neurones within the subjacent white matter. In summary, these changes were classified as FCD Type Ic (ILAE classification 2011; (Blümcke *et al.*, 2011)). There were no signs for tumour or any acute inflammation.

Microscopic findings in FCD ILAE Type Ic

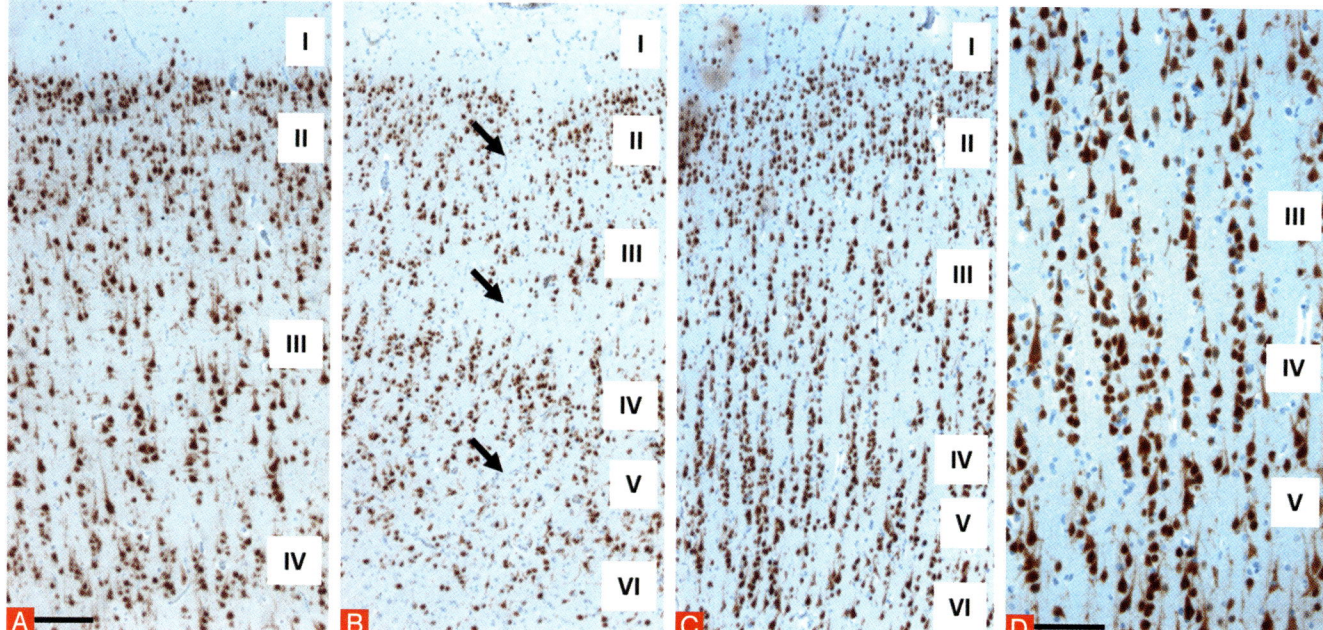

Figure 14

A. Regular six-layered cortical ribbon for comparison with findings in FCD ILAE Type Ic (B-D). Of note A-C are of same magnification. B. Six-layered, but overall thinned cortex with patchy neuronal cell loss (black arrows) within the supra- and infra-granular layers as well as blurred grey/white matter boundaries. C-D. In addition to this horizontal dyslamination there were areas showing a radial dyslamination with micro-columnar arrangement of the neocortex (C; higher magnification in D). A-D: NeuN immunohistochemistry. I-IV: cortical layers. Scale bar in A: 200 µm, applies also for B and C. Scale bar in D: 100 µm.

Focal cortical dysplasia ILAE Type IIa

Clinical history

9-year old boy with focal epilepsy arising from left anterior temporal lobe.

Histopathology and immunohistochemistry

We received two en bloc resections of the temporal lobe (I: 5 × 4 × 2 cm), and hippocampus (II: 2 × 2 × 1 cm). The cortical specimen had a characteristic surface gyration and blood vessel supply. Representative material was embedded in five paraffin blocks. Microscopic inspection of H&E stained sections revealed cortical grey and subcortical white matter with loss of hexaluminar cortical architecture and blurred grey/white-matter boundaries. This cortical dysplasia was pronounced in the depth of the sulcus and harboured many dysmorphic neurones (*Figure 15A, D, M*) characterized by prominent Nissl substance and lack of anatomical orientation (NeuN, MAP2, SMI32). We could not detect balloon cells, neither by H&E staining nor vimentin immunohistochemistry. Other areas of the neocortex revealed normal six-layering, though focal neuronal cell loss in layer IV often was encountered. Subcortical white matter showed focal areas of hypomyelination as well as small vessel disease with enlarged perivascular spaces.

Comments

Microscopic inspection of the tissue specimens revealed central nervous tissue with cortical disarray consisting of dysmorphic neurones but no balloon cells (immunohistochemically confirmed). We classified these findings as FCD ILAE Type IIa (ILAE classification 2011; [Blümcke et al., 2011]). The hippocampal specimen is not illustrated but showed neither dysmorphic neurones or segmental neuronal loss (no-HS; ILAE classification 2013; [Blümcke et al., 2013]). There were no signs of tumour or an acute inflammatory process.

Microscopic findings in FCD ILAE Type IIa

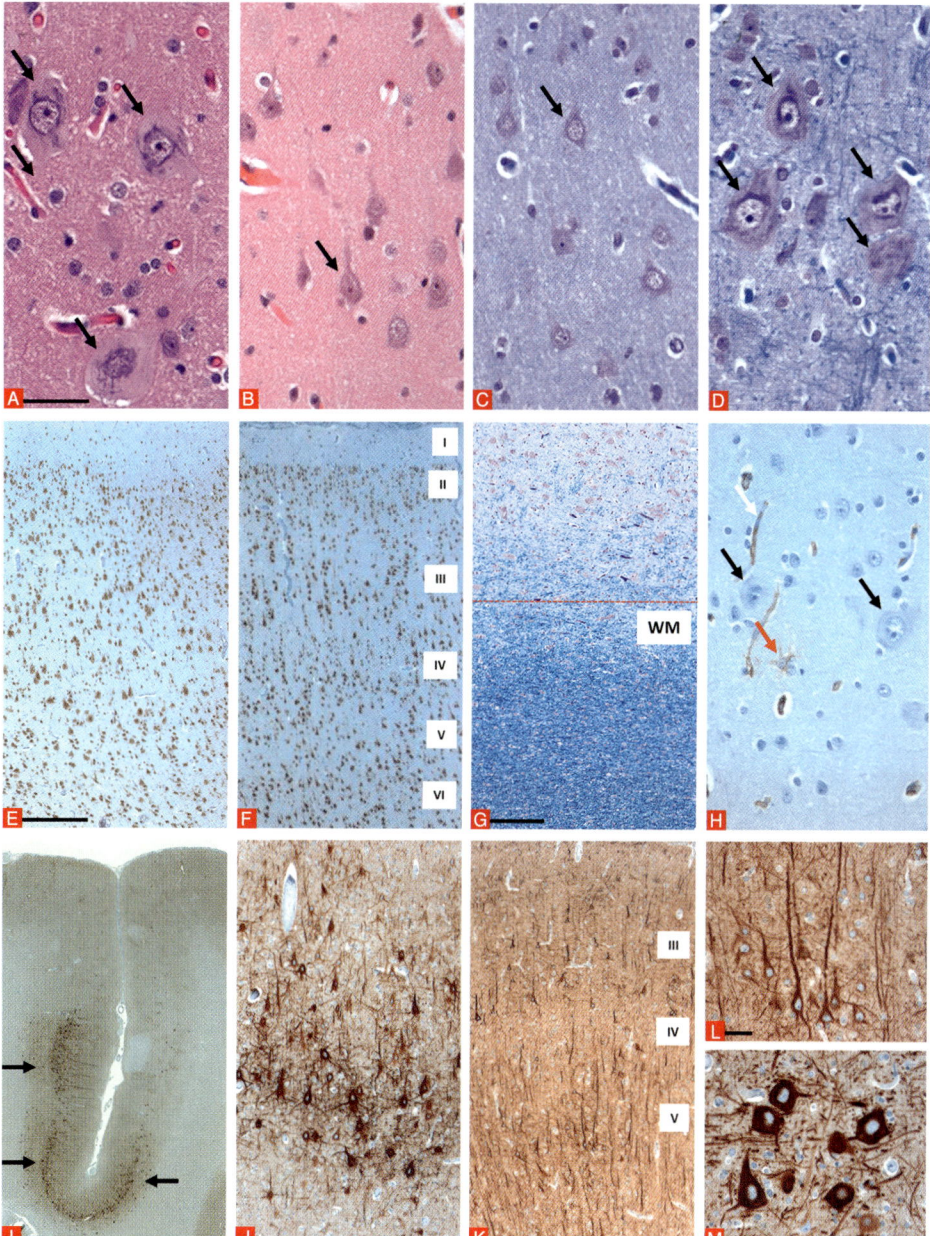

Figure 15

A-C. H&E staining showing several dysmorphic neurones with enlarged cell bodies as well as enlarged nuclei (black arrows) compared to regular-sized and oriented pyramidal neurones of layer III (black arrows in B: H&E staining; C: Nissl-LFB staining). D. Dysmorphic neurones with prominent accumulation of Nissl substance (black arrows; Nissl-LFB staining). E. Field of dysmorphic neurones and loss of hexalaminar cortical architecture. For comparison: F. Regular six-layered cortical ribbon (E & F: NeuN immunohistochemistry). G. Nissl-LFB staining at the grey/white matter junction with slight blurring but no distinct signs for hypo-/demyelination. H. Vimentin immunohistochemistry: Balloon cells were not detectable. This immunoreactivity labelled only vascular endothelium (white arrow) and single reactive astrocytes (red arrow). Dysmorphic neurones were negative (black arrows). I-M: SMI32 immunohistochemistry: I. Low magnification showing conglomerates of dysmorphic neurones with neurofilament-protein accumulation at the bottom of sulcus (black arrows). J. several dysmorphic neurones with neurofilament-protein accumulation and disoriented anatomical orientation (higher magnification in M) distributed unevenly in layers III-IV compared to regular labelling of normal-sized and regularly oriented pyramidal neurones in layers III and V (higher magnification in L). WM: white matter. I-IV: cortical layers. Scale bar in A: 50 µm, applies also for B-D & H. Scale bar in E: 500 µm, applies also for F. Scale bar in G: 200 µm. Scale bar in I: 2,000 µm. Scale bar in J: 200 µm, applies also for K. Scale bar in L: 50 µm, applies also for M.

Focal cortical dysplasia ILAE Type IIb

Clinical history

43-year old patient with focal epilepsy elicited from right frontal lobe with epilepsy onset at the age of 4. Presurgical MRI (T2 weighted image in *Figure 16A*) revealed a circumscribed thickening of the cortex in a deeper sulcus (white arrows) and a hyperintensity towards the lateral ventricle (transmantle sign; red arrows), suggesting FCD of the right inferior frontal gyrus.

Histopathology and immunohistochemistry

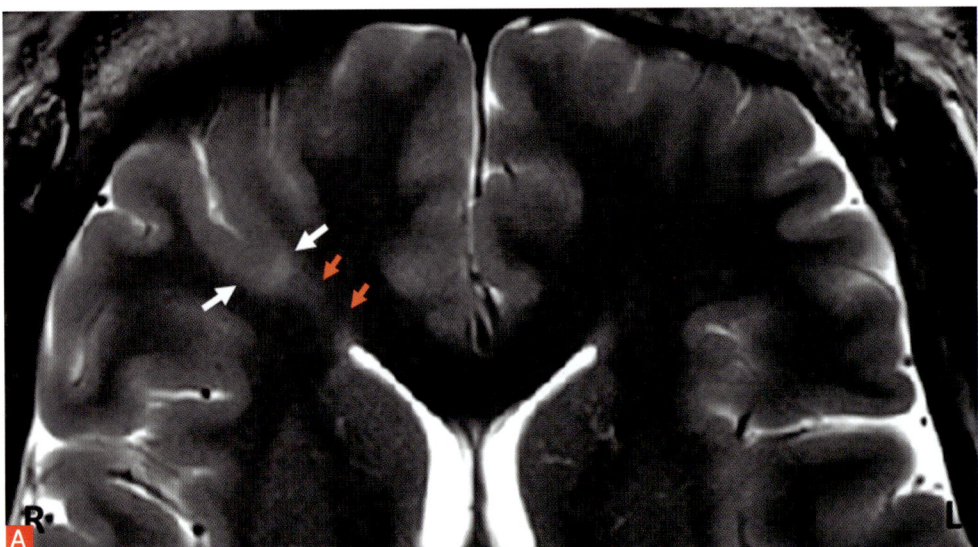

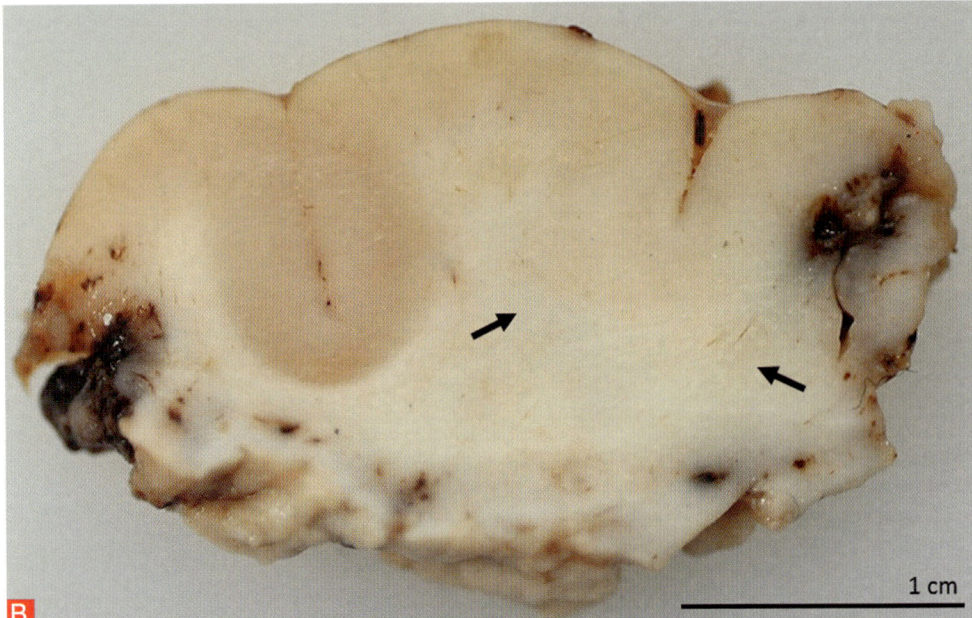

Figure 16

We received formalin-fixed grey to brownish and firm tissue with a size of 5.5 × 4 × 1.5 cm originating from the right frontal lobe. The surface presented with characteristic cortical relief and proper vasculature. The material was sliced completely and representative sections were embedded in nine paraffin blocks. Macroscopic inspection already revealed areas of pronounced thickening of the cortical ribbon and barely discernible grey/white matter boundaries (arrows in macroscopic photograph *Figure 16B*). Microscopic inspection revealed neocortex and subcortical white matter. Prominent cortical dyslamination was visible in several regions as increased cortical thickness without discrimination of individual layers (*Figure 17A, C*). Numerous dysmorphic neurones with enlarged nuclei and aggregates of Nissl substance lacking a regular anatomic orientation were demonstrated. Borders between grey and white matter were blurred. Balloon cells were detected in deep cortical layers as well in the underlying white matter, which was partially hypo-myelinated (Nissl-LFB staining). The balloon cells were characterized by a large cell body with opaque cytoplasm and occasionally multiple nuclei. No neoplasia or inflammatory infiltrates were evident. NeuN and MAP2 staining highlighted the architectural disturbance with loss of the hexalaminar organization of the cortex. There were foci containing dysmorphic neurones with intra-cytoplasmatic neurofilament-protein accumulation (SMI32). Balloon cells expressed vimentin and partially also GFAP within the subjacent white matter. There was a pronounced fibrillary gliosis (GFAP).

Comments

Microscopic inspection of the tissue specimen revealed fragments of central nervous tissue with a focal cortical dyslamination. The cortical ribbon was thickened and showed a loss of the six-layered architecture as well as blurring of grey/white-matter boundaries. Furthermore, clusters of dysmorphic neurones and balloon cells. These were typical histomorphological findings of a FCD Type IIb (ILAE classification 2011). There were no signs of inflammatory or neoplastic processes.

Microscopic findings in FCD ILAE Type IIb

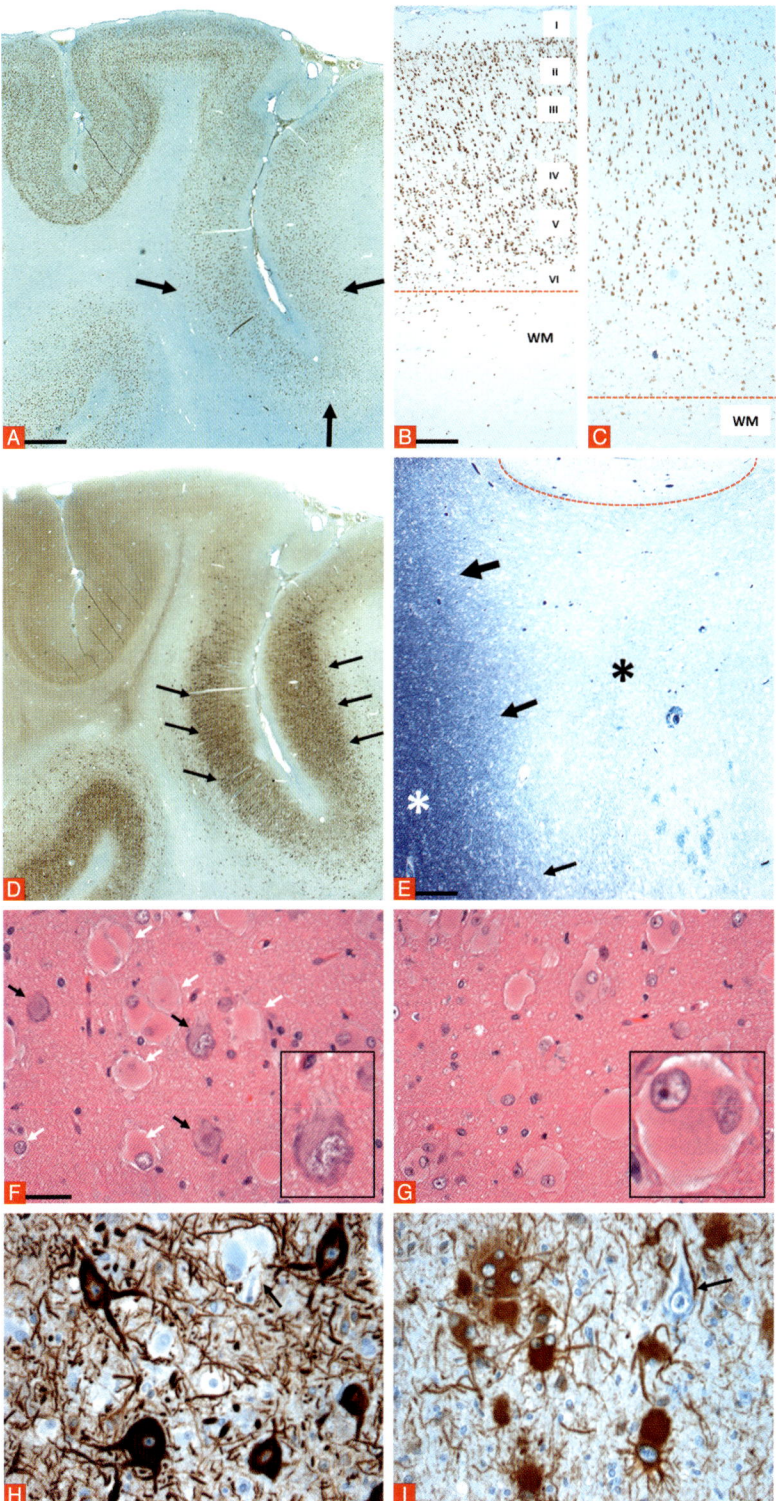

Figure 17

A. NeuN immunohistochemistry demonstrated already at low magnification cortical dyslamination in the depth of the sulcus (black arrows), confirmed at higher magnification in C. These areas showed a thickened cortical ribbon with loss of the cortical six-layering and blurred grey/white matter junctions. **B:** NeuN immunohistochemistry of a region with regular cortical architecture and normal width of the cortical ribbon, as well as sharp grey/white matter boundaries at the same magnification as C for comparison. **D:** Serial section of A incubated with an antibody against SMI32 indicated an increased density of neurofilament accumulating neurons in the area of cortical dyslamination (black arrows). **E:** Nissl-LFB staining highlighting hypomyelination of white matter (black asterisk; normal myelination white asterisk), most prominent at the bottom of a sulcus (red dotted delineation), fading (black arrows) towards the lateral ventricle as equivalent of the transmantle sign viewed on MRI. **F:** Cortical areas with dyslamination on H&E staining showing dysmorphic neurones with enlarged cell bodies, aggregates of Nissl substance, and enlarged nuclei (black arrows; one dysmorphic neurone at higher magnification in inset) intermingled with balloon cells (white arrows). **G:** H&E staining of the subjacent white matter demonstrated numerous balloon cells with large cell bodies and opaque cytoplasm (one bi-nucleated balloon cell at higher magnification in inset). **H:** SMI32 immunohistochemistry showing dysmorphic neurones with neurofilament-protein accumulation, but no immunoreactivity within balloon cells (black arrow). **I:** Balloon cells with vimentin immunoreactivity but without reactivity for dysmorphic neurones (black arrow). WM: white matter. I-IV: cortical layers. Scale bar in A: 2,000 μm, applies also for D. Scale bar in B: 500 μm, applies also for C. Scale bar in E: 500 μm. Scale bar in F: 50 μm, applies also for G-I.

Focal cortical dysplasia ILAE Type IIIa

Clinical history
28-year old male patient with left-sided temporal lobe epilepsy.

Histopathology and immunohistochemistry
We received a surgical brain tissue specimen with a total size of 4 × 3 × 2.3 cm resected from the temporal lobe (anterior pole, sample I.). The material was serially dissected and embedded into paraffin. Fraction II. was the hippocampus specimen (2 × 2 × 1.4 cm), sliced along the anterior-posterior axis and also embedded into paraffin. Microscopic inspection of the tissue specimen (sample I.) revealed cortical grey and subcortical white matter with horizontal dyslamination. Several areas showed reduced neuronal densities, predominantly affecting the upper cortical layers (layers II, III and IV). Layer II showed a focal abnormal band of small and clustered granular neurones (*Figure 18A*). No hypertrophic or dysmorphic neurones were detected. The white matter was normally myelinated (Nissl-LFB staining). The horizontal cortical dyslamination with variable reduction of neurones in cortical layers II and III was well demonstrated by NeuN staining. Here, pronounced reactive gliosis (GFAP staining). No hypertrophic nor dysmorphic neurones with intra-cytoplasmatic neurofilament-protein accumulation detectable (SMI32). Microscopic inspection of the hippocampal tissue specimen (fraction II) revealed segmental pyramidal cell loss affecting sectors CA1, CA3 and CA4 (*Figure 18E*). The granule cell layer showed focally decreased neuronal cell densities as well as granule cell dispersion.

Comments
Microscopic inspection revealed central nervous tissue originating from the temporal neocortex as well as from the hippocampal formation. Within the hippocampal formation (*Figure 18E*), we encountered neuronal cell loss within the hippocampal subfields CA1, CA3 and CA4 accompanied by reactive gliosis as well as granule cell dispersion (HS Type 1; ILAE classification 2013). Another striking finding was observed within the temporal neocortex. Here, a horizontal cortical dyslamination with variable neuronal reduction in layers II and III could be detected. These changes were associated with a laminar gliosis, consistent with a so-called temporal lobe sclerosis (TLS, Thom *et al.*, 2009). This specific type of cortical dyslamination can be observed in approx. 10% of patients with hippocampal sclerosis and is now classified as FCD Type IIIa (ILAE classification 2011). No acute inflammation or tumour was seen.

Microscopic findings in FCD ILAE Type IIIa (see *Figure 18*)

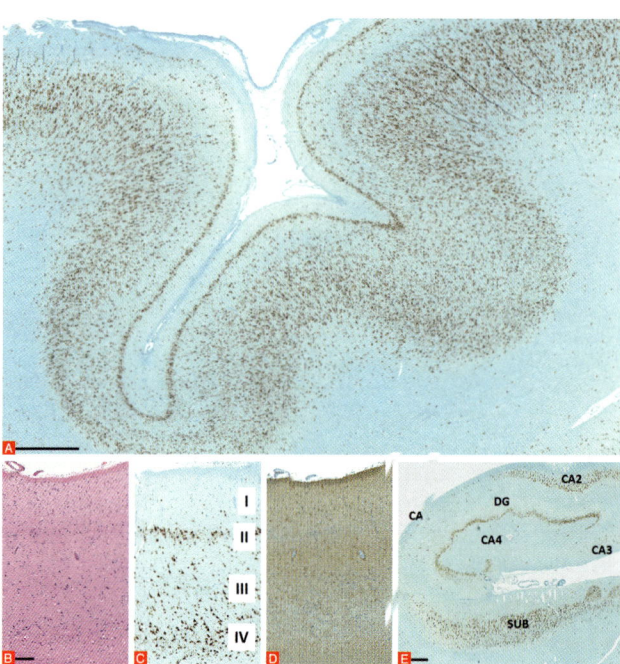

Figure 18

A. Lower magnification demonstrating horizontal cortical dyslamination over a long reach along the cortical ribbon with laminar cell loss in layers II-IV. B-D. Serial sections of temporal neocortex (fraction I., see above) stained with H&E (B), NeuN (C) and GFAP (D). The horizontal cortical dyslamination with variable neuronal reduction in layers II and III already well visible on H&E staining is highlighted by NeuN immunohistochemistry (C). Same area with pronounced reactive gliosis (D). E. The hippocampal formation (fraction II.) with segmental cell loss in sectors CA1, CA3 and CA4 (NeuN immunohistochemistry). I-IV: cortical layers. Scale bar in A: 1,000 μm, also applies to E. Scale bar in B: 200 μm, applies also for C and D.

Focal cortical dysplasia ILAE Type IIIb

Clinical history

4-year old girl with right temporal lobe epilepsy. MRI revealed a cystic tumour of the right temporo-occipital region and suspicious peri-lesional cortical dysplasia.

Histopathology and immunohistochemistry

We received two surgical specimens labelled as I: temporal lobe (6 × 4 × 2.5 cm), dissected into 5 mm thin slices and completely embedded into paraffin. Macroscopically, the grey/white matter boundary was difficult to identify. II: Occipital lobe (6 × 5 × 4 cm) with macroscopically normal appearance. Microscopic inspection of the H&E stained tissue specimen of sample I. revealed central nervous tissue with a glio-neuronal tumour. The tumour consisted of small isomorphic cells with round chromatin-rich nuclei in a fibrillary matrix and an increased capillary network. Tumour cells often were arranged in columns. Mature floating neurons could often be identified. No brisk mitotic activity, microvascular proliferation or necrosis. The tumour was classified as dysembryoplastic neuroepithelial tumour WHO I° (see also *Figure 19A, 33 and 34*). In both samples (I and II), neocortex revealed mostly a hexalaminar architecture and sharp grey/white matter boundaries. However, there were also areas with micro-columnar architectural disturbance (*Figure 19*) and increased heterotopic neurones in white matter. NeuN was most helpful to confirm the micro-columnar architectural dysplasia within the neocortex.

Comments

Microscopic inspection revealed a CD34 negative tumour with the characteristic histopathology pattern of specific glio-neuronal elements, consistent with the diagnosis of DNT (WHO I°). Nodular cortical growth and low proliferation were further histopathological hallmarks of this tumour entity. The adjacent neocortex revealed architectural abnormalities in its vertical organization with abundant micro-columns and heterotopic neurones in white matter. This pattern was classified as associated FCD Type IIIb according to the ILAE classification of FCD, rather than judged as independent cortical malformation (*i.e.* double pathology). There were no signs for an acute inflammatory process or neoplasia.

Microscopic findings in FCD ILAE Type IIIb

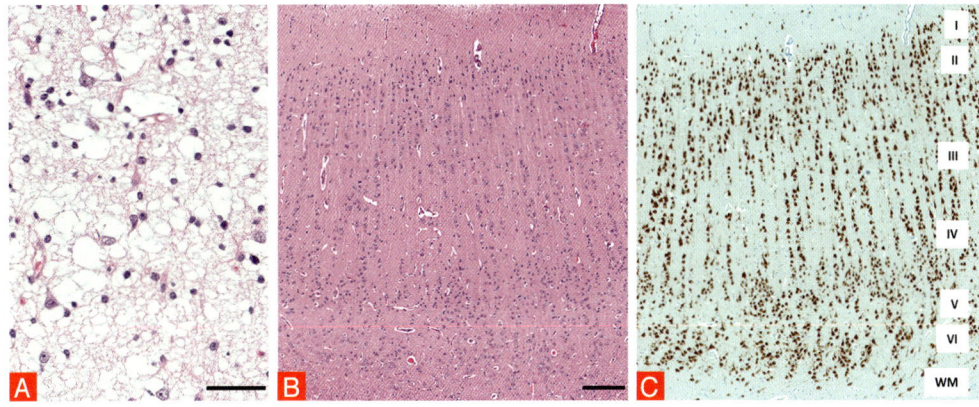

Figure 19

A. H&E staining showed a glio-neuronal tumour of moderate cellularity with micro-cystic structures and a specific glio-neuronal element with "floating" neurones. B & C. Serial sections of adjacent neocortex, without tumour infiltration, showing radial dyslamination with abundant micro-columns and focal neuronal cell loss in supra-granular layers (H&E staining in B, NeuN immunohistochemistry in C). Scale bar in A: 50 μm. Scale bar in B: 200 μm, applies also for C.

Focal cortical dysplasia ILAE Type IIIc

Clinical history

6-year old boy with Sturge-Weber syndrome and epilepsy onset at the age of 2 years with a large vascular lesion in the right fronto-parietal area.

Histopathology and immunohistochemistry

We received one fronto-parietal tissue specimen with a total size of 6.5 × 6 × 2.5 cm. The material was serially dissected and embedded in paraffin blocks. Histological examination of H&E staining showed cortical grey and subcortical white matter. There was a prominent vascular malformation of the leptomeninx with abundant small vessels (*Figure 20A*). The subjacent cortex revealed a thinned cortical ribbon (*Figure 20B*). In these regions, there was a pronounced laminar neuronal loss in layer III. In addition, focal cell loss in infra-granular layers and blurred grey/white matter boundaries with increased numbers of heterotopic neurones within the subjacent white matter. This cortical dyslamination was highlighted by NeuN immunohistochemistry. Reactive gliosis (GFAP staining) was pronounced within the areas of neuronal loss. There was no evidence for hypertrophic or dysmorphic neurones using SMI32 immunohistochemistry.

Comments

Microscopic inspection revealed a leptomeningeal vascular malformation consistent with a leptomeningeal angiomatosis in the setting of a clinically confirmed Sturge-Weber syndrome. The adjacent neocortex showed cortical dyslamination in terms of an associated FCD Type IIIc (ILAE classification, 2013). There were no signs for acute inflammation or a tumour.

Microscopic findings in FCD ILAE Type IIIc

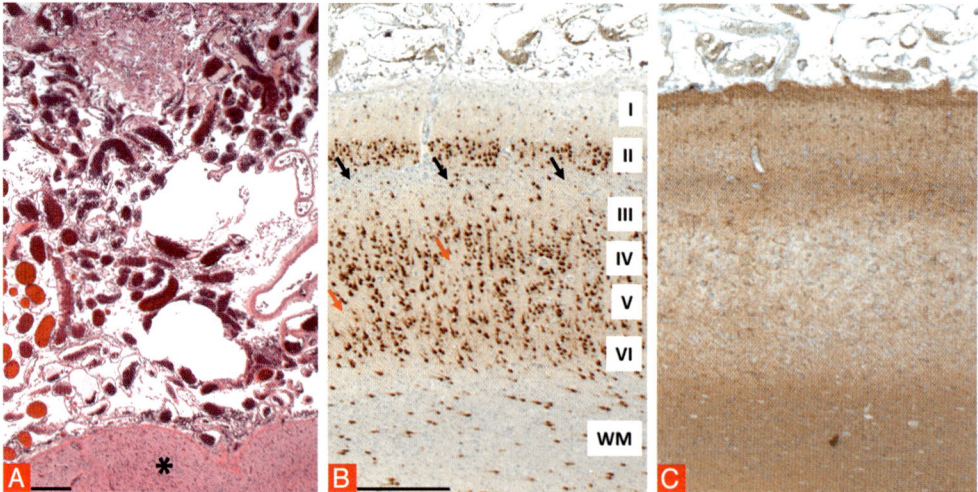

Figure 20

A. H&E staining showed a highly vascularised leptomeningeal angiomatosis (asterisk indicates cortical layer I). B. NeuN staining demonstrating thinning of the cortical ribbon and laminar neuronal loss predominantly in layer III (black arrows). In addition, focal cell loss in other layers (red arrow) and blurred grey/white matter junction. C. Serial section to B (GFAP immunohistochemistry) demonstrating laminar and also diffuse reactive gliosis. WM: white matter. I-IV: cortical layers. Scale bar in A: 500 μm. Scale bar in B: 500 μm. applies also for C.

Focal cortical dysplasia ILAE Type IIId

Clinical history
14-year old girl with focal temporal lobe epilepsy. She suffered from intrauterine middle cerebral artery infarction.

Histopathology and immunohistochemistry
We received three surgical specimen from the hippocampus (not shown), the temporal lobe (not shown), and the parieto-occipital lobe (7 × 6 × 4 cm) with characteristic gyral patterning of cerebral neocortex and an old pseudocystic lesion visible at parieto-occipital site (black arrow in macroscopic photograph, *Figure 21*). Adjacent tissue of darker brownish colour, indicative for stored haemosiderin pigments. Microscopic inspection of the H&E stained tissue specimen revealed cortical grey and white matter with a pseudocystic lesion located in the subcortical white matter and extended to the ventricle. The lesion was surrounded by prominent fibrillary gliosis and haemosiderin storage (*Figure 22B*). The latter was confirmed using Prussian blue staining. Adjacent cortical ribbon revealed focally a micro-columnar architectural disturbance as well as neuronal clusters close to the ventricle and adjacent hypoplastic neocortex. Cortical dysplasia became most evident using NeuN and MAP2 immunohistochemistry, confirming micro-columnar, hypoplastic as well as nodular architectural abnormalities (*Figure 22D-G*). Fibrillary gliosis was prominent and always detectable by GFAP staining. In addition, hypertrophic neurones with neurofilament accumulation were detectable (SMI32), but not regarded as dysmorphic.

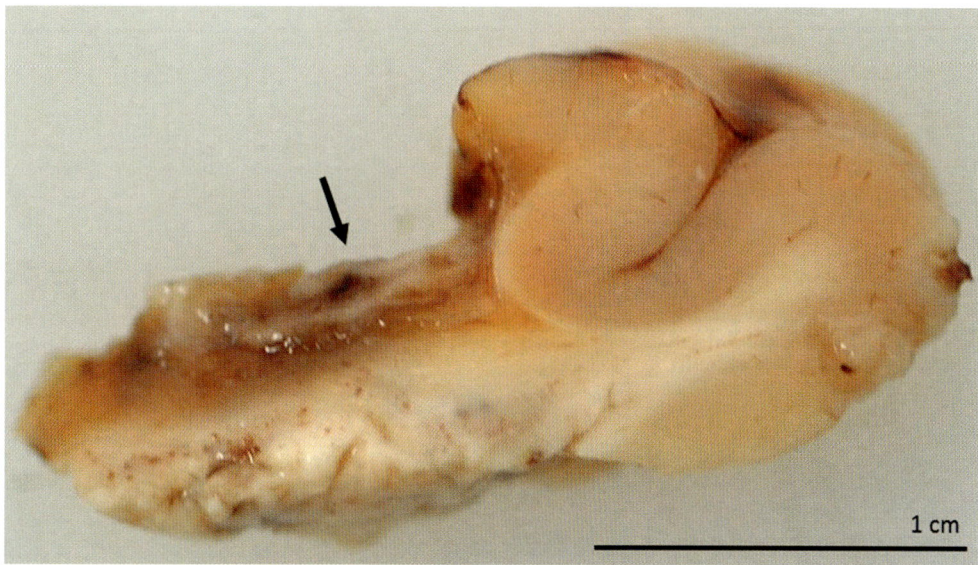

Figure 21

Comments
The surgical specimen from the parieto-occipital lobe revealed a glio-mesodermal scar with haemosiderin deposits, compatible with intrauterine MCA infarct (according to clinical information). Adjacent cortical tissue revealed a prominent FCD with micro-columnar architectural organization, neuronal cell clustering and hypoplastic cortical structure. This pattern was classified as FCD associated with a porencephalic cyst, *i.e.* FCD Type IIId according to the 2011 ILAE classification system. The hippocampal specimen showed a CA1 predominant sclerosis and granule cell dispersion and was classified as HS Type 2 according to the 2013 ILAE classification system (dual pathology).

Microscopic findings in FCD ILAE Type IIId

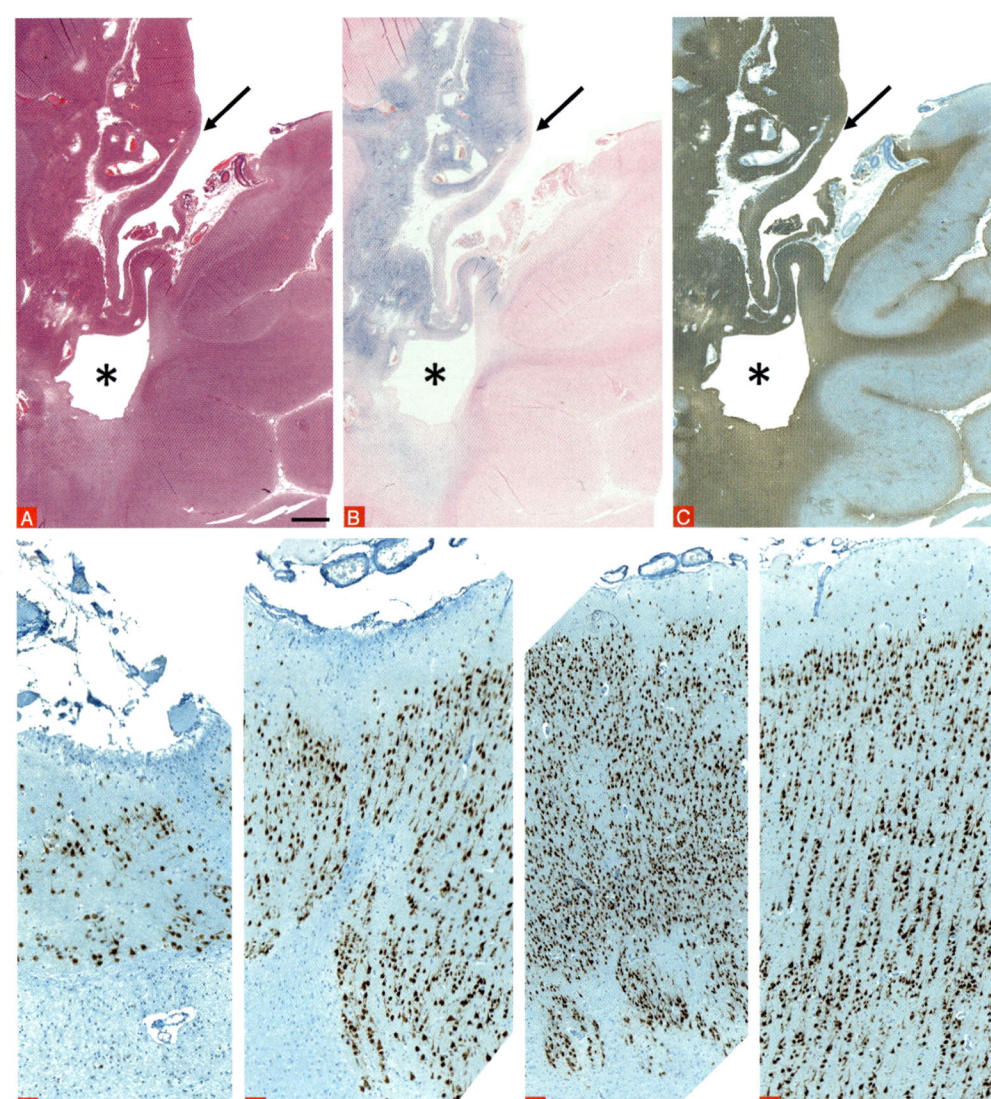

Figure 22

A–C. H&E staining (A) showing cortical grey and subcortical white matter with a pseudocystic lesion (arrows in A–C) extending to the ventricle (asterisks in A–C) and surrounded by haemosiderin storage (highlighted in B by Prussian blue staining) and prominent fibrillary gliosis (highlighted by GFAP immunohistochemistry in C). **D–G.** NeuN immunohistochemistry provides evidence of different patterns of cortical dyslamination with cortical hypoplasia (D & E), patchy neuronal cell loss and neuronal clustering (F) as well as micro-columnar architectural abnormalities (G). Scale bar in A: 2,000 μm, applies also for B and C. Scale bar in D: 200 μm, applies also for E–G.

Cortical tuber (genetically confirmed TSC)

Clinical history
2-year old boy with right frontal lobe epilepsy with genetically confirmed tuberous sclerosis complex (TSC) and several cortical tubers.

Histopathology and immunohistochemistry
We received a formalin-fixed surgical specimen with a total size of 7.5 × 6 × 2.5 cm. It was described as en bloc resection of the right frontal lobe. We recognized a typical neocortical surface and gyral patterning. One particular gyrus appeared large and lumpy (see macroscopic photographs, arrows in *Figure 23*). The entire specimen was sliced into 5 mm sections. Eleven samples (i.e. every 2nd) were embedded in paraffin and all additional material kept in formalin. Microscopic inspection of the specimen stained for H&E revealed neocortex and subcortical white matter. We observed a large cortical dysplasia affecting several gyri. They were all characterized by an increase cortical thickness without discrimination of individual cortical layers. There were many balloon cells, often clustered, throughout the neocortex and white matter, which was partially also hypo-myelinated (Nissl-LFB staining). Balloon cells were characterized by a large cell body with opaque cytoplasm and presented occasionally with multiple nuclei. These balloon cells cannot be distinguished from balloon cells in FCD Type IIb (case 18). Numerous dysmorphic neurones with enlarged nuclei and aggregates of Nissl substance lacked a regular anatomical orientation. Prominent micro-calcifications were present (*Figure 24*). NeuN and MAP2 staining highlighted the architectural abnormality with loss of hexalaminar organization of the cortical ribbon. There were many dysmorphic neurones with intracytoplasmatic neurofilament-protein accumulation (SMI32) throughout the neocortex, as well as a pronounced fibrillary gliosis (GFAP). Balloon cells showed prominent vimentin expression. CD34 labelled only endothelial cells. No signs of acute inflammation were seen.

Comments
Microscopic inspection revealed a histopathological lesion characterized by architectural dyslamination of the cortical ribbon, abundant dysmorphic neurones and balloon cells, as well as micro-calcifications, consistent with the diagnosis of a cortical tuber. However, this diagnosis is only possible with clinically and/or genetically conclusive information, as the histopathological pattern *per se* would only justify FCD Type IIb.

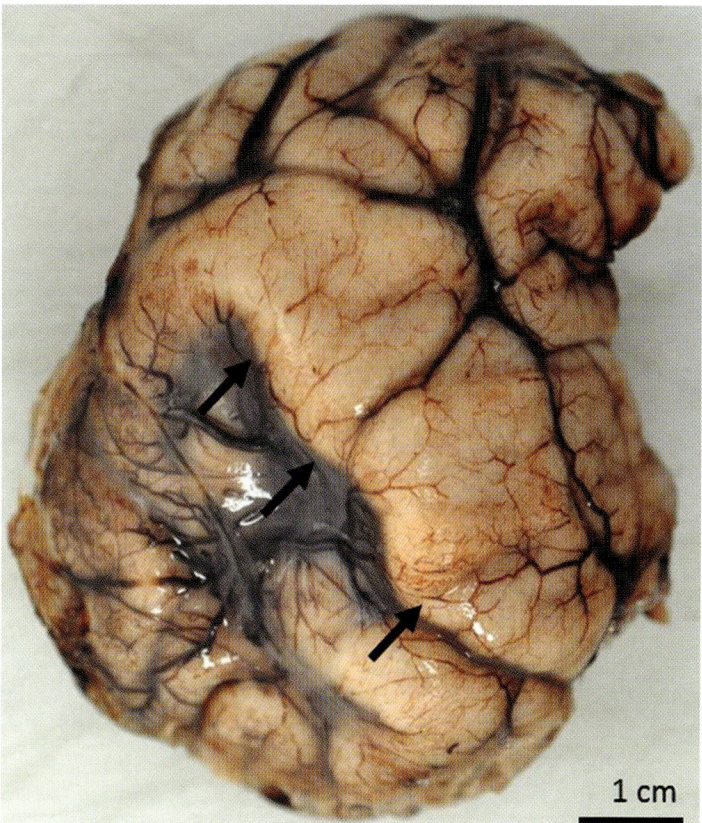

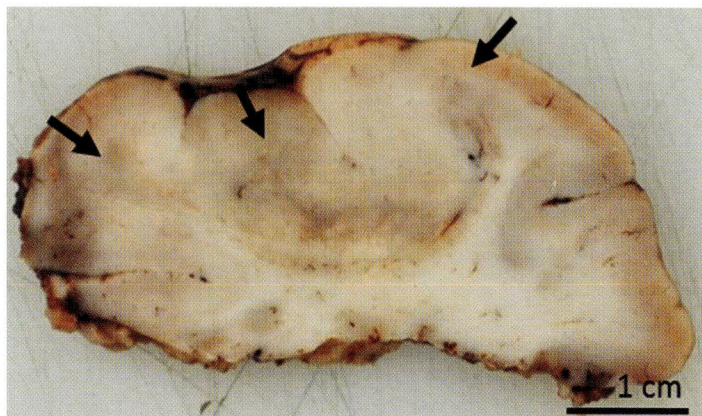

Figure 23

Microscopic findings in cortical tuber

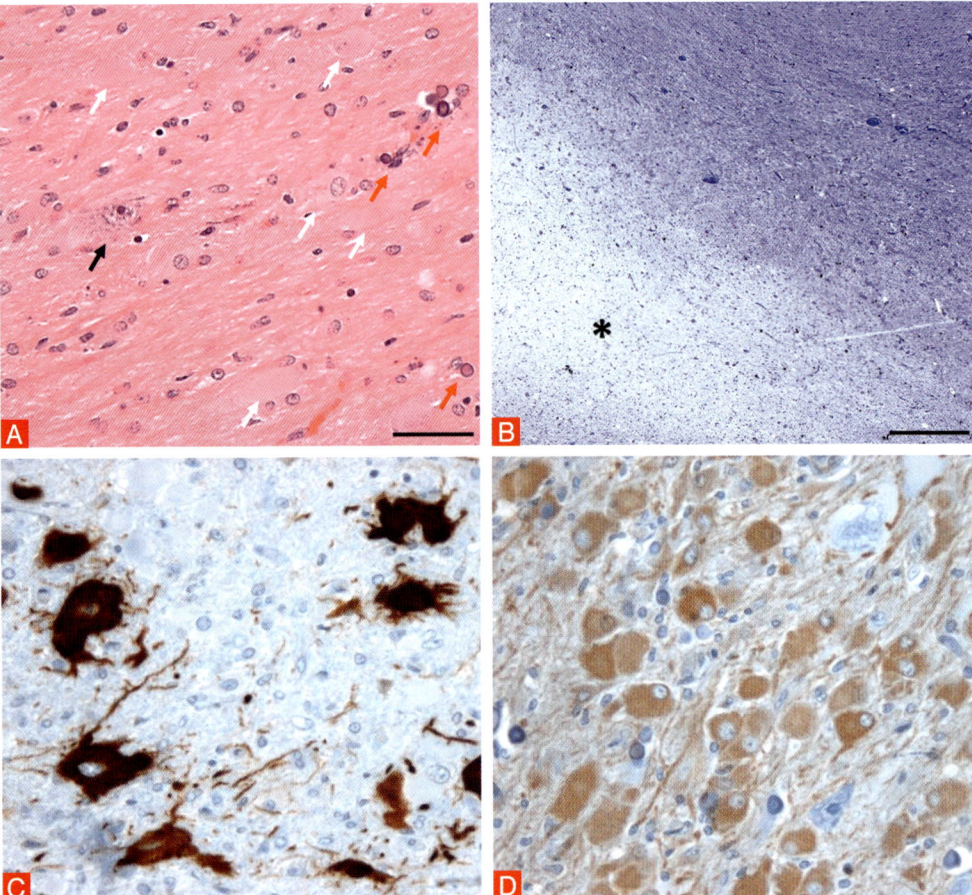

Figure 24

A. H&E staining showing numerous balloon cells with opaque cytoplasm, some bi-nucleated (white arrows), a dysmorphic neurone (black arrow) with enlarged nucleus and aggregates of Nissl substance, as well as micro-calcifications (red arrows). B. Nissl-LFB staining highlighting patchy hypo-myelination of white matter (asterisk). C. Dysmorphic neurones with intra-cytoplasmatic neurofilament-protein accumulation (SMI32 immunohistochemistry). D. Numerous balloon cells with vimentin immunoreactivity. Scale bar in A: 50 μm, applies also for C and D. Scale bar in B: 200 μm.

Hemimegalencephaly (HME)

Clinical history
3-year old girl with hemimegalencephaly of the right hemisphere.

Histopathology and immunohistochemistry
We received four different formalin fixed specimens described as I. Temporal lobe (6 × 3 × 2 cm), II. Hippocampus (2.5 × 2 × 1.5 cm); III. Gyrus frontalis inferior (6 × 4 × 4 cm), and IV. Gyrus frontalis medius (4 × 2 × 2 cm). All specimens were sliced and representative samples embedded in paraffin. The inferior frontal gyrus is shown. H&E staining revealed a broad histopathological spectrum of cortical malformations. Hexalaminar cortical architecture was not demarcated; cytoarchitectural dysplasia also was evident, *i.e.* dysmorphic neurones and balloon cells (*Figure 25*). These cellular populations also were readily visible using NeuN, SMI32 and vimentin immunohistochemistry. Gyral fusion was another histopathological hallmark of this specimen, further supported by NeuN immunohistochemistry. In the white matter, there were zones of decreased myelination as detected by Nissl-LFB stains. No micro-calcifications were seen.

Supplementary special techniques to further confirm the diagnosis of HME reveal additional findings (not shown here): activation of the mTOR signalling pathway and up-regulation of abnormally phosphorylated tau protein (see textbook).

Comments
Surgical specimens from the frontal lobe showed a histopathologically complex malformation of cortical development including areas without any hexalaminar cortical architecture, dysmorphic neurones and balloon cells as well as polymicrogyria. The temporal lobe showed less prominent histopathology changes, although micro-columnar architectural dysplasia was encountered (not shown here). The hippocampus specimen showed no segmental neuronal loss, or any other structural abnormality in the dentate gyrus; it was classified as no-HS according to the 2013 ILAE classification system. This complex histopathological pattern is compatible with the clinical diagnosis of hemimegalencephaly when imaging findings were conclusive.

Microscopic findings in hemimegalencephaly

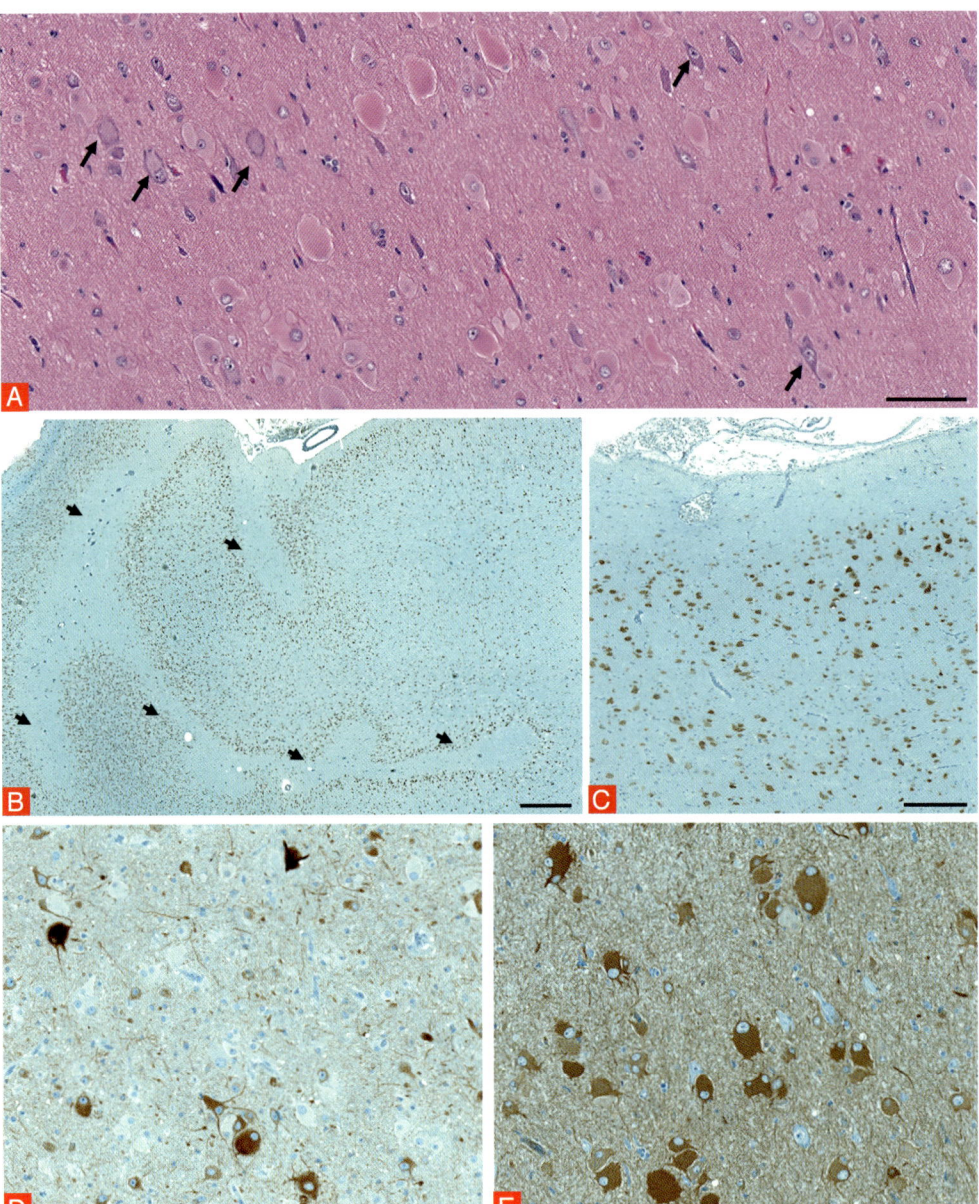

Figure 25

A. H&E staining showing numerous balloon cells with opaque cytoplasm, some bi- or multi-nucleated. Dysmorphic neurones with accumulation of Nissl substance (arrows) were intermingled. B. NeuN immunohistochemistry shows gyral fusion (arrows). C. Dyslamination of the cortical ribbon (NeuN immunohistochemistry). D. Dysmorphic neurones contain intra-cytoplasmatic neurofilament-protein accumulation (SMI32 immunohistochemistry). E. Numerous balloon cells with Vimentin immunoreactivity. Scale bar in A: 100 µm. Scale bar in B: 1,000 µm. Scale bar in C: 200 µm. Scale bar in D: 100 µm, applies also for E.

Polymicrogyria (PMG) and nodular heterotopia

Clinical history
14-year old girl with left frontal lesion (gyrus frontalis superior), clinically suspected FCD or glio-neuronal tumour.

Histopathology and immunohistochemistry
We received formalin-fixed surgical brain tissue with a total size of 6 × 4.8 × 2 cm. The cortical surface appeared polymicrogyric in the central parts of the specimen (arrows in *Figure 26*).

Representative tissue was embedded in 8 paraffin blocks. Microscopic inspection revealed central nervous tissue with disruption of the cortical architecture. Numerous adjacent gyri were fused (*Figure 27*). The cortical ribbon was thinned. There was prominent abnormal dyslamination with areas showing a four-layered cortex. The grey/white matter boundaries were blurred with increased numbers of heterotopic neurones in the white matter. Here, multiple nodular heterotopia (already visible macroscopically, see also macroscopic photograph). Smaller lentiform heterotopia as well as areas of hypo-myelination were also visible using Nissl-LFB staining. Immunohistochemical reactivities with antibodies against NeuN and MAP2 high-

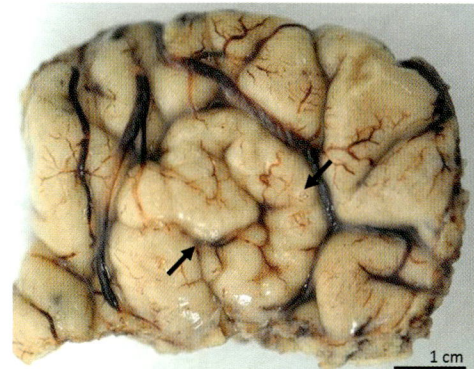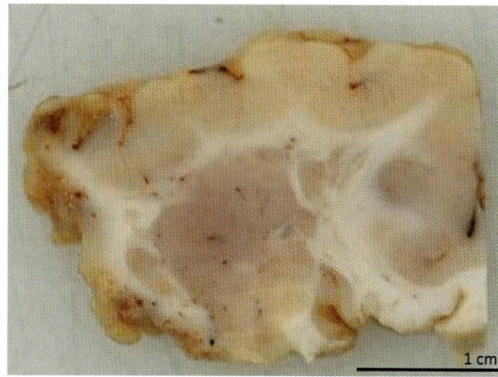

Figure 26

lighted the cortical malformation with a thinned, malformed cortical ribbon, blurred grey/white matter boundaries as well as pronounced nodular and also lentiform heterotopia within the white matter. No dysmorphic neurones with neurofilament-protein accumulation (SMI32 immunohistochemistry). GFAP revealed abundant reactive astrocytes.

Comments
Microscopic inspection of the tissue specimen revealed central nervous tissue with a complex cortical malformation, characterized by numerous fused adjacent gyri without physiological separation of the surfaces of apposed molecular zones. Furthermore, there was an abnormally thinned cortical ribbon with loss of the six-layered architecture. These histomorphological features are consistent with the diagnosis of a polymicrogyria. Another feature of this complex malformation was the presence of prominent nodular and lentiform heterotopia within the subcortical white matter. There were no signs of acute inflammation or tumour.

Microscopic findings in polymicrogyria

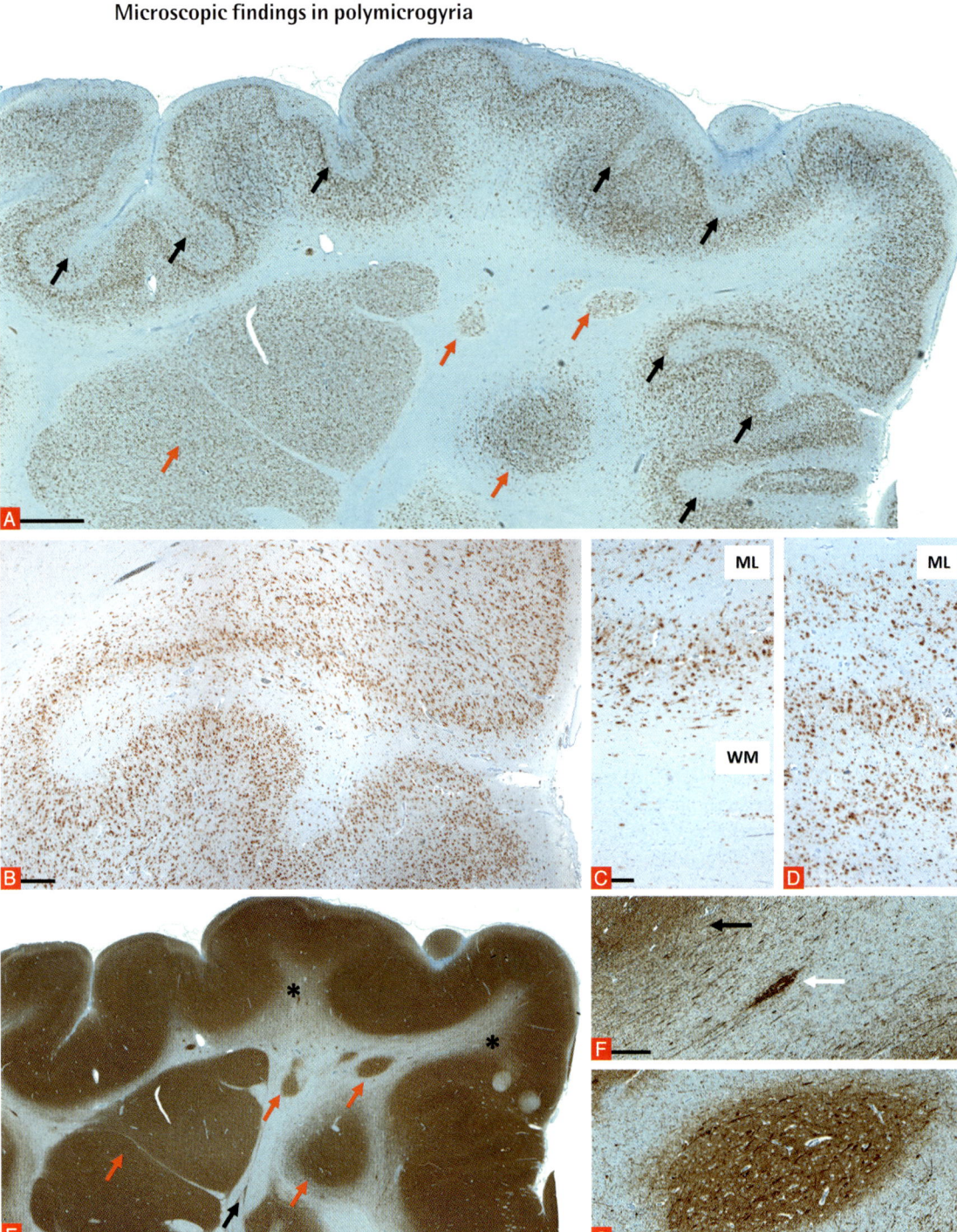

Figure 27

A. NeuN immunohistochemistry showing already at low magnification the prominent malformation with numerous fused adjacent gyri (black arrows) and distinct nodular heterotopia within the white matter (red arrows). **B.** NeuN immunohistochemistry in higher magnification provide additional evidence of fused gyri. **C & D.** Different patterns of severe cortical dyslamination (NeuN immunohistochemistry. **E.** Serial section to A stained with MAP2 illustrating several areas with blurred grey/white matter boundaries (asterisks) as well as nodular (red arrows) and lentiform (black arrow) heterotopia. **F.** Blurred grey/white matter junction (black arrow) and lentiform heterotopia in subjacent white matter (white arrow). **G.** Example of a nodular heterotopion at higher magnification. (F & G: MAP2 immunohistochemistry). ML: molecular layer. WM: white matter. Scale bar in A: 2,000 μm. Scale bar in B: 500 μm. Scale bar in C: 200 μm, applies also for D. Scale bar in E: 2,000 μm. Scale bar in F: 200 μm, applies also for G.

Ganglioglioma (WHO I°)

Clinical history

27-year old male patient suffering from symptomatic epilepsy since age 13. MRI revealed a left temporal cystic lesion. T2 weighted images were shown in *Figure 28A & B*. Homogeneous contrast enhancement of the solid parts (*Figure 28C*: T1 weighted image). The imaging findings were suspicious for a low-grade ganglioglioma.

Histopathology and immunohistochemistry

We received formalin-fixed cortical tissue with a total size of 6 × 3 × 1 cm. A tumorous lesion could be identified already macroscopically affecting the cortical ribbon (arrow in *Figure 29*). The material was sliced and embedded in paraffin.

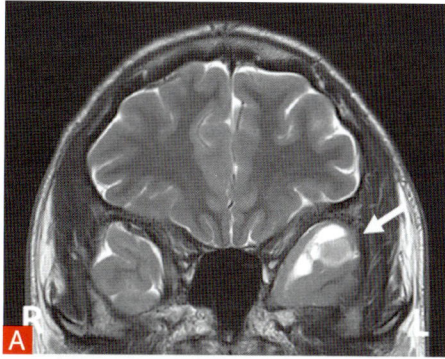
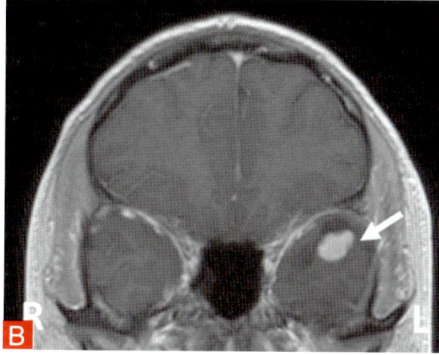
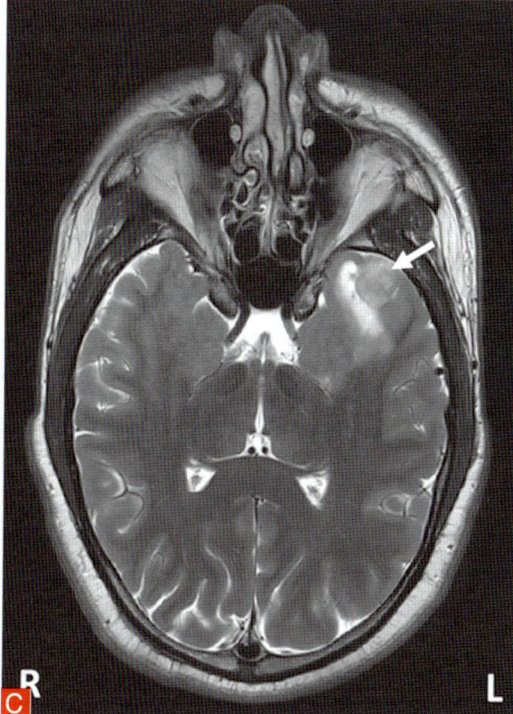

Figure 28

Microscopic inspection of the H&E stained specimen revealed cortical grey and subcortical white matter with infiltration by a glio-neuronal tumour of moderate cellularity (*Figure 30*). The predominant glial tumour component showed small to mid-sized nuclei with dense to speckled chromatin. No mitoses were recognized. The cytoplasm was faintly eosinophilic. Tumour cells showed predominantly fine arborisation. Tumour cells with clear cytoplasm also were found. This glial cell population can be regarded as neoplastically transformed component of the tumour. In addition, few dysplastic neurones were detected within the glial matrix; some were bi-nucleated. Focal micro-calcifications were present. Circumscribed areas with perivascular lymphocytic infiltrates were seen. No micro-vascular proliferation (though increased capillary networks noted) or necrosis was visible. Cortical areas not infiltrated by this tumour showed a regular architecture without dyslamination. The tumour also invaded the subarachnoidal space. Some cortical areas showed a blurred grey/white matter boundary.

The tumour was characterized by its CD34 immunoreactivity (Blümcke *et al.*, 1999), which also labelled cortical infiltration of clustering tumour satellites (Blümcke *et al.*, 2014). The glial tumour cell component was specifically reactive to an antibody directed against GFAP, without co-expression of MAP2 (Blümcke *et al.*, 2001). MAP2 labelled few dysplastic neurones within the tumour matrix. No IDH1 mutation was found. Faint nuclear accumulation of p53 did not exceed 5% of tumour cells. The proliferative index by MIB1/Ki-67 immunohistochemistry was low, with only 1-2% reactive nuclei. NeuN did not reveal any signs of cortical dyslamination in regions adjacent to the tumour.

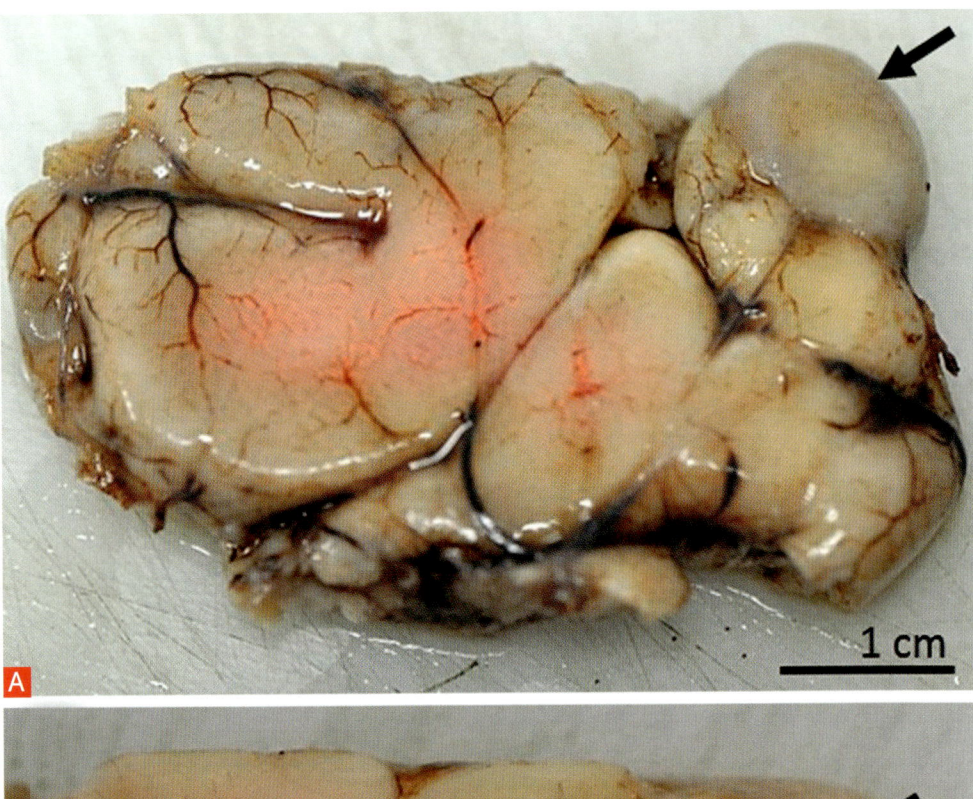

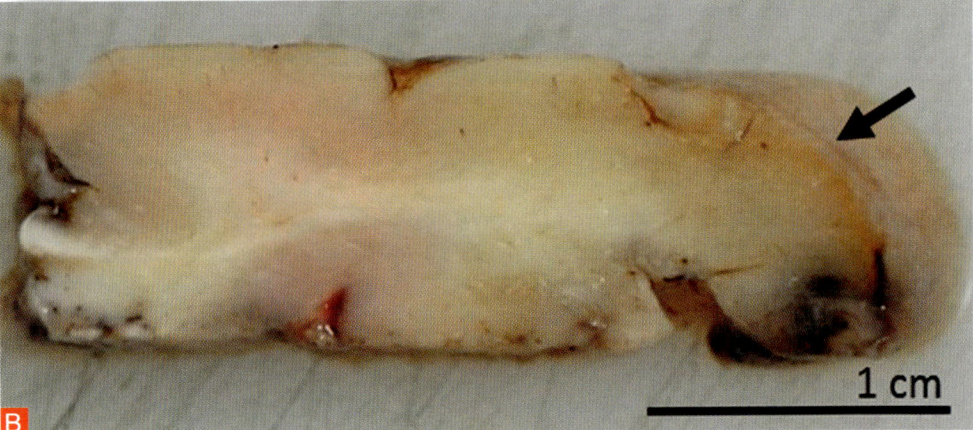

Figure 29

Comments

The microscopic inspection of the specimen revealed a diffusely infiltrating, mixed glio-neuronal tumour with histomorphological characteristics of ganglioglioma. The expression of CD34, detected in numerous tumour cells, further supported this diagnosis (Blümcke and Wiestler, 2002). The biological behaviour of this tumour corresponds to WHO° I Grade I. No frank signs of atypia or anaplasia were found, i.e. mitotic activity in the glial cell component, vascular proliferation or necrosis. Acute inflammation and associated FCD were not demonstrated.

Gangliogliomas represented the 2nd most frequent lesion (10.8%) in our series of epilepsy surgery specimens (see chapter 8 "Tables", *Table I*). They were predominantly located in the temporal lobe (85%), and patients had seizure onset at a mean age of 12.7 years.

Microscopic findings in a ganglioglioma (WHO I°)

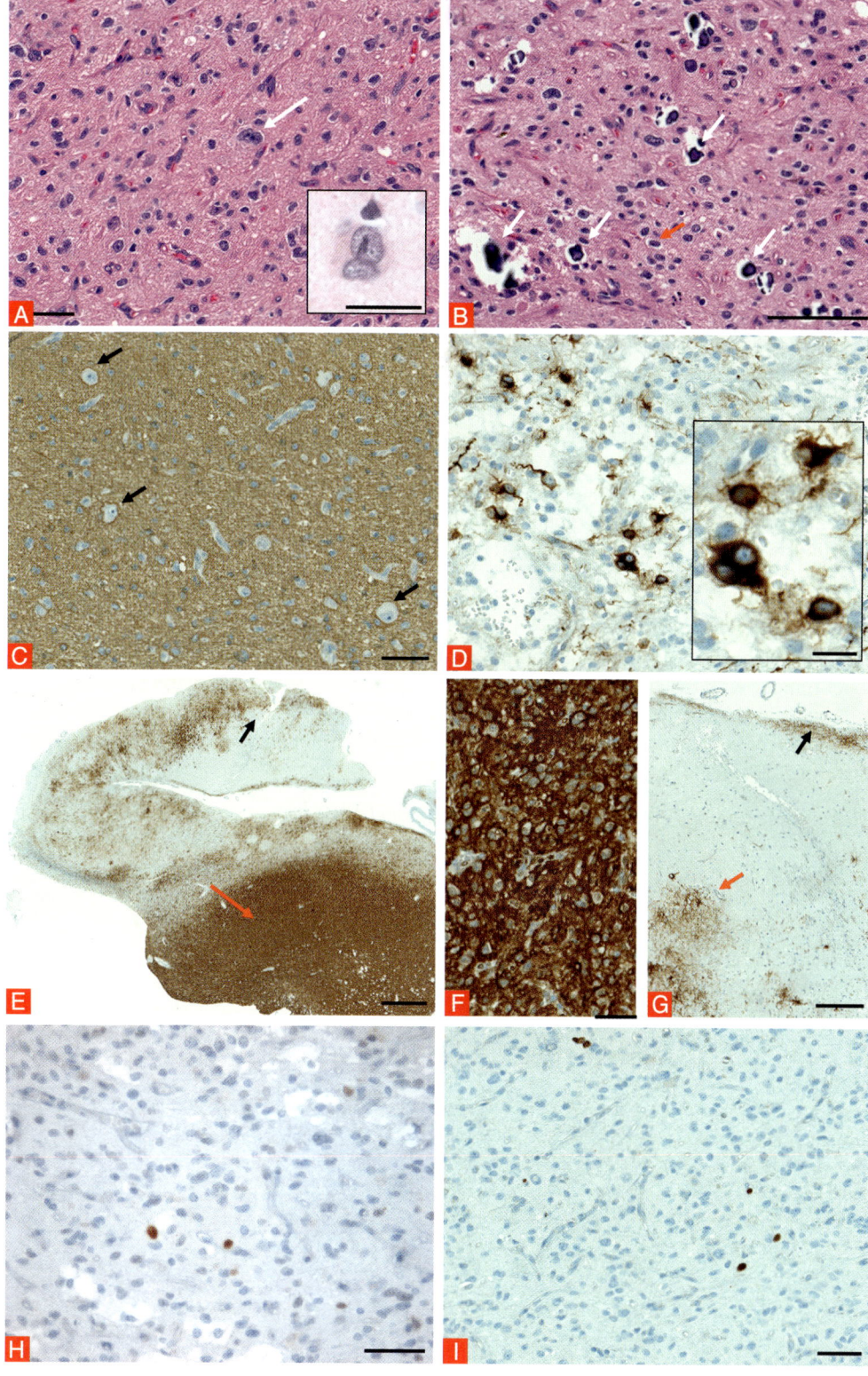

Figure 30

A & B. H&E staining showing a glio-neuronal tumour of moderate cellularity with dysplastic neurones (white arrow in A) within a fibrillary glial tumour matrix. Inset in A: Higher magnification of a bi-nucleated dysplastic neurone. Within the tumour matrix were foci of micro-calcification (white arrows in B). Glial tumour cells with clear cell cytoplasm (red arrow in B) were seen focally. C. The glial tumour matrix showed strong immunoreactivity for GFAP. Dysplastic neurones within the tumour matrix were not labelled (arrows). D. Dysplastic neurones with MAP2 expression, some also bi-nucleated (higher magnification in inset in D). Of note: no significant MAP2 immunoreactivity within the glial tumour component. E-G. Characteristic CD34 pattern of a ganglioglioma with strong immunoreactivity of the tumour mass (antibody QBend10; red arrow in E; see also higher magnification of this area in F) as well as detectable CD34 immunoreactive tumour cell satellites in adjacent tissue (black arrow in E). G: Higher magnification showing tumour cell satellites within adjacent deep cortical areas (red arrow) and highlighting tumour spread along the cortical surface. H. Focally, tumour cells with nuclear p53 expression were found. I. Low proliferative activity (MIB1/Ki-67 labelling). Scale bar in A: 50 µm. Inset in A: 20 µm. Scale bar in B: 100 µm. Scale bar in C: 50 µm, applies also for D. Inset in D: 20 µm. Scale bar in E: 1,000 µm. Scale bar in F: 50 µm. Scale bar in G: 200 µm. Scale bar in H: 50 µm, applies also for I.

Anaplastic ganglioglioma (WHO III°)

Clinical history
9-year old girl with focal epilepsy and a right temporal tumour with irregular contrast enhancing areas.

Histopathology and immunohistochemistry
We received several formalin-fixed tissue fragments of temporal origin with a total size of 1.3 × 0.7 × 0.2 cm, which were entirely embedded in paraffin.

Microscopic inspection of the H&E-stained specimen revealed fragments of a pleomorphic, glio-neuronal tumour with alternating cellularity (*Figure 31*). Glial tumour cells showed small to mid-sized nuclei with dense to speckled chromatin, fine arborisation and also coarse processes. Some tumour cells displayed a clear cell cytoplasm. There were areas with increased cellularity and increased mitotic activity. Bi-nucleated and dysplastic neuronal cells were also observed. In addition, there was micro-vascular proliferation, thrombotic vascular occlusions and circumscribed foci of necrosis. No reticulin fibre meshwork was visible using Gomori trichrome staining.

The tumour was characterized by its strong CD34 immunoreactivity. The majority of tumour cells showed immunoreactivity for GFAP but no co-expression with MAP2. Few intermingled dysplastic neurones with immunoreactivity for MAP2 and synaptophysin. No immunoreactivity with mutation-specific IDH1-antibodies. Up to 25-30% of tumour cells had a nuclear accumulation of p53. The proliferation activity, as indexed by MIB1/Ki-67 immunohistochemistry, was increased and exceeded focally 10%.

Comments
The microscopic inspection of the specimen revealed a bi-phasically differentiated glio-neuronal tumour with malignant transformation, *i.e.* increased pleomorphism and cellularity with mitotic activity, micro-vascular proliferation and small foci of necrosis. The tumour was immunohistochemically characterized by its prominent CD34 immunoreactivity and would classify, therefore, as anaplastic ganglioglioma (WHO III°).

Microscopic findings in an anaplastic ganglioglioma (WHO III°)

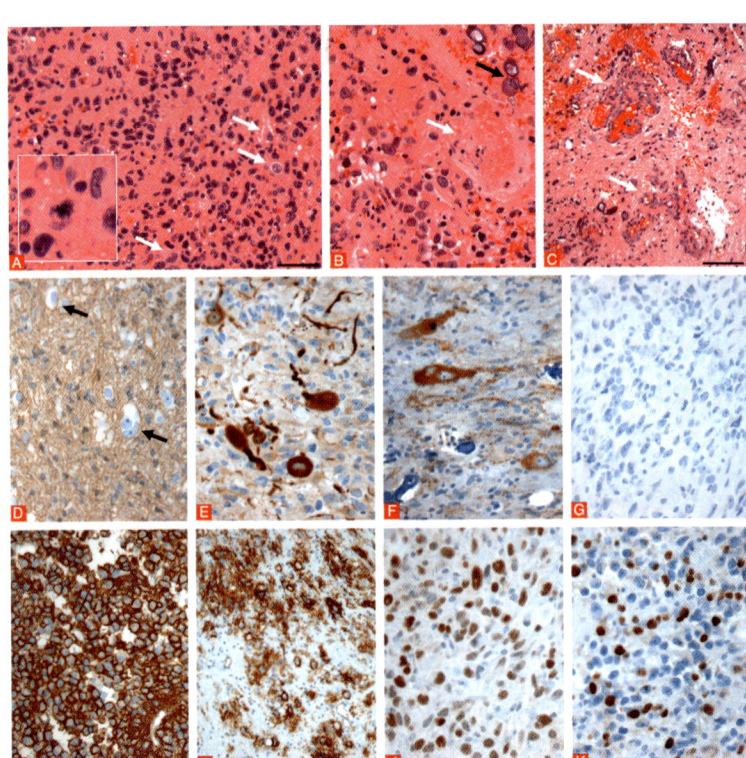

Figure 31

A-C. H&E stainings showed a pleomorphic tumour with increased cellularity (A) composed of a predominant glial component and few dysplastic neurones (white arrows in A). Inset in A: higher magnification of a mitotic figure. In addition, areas with thrombotic occlusions of vessels (white arrow in B) and micro-vascular proliferation (white arrows in C). Note foci of calcifications (black arrow in B). D. Glial tumour cells with immunoreactivity for GFAP (no expression of GFAP in dysplastic neurones: black arrows in D). E-F. MAP2 (E) and synaptophysin (F) immunoreactivity in dysplastic neurones but not the glial tumour component. G. No IDH-1 mutation. H-I. Strong CD34 immunoreactivity of the tumour mass (H) as well as tumour cell satellites in adjacent tissue (I). J. Prominent nuclear accumulation of p53. K. Significantly increased proliferation activity (MIB1/Ki-67 labelling). Scale bar in A: 50 μm, applies also for B, D-G, J & K. Scale bar in C: 100 μm, applies also for H & I.

Dysembryoplastic neuroepithelial tumour (WHO I°)

Clinical history

34-year old male patient with right temporal epilepsy since age of 29 years. MRI showed a tumour of the right amygdala, hyperintense on T2/FLAIR (*Figure 32A, B*, white arrows) and non-contrast enhancing on T1 (*Figure 32C*, white arrow).

Histopathology and immunohistochemistry

We received a soft surgical tissue specimen from the temporal lobe with a total size of 7 × 4 × 2 cm. Serial sections revealed a microcystic tumour without clear demarcation between grey and white matter. Microscopic inspection of the tissue specimen showed a predominantly isomorphic, glio-neuronal tumour of moderate cellularity (*Figure 33*). The tumour cells typically had small, round nuclei and dense chromatin. Cytoplasm was sparse. Focally cells showed clear cellular cytoplasm. Within the tumour matrix were small cystic structures with mucinous content in which several neurones were embedded (so-called "floating neurones"). No mitoses were detected. No microvascular proliferation or necrosis was seen. There was alternating immunoreactivity for GFAP, foremost focally within the tumour matrix. MAP2 highlighted neuronal cells within the tumour as well as scattered small tumour cells. NeuN labelled "floating" neurons. Immunoreactivities with antibodies against IDH-1 and p53 were negative. CD34 reactivity was restricted to endothelial cells. No CD34-positive tumour cells or satellite cells were detectable. Proliferative activity (MIB1/Ki-67) remained below 2%.

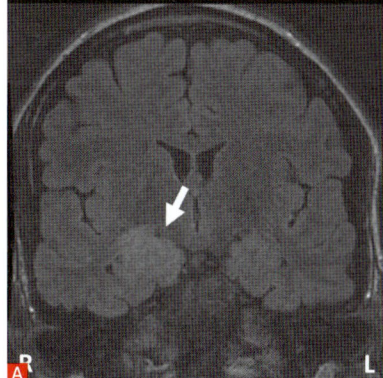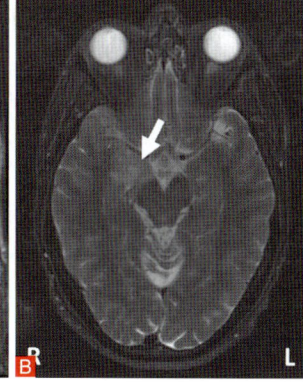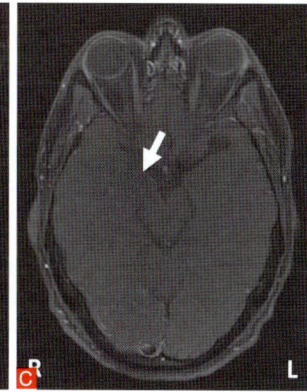

Figure 32

Comments

Microscopic inspection of the tissue specimen revealed fragments of neocortical tissue infiltrated by a relatively isomorphic tumour with characteristic histomorphological differentiation and immunohistochemical patterns of dysembryoplastic neuroepithelial tumour (DNT), corresponding to WHO° I Grade I. The lack of a multinodular architecture may qualify as a simple DNT variant according to the 2007 WHO classification system of brain tumours. However, the subclassification of DNT variants is controversial and does not correlate with clinical features or post-surgical outcome (Blümcke *et al.*, 2014, Thom *et al.*, 2012, Thom *et al.*, 2011).

Microscopic findings in a DNT (WHO I°)

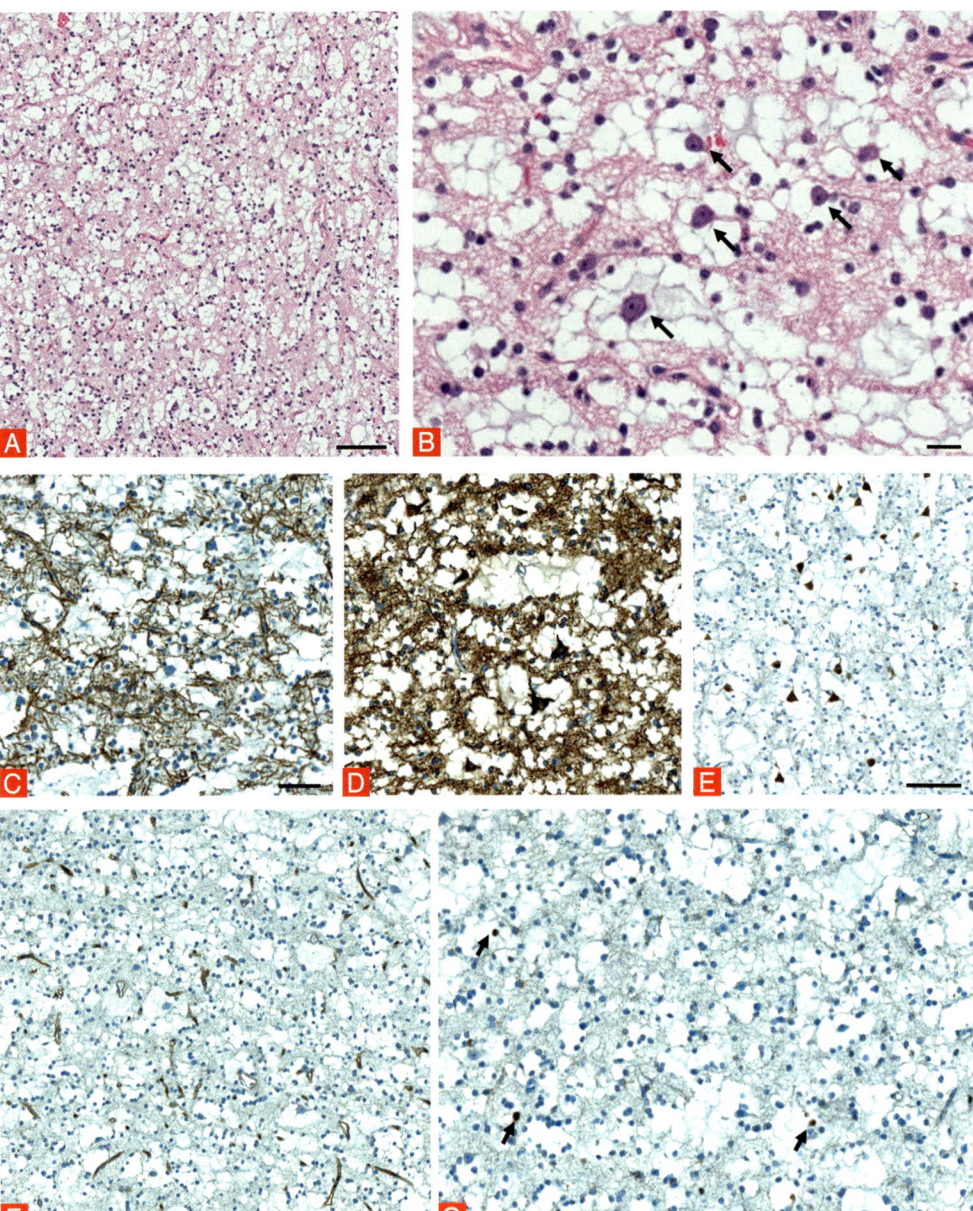

Figure 33

A & B. H&E staining showing an isomorphic, glio-neuronal tumour of moderate cellularity with micro-cystic structures and a mucinous content. Within the micro-cysts are so-called "floating" neurones (arrows in B). C. Alternating immunoreactivity for GFAP. D. MAP2 highlighted neurones within the tumour matrix, as well as small glial tumour cells. E. Floating neurones within the tumour matrix were highlighted by NeuN immunoreactivity. F. CD34 was restricted to endothelial cells. No CD34-positive tumour cells or tumour cell satellites were detectable. G. Proliferative activity (MIB1/Ki-67) remained below 2% (arrows). Scale bar in A: 100 μm. Scale bar in B: 20 μm. Scale bar in C: 50 μm, applies also to D. Scale bar in E-G: 100 μm.

Dysembryoplastic neuroepithelial tumour (WHO I°)/variant

Clinical history

15-year old girl with epilepsy and a suspected low-grade tumour of the right temporal lobe. Clinical suspicion of ganglioglioma.

Histopathology and immunohistochemistry

We received soft to firm light-brownish tissue (size 3 × 2 × 1.8 cm, *Figure 34A*), which was dissected and entirely embedded in paraffin. On H&E-stained sections, microscopic inspection revealed cortical grey and subcortical white matter with infiltration of an unusually configured glio-neuronal tumour. The tumour showed a diffuse infiltrative pattern with prominent clear-cell morphology and few branching processes. Furthermore, we observed nodular tumour growth (*Figure 34B*) within a mucinous micro-cystic matrix, glial-like cells with small round nuclei and few "floating" neurones. The capillary network didn't reveal excessive branching. This pattern can be classified as a specific glio-neuronal element. There were no mitotic spindles seen and no signs of acute inflammation.

GFAP-immunoreactivity showed numerous reactive astrocytes in the adjacent neocortex as well as the glial tumour component. MAP2-labelling recognized scattered neuronal elements within the tumour as well as a small tumour cell component. Neurofilament-protein and synaptophysin immunoreactivity labelled neuronal cell processes in the tumour. CD34-immunoreactivity was restricted to endothelial cells. CD34-positive tumour cells or tumour cell satellites were not detectable in the adjacent neocortex. Immunoreactivity with antibodies against IDH-1 and p53 were negative. The proliferation rate (as indexed by MIB1/Ki-67 immunoreactivity) was low and did not exceed 2%.

Comments

The microscopic inspection of the surgical specimen revealed fragments of neocortex with a glio-neuronal tumour and different patterns of differentiation. On the one hand, the tumour showed a mucinous matrix, oligodendroglia-like cells and floating neurones. Other areas of this tumour showed a diffuse infiltrative pattern. In summary we classify this tumour as dysembryoplastic neuroepithelial tumour (DNT), corresponding to WHO° I Grade I. Based on the different patterns of differentiation the lesion could represent a complex DNT variant, but this sub-classification has no clinical or therapeutic implications (Thom *et al.*, 2011). The specific glio-neuronal element and lack of CD34 expression also did not support the clinically suspected ganglioglioma. There were no signs for atypia or anaplasia.

Macroscopic and microscopic findings in a DNT (WHO I°) (see *Figure 34*)

Figure 34

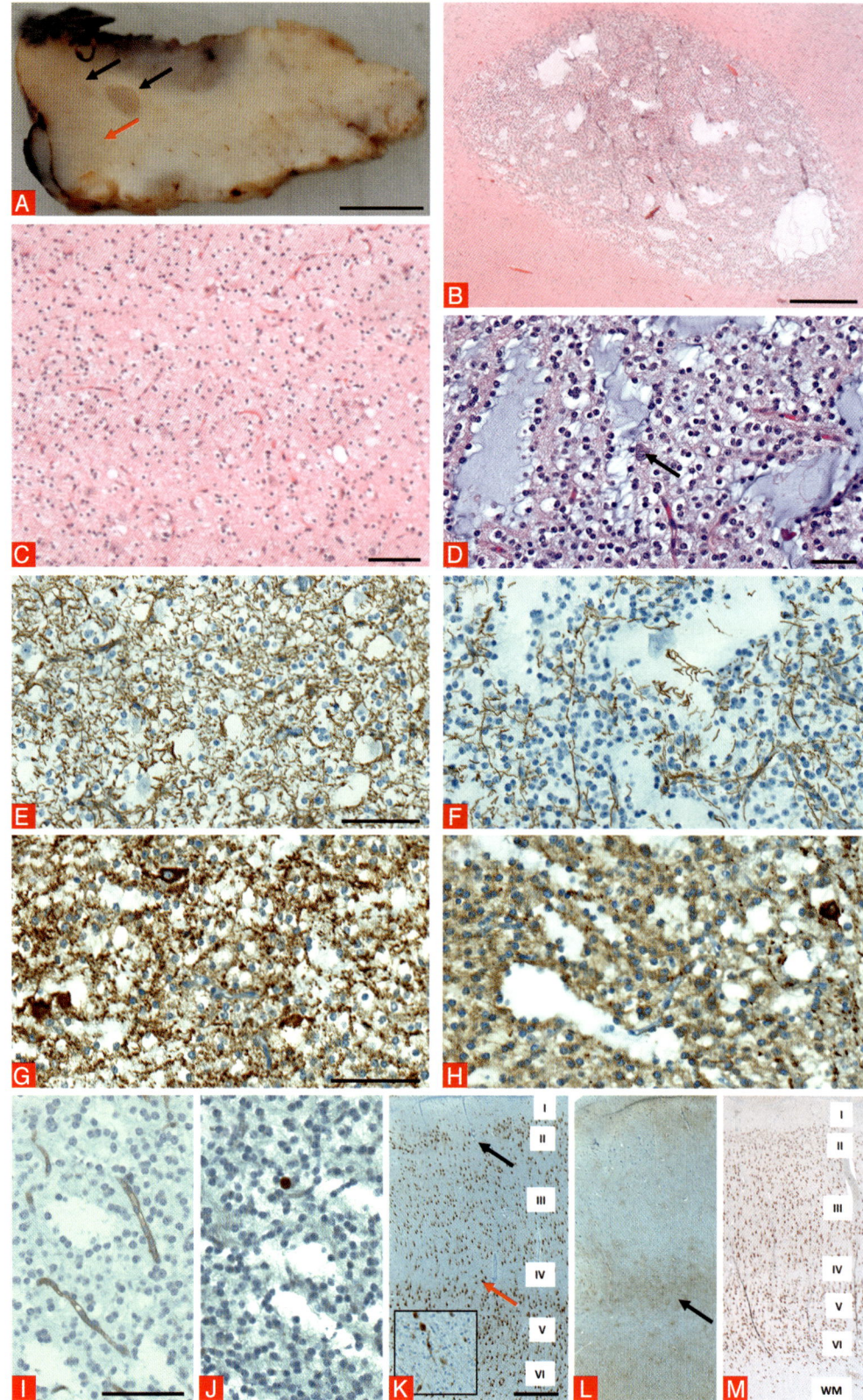

A. Macroscopic inspection revealed a thickened cortical ribbon (red arrow) without visible grey/white matter boundaries (histology of these areas is depicted in C, E and G). In addition, multiple nodules (black arrows) at the grey/white matter junction as well as in the subcortical white matter (histology of these areas is depicted in B, D, F and H). B & D. Nodular tumour growth with a predominant mucinous matrix, glial-like cells with small round nuclei and few "floating" mature neurones (arrow in D). C. Diffuse cortical infiltration patterns with a clear-cell morphology. E & F. GFAP immunohistochemistry and G & H. MAP2 immunohistochemistry characterising different growth pattern components. I. no CD34 immunoreactivity (positive endothelial staining served as control). J. proliferation activity was low (Ki-67 staining). K. Cortical ribbon in close vicinity to the tumour appeared dyslaminated with patchy neuronal loss in layer II (black arrow) and laminar neuronal cell loss in layer IV (red arrow). However, higher magnification (inset from red arrow region) showed infiltrating tumour cells with concomitant astrogliosis (serial section in L stained for GFAP). M. Adjacent cortical ribbon not infiltrated by tumour always showed a regular architecture without distinct signs for an associated focal cortical dysplasia Type IIIb (ILAE classification). I-IV: cortical layers. WM: white matter. Scale bar in A: 0.5 cm. Scale bar in B: 500 µm. Scale bar in C: 100 µm. Scale bar in D: 50 µm. Scale bar in E: 100 µm, applies also for F. Scale bar in G: 100 µm, applies also for H. Scale bar in I: 100 µm, applies also for J. Scale bar in K: 500 µm, applies also for L and M.

Pilocytic astrocytoma (WHO I°)

Clinical history

9-year old male patient with epilepsy starting at age of 8 years. MRI revealed a right parietal tumour with a huge cyst and contrast enhancing nodule (black arrow in *Figure 35A*: T2/FLAIR MRI). Suspected pilocytic astrocytoma.

Histopathology and immunohistochemistry

We received unfixed tissue with a total size of 6 × 4 × 1.5 cm. Macroscopically, we observed a regular gyral surface (*Figure 35B*). A cystic lesion (white arrow in D) with a mural nodule (black arrows in *Figure 35C & D*; C: flipside of B) was visible at the flipside. The material was sliced and embedded in 11 paraffin blocks.

Microscopic inspection of the specimen revealed cortical grey matter with regular lamination and subcortical white matter. There were areas with a pseudocystic lesion and adherent tumour of moderate cellularity. The tumour cells showed astrocytic differentiation with piloidal processes (*Figure 36*). The nuclei were small to mid-sized, had round to oval nuclei and fine speckled chromatin. The tumour showed a bi-phasic growth pattern. On the one hand, a loose tumour matrix with micro-cysts and multipolar tumour cells. On the other hand, compact areas with bipolar cells. Rosenthal fibres and eosinophilic granular bodies were visible in several areas. Blood vessels in the tumour matrix were focally thickened. However, there was no distinct micro-vascular proliferation or tumour necrosis. Adjacent neocortical areas showed always a regular layering.

Tumour cells labelled strongly with an antibody against GFAP as well as co-expression of MAP2. CD34 immunoreactive tumour cells or tumour cell satellites were not detectable. Immunoreactivity with antibodies against IDH-1 was negative. 1-2% of tumour cells with a faint p53 nuclear accumulation. The proliferation activity, as indexed by MIB1/Ki-67 labelling reaches 2-3%. NeuN immunohistochemistry revealed no associated cortical dyslamination in adjacent neocortical fields.

Comments

Microscopic inspection of the specimen revealed cortical grey and subcortical white matter with a well differentiated astrocytic tumour. The tumour showed histomorphological features and an immunohistochemical profile characteristic for a pilocytic astrocytoma (PA), corresponding to WHO° I Grade I. There were no signs for malignancy.

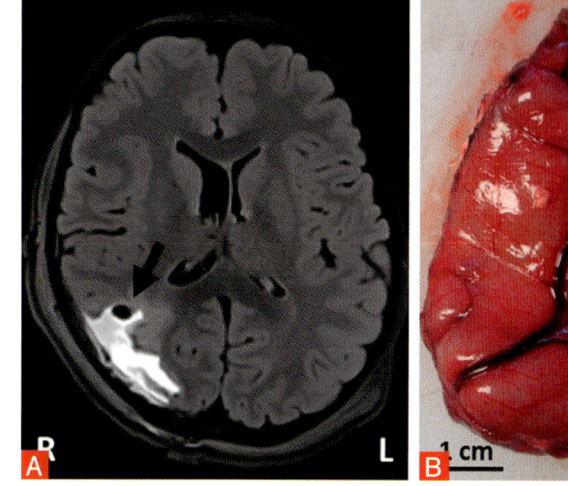
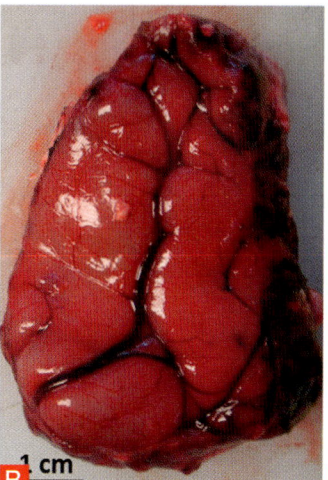
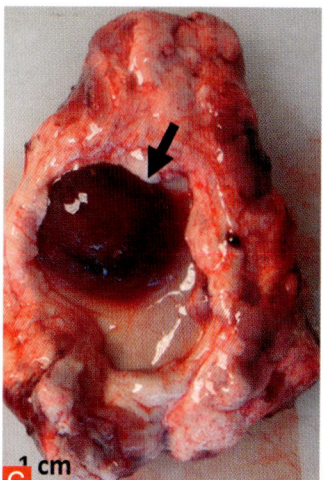
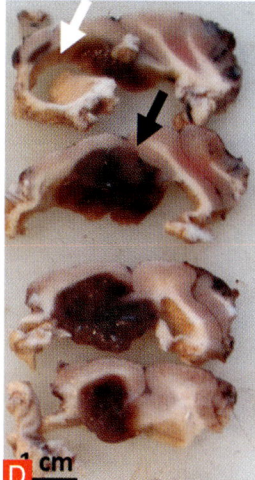

Figure 35

Supratentorial PAs were observed in 1.2% of patients submitted to epilepsy surgery in our series (see *chapter 8, Table I*). They were predominantly located in the temporal lobe (69%), and patients had seizure onset at a mean age of 15 years.

Microscopic findings in a pilocytic astrocytoma (WHO I°)

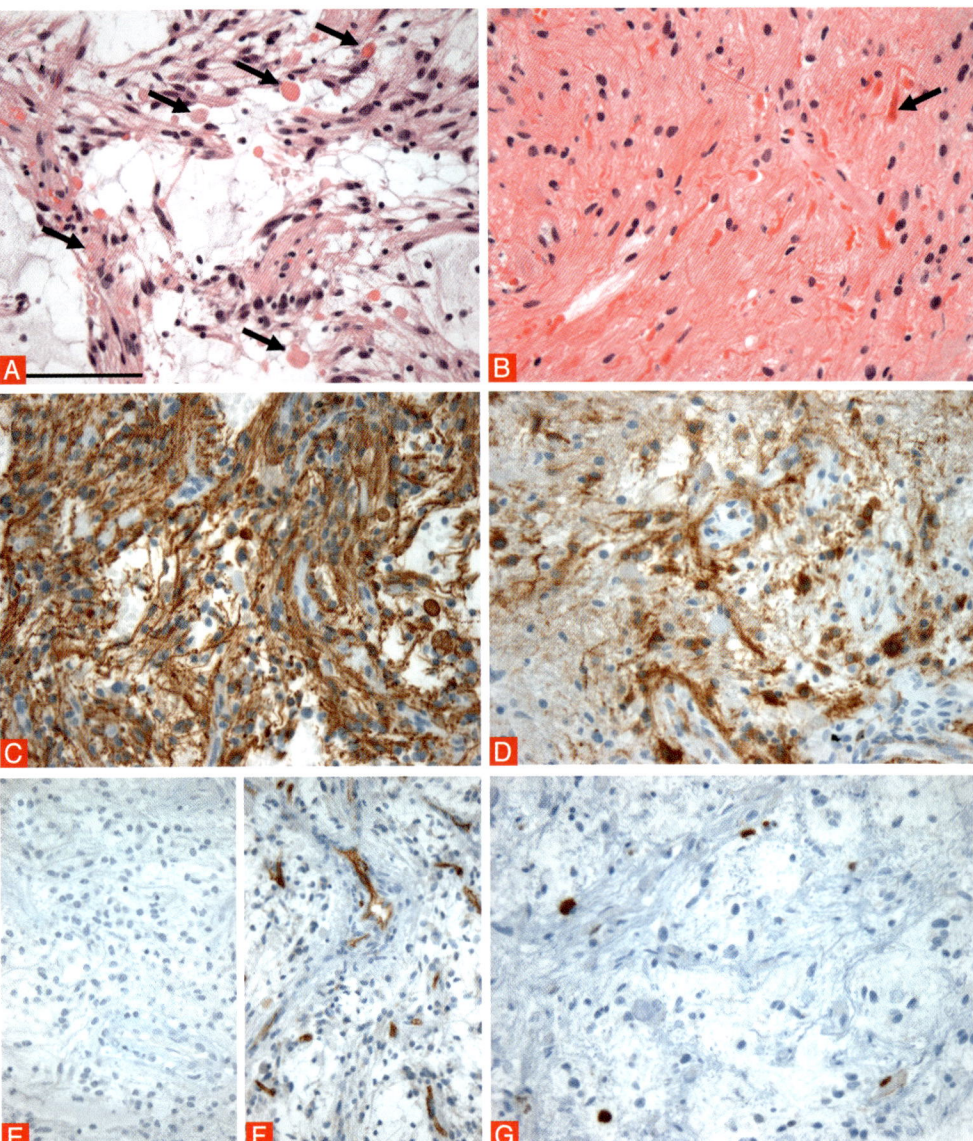

Figure 36

A–B. H&E staining showing an astrocytic tumour with a biphasic growth pattern. **A:** micro-cystic areas with bi-polar tumour cells, eosinophilic granular bodies and hyaline droplets (black arrows in A) next to more compacted piloidal regions with numerous Rosenthal fibres (black arrow in B) as shown here in B. **C–D.** The tumour cells showed co-expression of GFAP (in C) and MAP2 (in D). **E.** No IDH-1 mutation (E). **F.** CD34 immunohistochemistry highlighted only vascular endothelia but no tumour cells or tumour cell satellites. **G.** Proliferation activity (MIB1/Ki-67 staining) was low and did not exceed 3%. Scale bar in A: 100 μm, applies also for B-D & G. Scale bar in E: 100 μm, applies also for F.

Isomorphic astrocytoma variant (analogue WHO I°)

Clinical history

6-year old boy with complex partial seizures. Imaging revealed a lesion in the right temporal lobe without peripheral oedema or contrast enhancement (white arrow in *Figure 37A*; T1 weighted image).

Histopathology and immunohistochemistry

We received a white to greyish, partly light brownish, soft tissue specimen with a total size of 4 × 2.5 × 2.5 cm. Representative material was embedded in four paraffin blocks. Macroscopic inspection revealed predominantly white matter alterations with softened tissue (black arrows in B). Microscopic inspection of the four specimens showed cortical grey and subcortical white matter. There was a moderate increase of cellularity affecting the subcortical white matter. The cells showed small, round to oval nuclei with a predominantly dispersed chromatin structure. No mitotic figures were detectable. Cellular processes showed fine arborisation giving rise to a fibrillary matrix. Micro-vascular proliferation or necrosis was not detectable. We also identified heterotopic neurones in these areas. A dysplastic neuronal component could not be verified. We classify this astroglial cell population as isomorphic variant of a diffusely infiltrating astrocytoma (Schramm *et al.*, 2004; Blümcke *et al.*, 2004). The tumour infiltrates were predominantly in the white matter. However, at circumscribed sites, there was also a diffuse cortical infiltration. Areas of the cortical ribbon, apparently not infiltrated by the tumour showed a regular architecture without any signs of a disturbed layering. Several regions showing blurred grey/white matter boundaries.

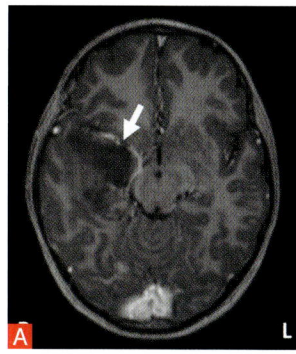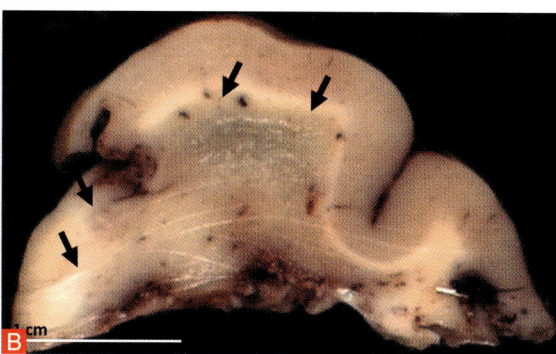

Figure 37

Figure B: Courtesy of Dr. V. Hans, Bielefeld-Bethel, Germany.

The glial tumour cell component was immunoreactive for GFAP without MAP2-(co)expression (*Figure 38*). No dysplastic neuronal tumour component, neither detectable by MAP2 or synaptophysin. CD34 immunoreactivity was restricted to vascular endothelia. CD34 immunoreactive tumour cells or tumour cell satellites were not detectable. Immunoreactivity with antibodies against IDH-1 and p53 were negative. The proliferation activity, as indexed by MIB1 (Ki-67) immunoreactivity was low and did not exceed 1-2%. No evidence was demonstrated for horizontal or radial dyslamination (NeuN).

Comments

Microscopic inspection revealed central nervous tissue with infiltration by an isomorphic, astrocytic tumour of low to moderate cellularity. The tumour was characterized by strong GFAP-expression, lack of MAP2- and CD34-immunoreactivity as well as absent nuclear p53 accumulation, no IDH-1 mutation and low mitotic/proliferation activity. In summary, we classified this tumour as a low-grade-astrocytoma (isomorphic subtype, analogous to WHO Grade I; [Blümcke *et al.*, 2004]). There were no clues for atypia or malignancy.

Isomorphic astrocytoma variants are rare, representing 0.3% of cases submitted to epilepsy surgery (see *chapter 8, Table I*). Their preferred localization is the temporal and occipital lobe, and patients had seizure onset at a mean age of 14.6 years.

Microscopic findings in an isomorphic astrocytoma variant

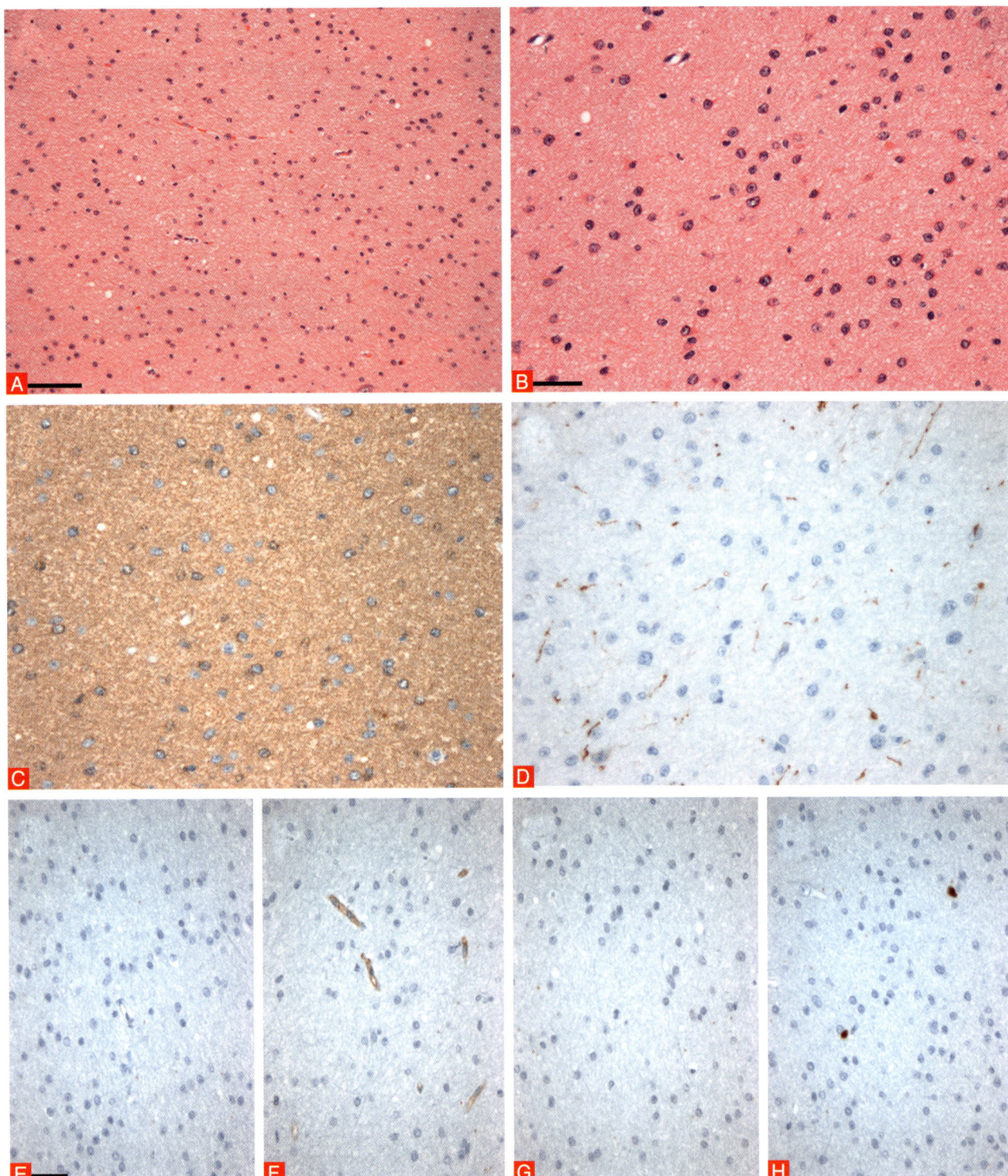

Figure 38

A & B. H&E stainings showing an isomorphic, astrocytic tumour of low to moderate cellularity with a dense fibrillary matrix. **C.** The tumour cells were labelled with an antibody directed against GFAP. **D.** No co-expression with MAP2, thereby also excluding any neuronal tumour component. **E.** No IDH-1 mutation. **F.** CD34-immunoreactivity was restricted to endothelial cells. No CD34-positive tumour cells or tumour cell satellites were visible. **G.** No nuclear p53 staining. **H.** Proliferation activity (MIB1/Ki-67 staining) was low. Scale bar in A: 100 μm. Scale bar in B: 50 μm, applies also for C & D. Scale bar in E: 50 μm, applies also for F-H.

Angiocentric glioma (WHO I°)

Clinical history

28-year old female patient with drug-resistant epilepsy. MRI revealed a tumour in the right temporal lobe. (*Figure 39A*, B: T1 weighted image, C: T2 weighted image). Suspected ganglioglioma. Differential diagnosis: pilocytic astrocytoma.

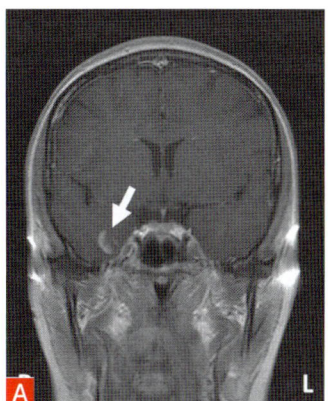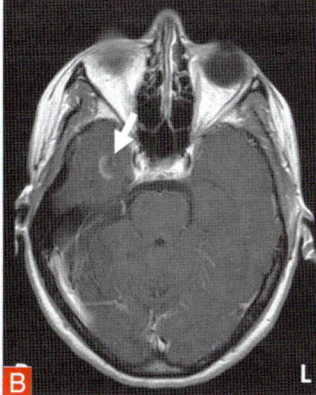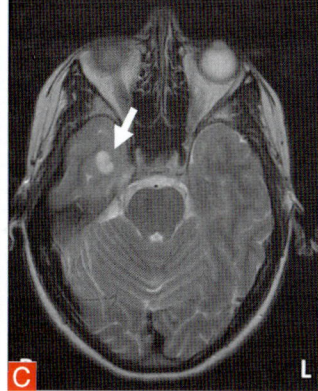

Figure 39

Histopathology and immunohistochemistry

We received white to greyish, partly brownish, soft tissue fragments with a total size of 3 × 2.3 × 0.6 cm. Microscopic inspection of the tissue specimen revealed fragments of central nervous tissue infiltrated by a relatively well differentiated neuroepithelial tumour. The spindle-shaped tumour cells showed small to mid-sized, predominantly oval nuclei with granular chromatin and nucleoli. No significant mitotic activity was seen. The tumour cells formed processes, several areas showing elongated bi-polar processes. There were micro-cystic loose areas next to regions with a more compact growth pattern. In several areas tumour cells were arranged around blood vessels (perivascular pseudorosettes; *Figure 40B*). Focally, an ependymal-like lining was observed. No tumour necrosis or distinctive microvascular proliferation were found. The tumour showed no dense reticulin fibre network (Gomori staining). Tumour cells showed a homogeneous expression of GFAP. No significant co-expression with MAP2. MAP2 labelled only fragments of the central nervous tissue. Focally, tumour cells exhibited small dot-like, EMA-positive intra-cytoplasmatic inclusions. CD34 labelled only vascular endothelium. CD34 immunoreactive tumour cells or tumour cell satellites were not detectable. No IDH1 mutation (negative immunoreactivity for mutation-specific IDH1 antibody). The tumour cells showed no synaptophysin or pan-cytokeratin (KL-1) expression. A predominantly faint nuclear p53 accumulation was seen in 10-15% of tumour cells. The proliferation activity (Ki-67 labelling) was low and focally reached only 1-2%.

Comments

Microscopic inspection revealed fragments of a well differentiated, neuroepithelial tumour. The histomorphological aspect and the immunohistochemical pattern indicate an angiocentric glioma, also termed as angiocentric neuroepithelial tumour (ANET), corresponding to WHO Grade I (Lellouch-Tubiana *et al.*, 2005, Wang *et al.*, 2005). No signs for atypia or anaplasia were demonstrated. We also considered ependymoma in the differential diagnosis. However, there were no further clues for ependymoma, ganglioglioma or pilocytic astrocytoma.

Angiocentric gliomas are rare, representing 0.1% of cases submitted to epilepsy surgery (see *chapter 8, Table I*). Half of all angiocentric gliomas were observed in the temporal lobe (50%), and patients had seizure onset at a mean age of 7 years.

Microscopic findings in an angiocentric glioma (WHO I°)

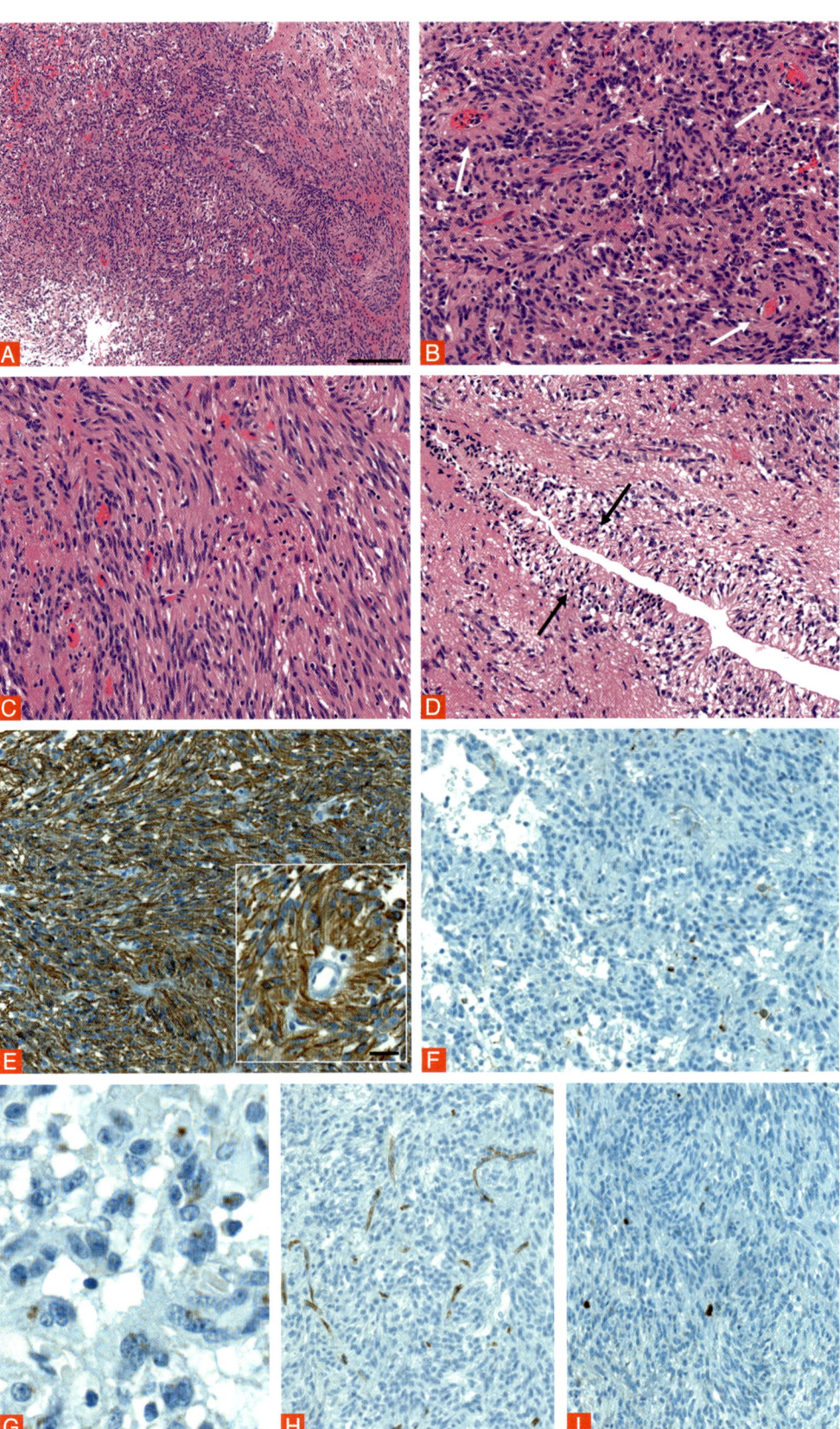

Figure 40

A–D. H&E staining showed a well differentiated spindle-shaped tumour (C) with tumour cells arranged around blood vessels (white arrows in B). Focally, there was an ependymal-like lining (arrows in D). **E.** Tumour cells with homogeneous expression for GFAP. Inset in E: Tumour cells in perivascular pseudorosettes expressed GFAP. **F.** No significant co-expression with MAP2. **G.** Focally, tumour cells with small dot-like, EMA-positive intra-cytoplasmatic inclusions. **H.** CD34 labelled vascular endothelium only. No detectable CD34 immunoreactive tumour cells or tumour cell satellites. **I.** Low proliferation activity (Ki-67 labelling). Scale bar in A: 200 µm. Scale bar in B: 50 µm, applies also for C–F. Inset in E: 20 µm. Scale bar in G: 20 µm. Scale bar in H: 50 µm, applies also for I.

Pleomorphic xanthoastrocytoma (WHO II°)

Clinical history

31-year old male patient with drug-resistant epilepsy starting at age of 19 years. MRI revealed a right parieto-occipital tumour with partial contrast enhancement suspicious for pilocytic astrocytoma.

Histopathology and immunohistochemistry

We received several white to brownish and yellowish tissue fragments with a total size of 3 × 2.5 × 1 cm. The material was embedded entirely in two paraffin blocks. Microscopic inspection revealed a cellular, pleomorphic tumour. The tumour showed a superficial cortical infiltration and invaded the subarachnoid space (*Figure 41*). The tumour cells presented with nuclei of variable size were multinucleated. The majority of tumour cells had elongated processes. We also observed eosinophilic granular bodies, and foamy, vacuolated cells. Few mitoses were visible. Perivascular lymphocytic cuffing was focally detected. Several areas revealed a fascicular architecture and a dense reticulin fibre meshwork (best visible by Gomori staining). There was no tumour necrosis visible.

The tumour cells showed alternating co-expression of GFAP and MAP2. However, several areas also showed tumour cells immunoreactive for CD34, whereas synaptophysin and NeuN immunoreactivity did not identify a dysplastic neuronal component. Immunoreactivity with antibodies against IDH-1 and p53 were negative. The proliferation activity (Ki-67 labelling) was low and did not exceed 5%.

Comments

Microscopic inspection revealed a pleomorphic tumour with differentiation patterns and an immunohistochemical profile characteristic for a pleomorphic xanthoastrocytoma (PXA), corresponding to WHO II°. There were no signs for anaplastic transformation. The differential diagnoses should always consider a pilocytic astrocytoma or ganglioglioma. This tumour entity shares CD34 immunoreactivity with ganglioglioma (Reifenberger *et al.*, 2003), and is regarded as semi-benign.

PXAs are rare, representing 0.5% of cases submitted to epilepsy surgery in our series (see *chapter 8, Table I*). Their preferred localisation is in the temporal lobe (73.1%), and patients had seizure onset at a mean age of 18.8 years.

Microscopic findings in a pleomorphic xanthoastrocytoma (WHO II°)

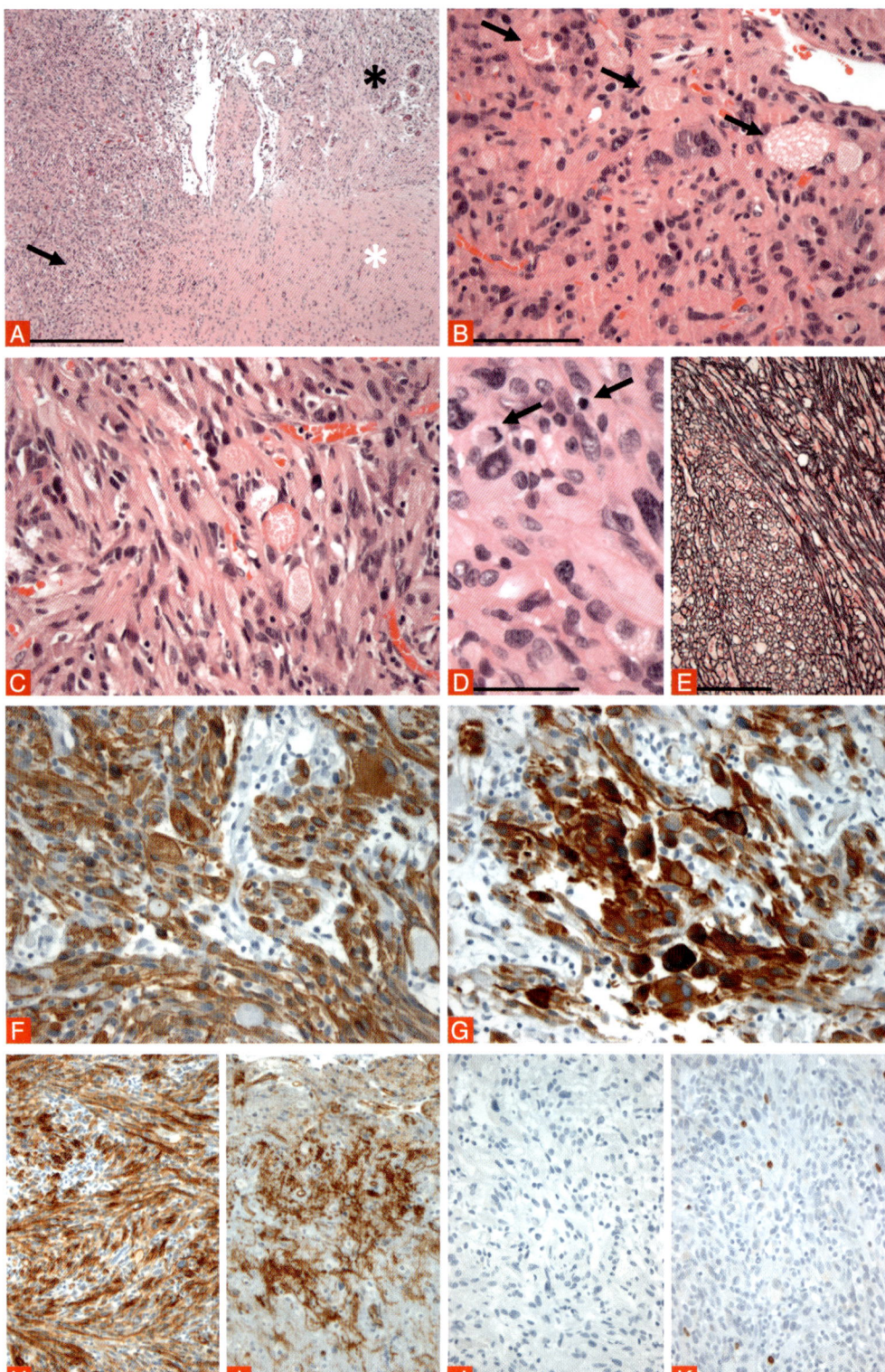

Figure 41

A. Overview (H&E staining) demonstrating a cellular tumour with growth into subarachnoid space (black asterisk; white asterisk indicates superficial neocortex) and cortical infiltration (black arrow). **B.** Higher magnification showing a pleomorphic glial tumour with bi- as well as multi-nucleated tumour cells intermingled with xanthomatous cells and granular bodies (black arrows). **C.** Fascicular growth pattern with a dense reticulin fibre meshwork (Gomori histochemical staining shown in E). **D.** Quantitative assessment revealed 5 mitoses per 10 high power fields. **F-G.** Co-expression of GFAP (F) and MAP2 (G). **H-I.** Areas with strong CD34 immunoreactivity (H) and CD34-positive tumour satellites infiltrating cortical regions (I). **J.** No IDH-1 mutation. **K.** Low proliferation activity (MIB1/Ki-67 labelling) < 5%. Scale bar in A: 500 µm. Scale bar in B: 100 µm, applies also for C, F & G. Scale bar in D: 50 µm. Scale bar in E: 200 µm. Scale bar in H: 100 µm, applies also for I. Scale bar in J: 50 µm, applies also for K.

Papillary glio-neuronal tumour (WHO I°)

Clinical history

27-year old male patient with tumour-associated epilepsy and two generalized seizures. A lesion was detected in the right temporal lobe, suspicious for astrocytoma, ganglioglioma or neurocytoma.

Histopathology and immunohistochemistry

We received several small, soft, grey and white tissue fragments with a total size of 1 × 1 × 0.5 cm. The material has been embedded entirely in one paraffin block. In routine H&E staining, small fragments of a glio-neuronal tumour could be identified. The cell number was not particularly high. Most cells displayed a round and small nucleus. Cells with fibrillary processes were considered as glial component, whereas other cells resemble small immature neurones. The matrix was mostly loose and a little mucinous with many capillaries and blood vessels. A hallmark of this peculiar tumour was that many (neuronal) tumour cells are located around small blood vessels, which gave rise to a predominant "papillary" architecture (*Figure 42B*). In addition, few small fragments of neocortex were attached. No evidence for necrosis or inflammation.

The glial component of the tumour could be identified using antibodies against GFAP, whereas neuronal cells were immunoreactive for neuronal markers NeuN and MAP2. Most importantly, the papillary architecture contained a dense synaptophysin expression. The proliferation activity (immunoreactivity for MIB1/Ki-67) was low (< 2%). Immunoreaction for CD34 and p53 did not show any specific labelling pattern.

Comments

The surgical specimens revealed a benign tumour with glio-neuronal differentiation. Due to the characteristic perivascular and papillary architecture, it should be classified as papillary glio-neuronal tumour (PGNT), corresponding to WHO I°. The differential diagnosis should comprise DNT as well as a ganglioglioma. However, both entities usually present with a different cellular and immunoreactivity pattern. The histopathological aspect did not match that of a (clinically discussed) neurocytoma or astrocytoma. The neuronal character of perivascular cells excluded the now obsolete designation of "astroblastoma".

PGNT are rare, with only 2 examples identified in our series of 5,603 patients submitted to epilepsy surgery (see *chapter 8, Table I*). Both tumours were observed in the temporal lobe, and patients had late seizure onset at age of 31 years.

Microscopic findings in a papillary glio-neuronal tumour (WHO I°)

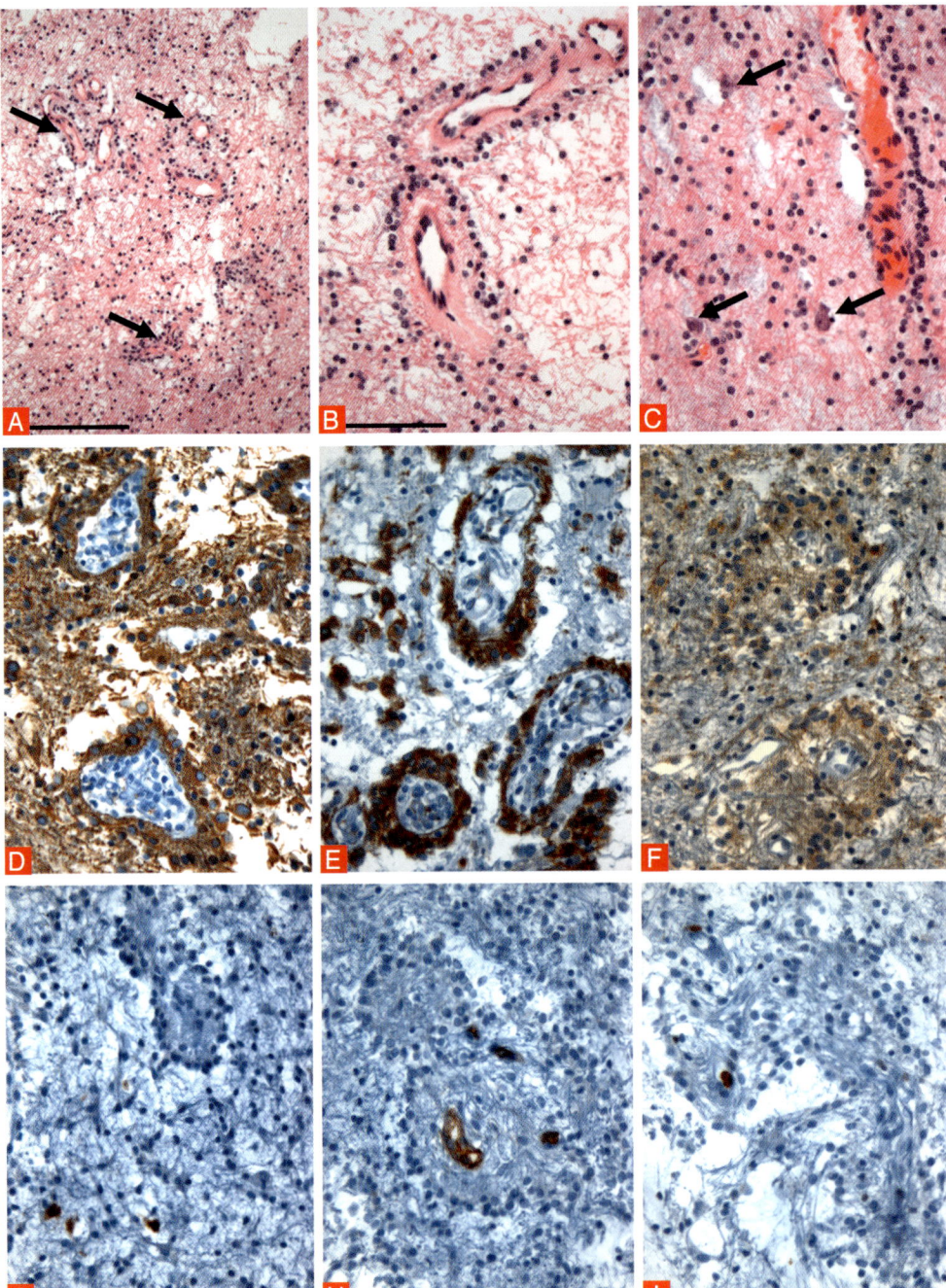

Figure 42

A-C. H&E stainings showing a tumour with perivascular pseudo-papillae (arrows in A) and small hyalinised vessels with a (single) layer of surrounding small and cuboidal cells (higher magnification in B). Small neurocytic cells as well as larger ganglion-like cells were visible between papillae (arrows in C). D. GFAP immunoreactive cells around vessels as well as between papillary structures. E-F. Co-expression of MAP2 (E) and synaptophysin (F). G: ganglion-like cells with NeuN immunoreactivity. H. CD34 immunohistochemistry highlighted vascular endothelia but no CD34 immunoreactive tumour cells. I. Proliferation activity was low (MIB1/Ki-67 staining). Scale bar in A: 200 µm. Scale bar in B: 100 µm, applies also for C-I.

Multinodular and vacuolating neuronal tumour (analogue WHO I°)

Clinical history

29-year old male patient with drug-resistant epilepsy. MRI revealed a lesion in the right temporal lobe with hyperintense subcortical signal alterations (arrows in *Figure 43A and B*). Differential diagnosis was principally between glioma and FCD.

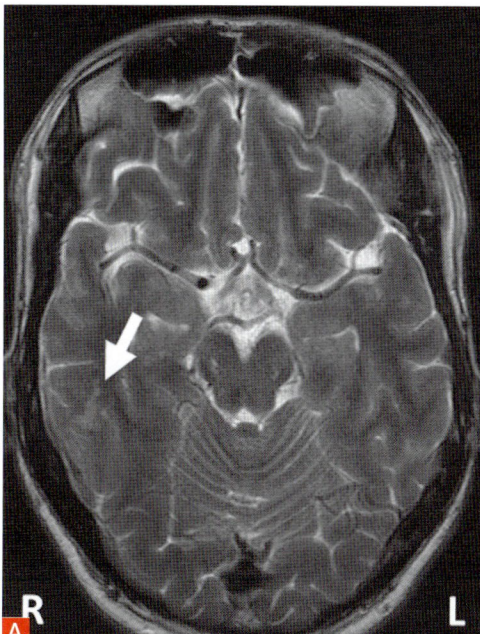
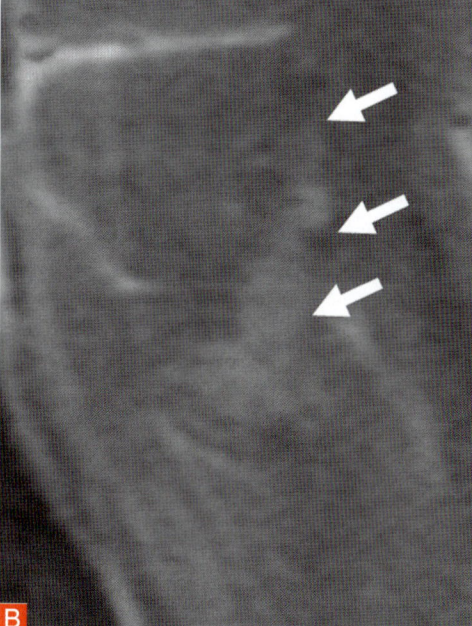

Figure 43

Histopathology and immunohistochemistry

We received white to greyish formalin-fixed tissue with a total size of 3 × 2 × 0.2 cm. The material was entirely embedded in one paraffin block. Microscopic inspection revealed fragments of cortical grey and subcortical white matter. The cortical ribbon showed a regular architecture without signs for cortical dyslamination. The white matter presented with a multinodular sharply delineated tumorous lesion (*Figure 44*). The nodules were separated by myelinated white matter bundles and contained neuronal elements with vesicular nuclei, eosinophilic cytoplasm and vacuolation in an otherwise astroglial matrix. A few cells also showed enlarged granular cytoplasm. No mitotic figures, microvascular proliferation or tumour necrosis were visible. The tumour matrix, as well as several cells, showed prominent vacuolation.

The astroglial matrix was labelled with an antibody against GFAP. The cell elements in nodules showed co-expression of neuronal markers (SMI32, MAP2, synaptophysin and NeuN). There was no CD34 expression in tumour cells or tumour cell satellites. Cell proliferative activity (MIB1/Ki-67 immunohistochemistry) was low (< 1%).

Comments

Microscopic inspection revealed cortical grey and subcortical white matter with a sharply demarcated tumorous lesion with nodular architecture in the white matter. We detected several neuronal elements in these areas which were characterized by cell and matrix vacuolation. There were no signs for atypia or anaplasia. In summary, the histomorphological aspect together with the immunohistochemical profile were compatible with the recently described entity of "multinodular and vacuolating neuronal tumour" (Fukushima *et al.*, 2014; Huse *et al.*, 2013; Bodi *et al.*, 2014). This entity has not yet been introduced into the WHO classification of tumours of the central nervous system (2007). However, published work describing this distinct clinico-pathological entity indicate that the biological behaviour of this tumour should be judged analogous to WHO I°. There was no evidence for an associated FCD or an inflammatory process.

Microscopic findings in multinodular and vacuolating neuronal tumour

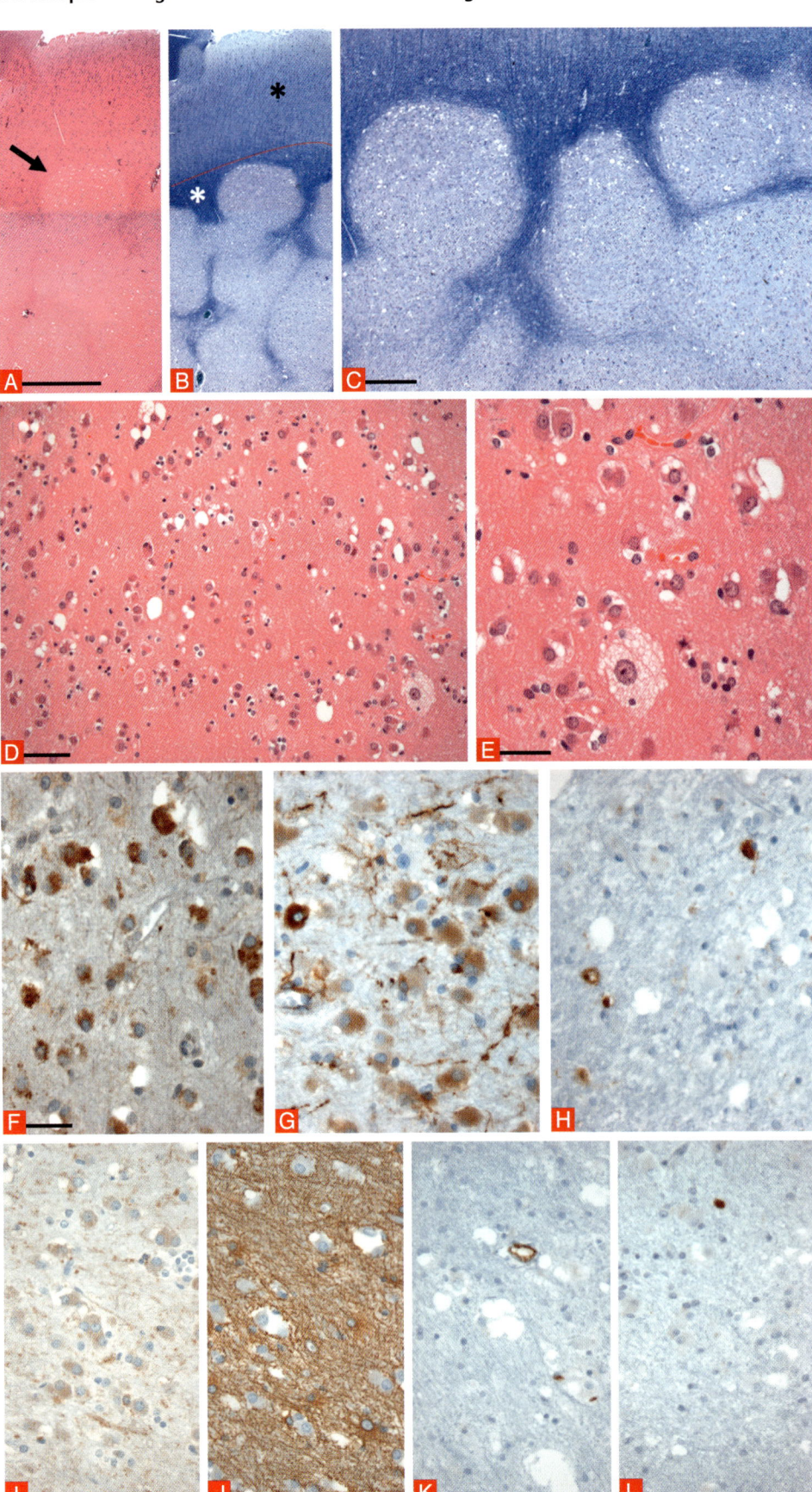

Figure 44

A. H&E staining at low magnification already suggested a tumorous lesion of the white matter with a nodular aspect. **B.** Serial section to A stained with Nissl-LFB highlighting the nodular configuration of the lesion in white matter (white asterisk) without infiltration of the cortical ribbon (black asterisk; red dotted line indicates the grey/white matter boundary). **C.** Higher magnification of B. **D-E.** Higher magnification of H&E stained nodules showing collections of neuronal elements with eosinophilic cytoplasm, few also with a granular cytoplasm as well as cell and matrix vacuolation. **F-I.** Neuronal elements were immunoreactive for neurofilament-protein (SMI32 immunohistochemistry in F) and MAP2 (G) with few showing expression of NeuN (H) and faintly synaptophysin (I). **J.** GFAP labelled an astroglial matrix with reactive cells but no distinct glial tumour component. **K.** CD34 expression visible only in vascular endothelia. **L.** Only single cells with proliferation activity (MIB1/Ki-67). Scale bar in A: 2,000 μm, applies also for B. Scale bar in C: 500 μm. Scale bar in D: 100 μm. Scale bar in E: 50 μm. Scale bar in F: 50 μm, applies also for G & H. Scale bar in I: 100 μm, applies also for J-L.

Rasmussen encephalitis

Clinical history

3-year old girl with seizure onset at the age of one year, suffering from right hemispheric epilepsia partialis continua and absence-like seizures. AED trials with LEV, VPA, OXC and TPM were unsuccessful. Serial MRI showed progressive uni-hemispheric atrophy.

Histopathology and immunohistochemistry

We received a firm surgical tissue specimen with a total size of 3 × 1.5 × 1.5 cm of fronto-central origin (according to accompanying clinical data). The sample was dissected and completely embedded in paraffin. H&E staining revealed the characteristic anatomy of cortical grey and white matter. Cortical ribbon was only focally hypoplastic and revealed an associated FCD ILAE Type IIId (Blümcke *et al.*, 2011, Wang *et al.*, 2013). There were many activated microglial cells visible (CD68 positive), also forming small nodules located in grey matter (*Figure 45*). In addition, lymphocytic infiltrates along small blood vessels but also within brain parenchyma (predominately CD3/CD8 positive T-cells). The T-cells also attack neurons and the cortical ribbon showed several areas with reduced neuronal densities (NeuN). No neurofilament-accumulating dysmorphic neurons (SMI32). GFAP revealed activated astrocytes in grey matter as well as in white matter, associated with otherwise normal myelination (Nissl-LFB staining). CD20-immunopositive B-lymphocytes represented a minority of infiltrating cells. Proliferation activity (as detected by MIB1/Ki-67) was mostly confined to activated microglia.

Comments

Histopathological hallmarks in these specimens were characterized by activated microglia forming microglial nodules in grey and white matter as well as T-lymphocytes along blood vessels also infiltrating brain parenchyma (> 10/mm^2), consistent with the diagnosis of Rasmussen encephalitis (in keeping with clinical and radiological criteria of a uni-hemispheric disease process). These CD8-positive T-lymphocytic "killer cells" have been previously shown to attack and destroy neurones (Bien *et al.*, 2002, Bien *et al.*, 2005). Affected areas showed prominent astrogliosis.

Microscopic findings in Rasmussen encephalitis

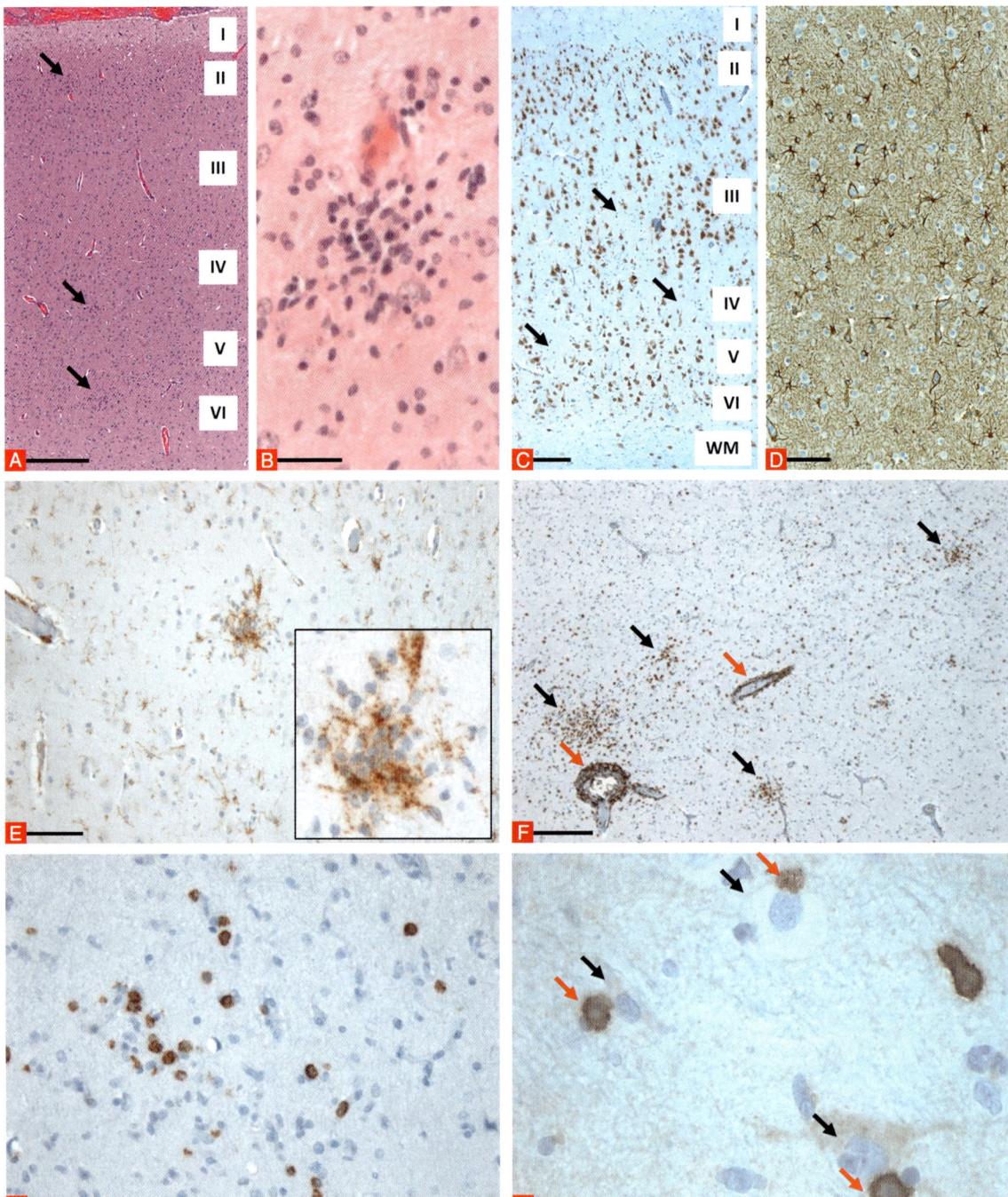

Figure 45

A & B. H&E staining: increased cellular density within the cortical ribbon, diffuse and nodular. B. Higher magnification of A with microglia nodule. C. Focally hypoplastic cortical ribbon with patchy neuronal loss (C: NeuN immunohistochemistry). Differentiation of cortical layers was difficult to recognize in this field, *i.e.* FCD IIId. D. Prominent astrogliosis was visible using GFAP immunohistochemistry. E. Diffuse microglial activation (CD68 immunohistochemistry) as well as microglia nodules (inset in E: higher magnification of microglia nodule). F. T-lymphocytic infiltrates (CD3 immunohistochemistry) along small blood vessels (red arrows) but also within brain parenchyma (black arrows). G. Accumulation of T killer cells (CD8 immunohistochemistry) H. Neurones (black arrows) receiving the "kiss of death" by CD8-positive cytotoxic T cells (red arrows). I-IV: cortical layers. WM: white matter. Scale bar in A: 500 μm. Scale bar in B: 40 μm. Scale bar in C: 200 μm. Scale bar in D: 100 μm. Scale bar in E: 100 μm. Scale bar in F: 250 μm. Scale bar in G: 50 μm. Scale bar in H: 20 μm.

MRI, macroscopic and microscopic findings in different stages of Rasmussen encephalitis

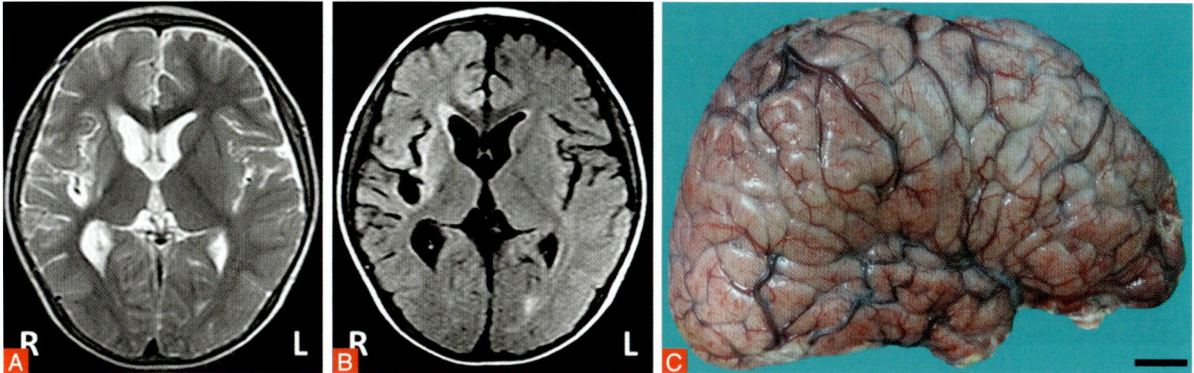

Figure 46

3-year old boy with a two year history of intractable seizures (courtesy of Dr. Dandan Wang, Beijing, China). MRI (**A**. T2 weighted; **B**. FLAIR) revealed signal abnormalities involving the right insular and right frontal lobe. **C**: Macroscopic surgical specimen after modified anatomical hemispherectomy (Scale bar in C = 2 cm). Corresponding histological findings are shown in D-K (*Figure 47*).

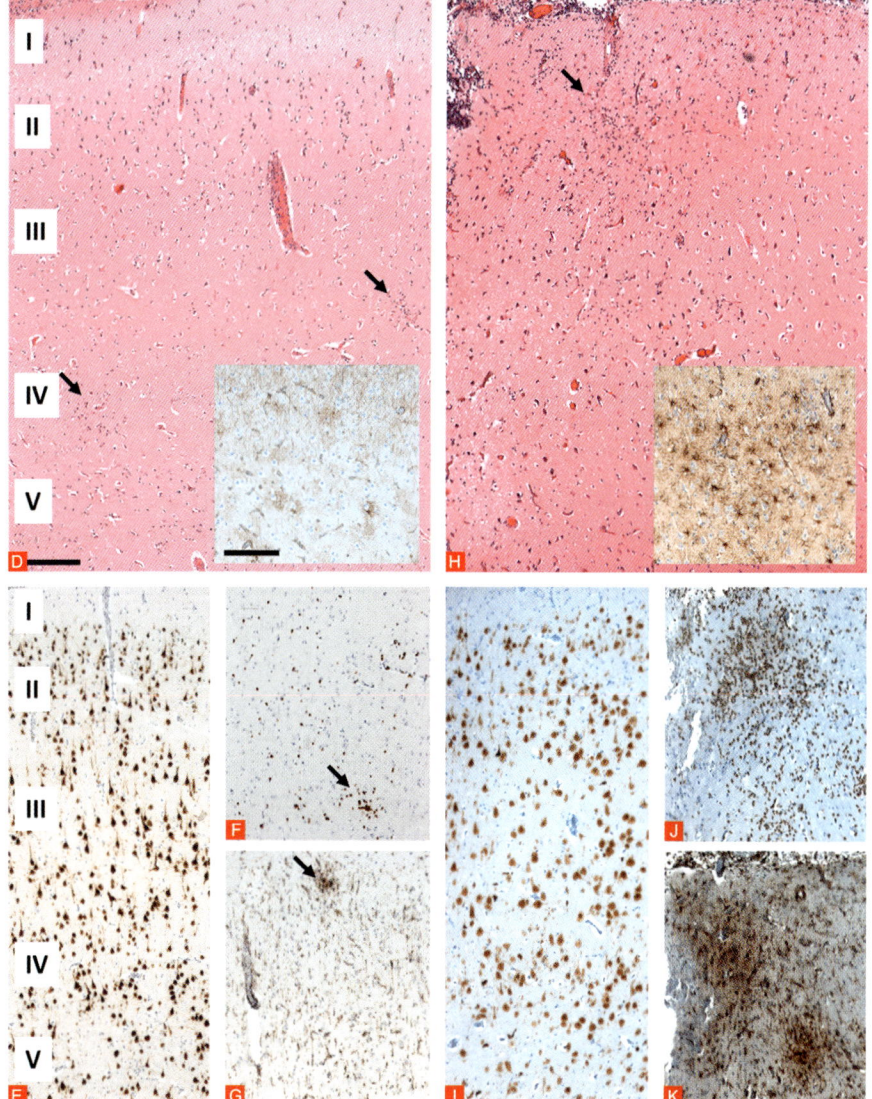

Figure 47

Co-occurring early (D, E-G) and intermediate (H, I-K) stages of Rasmussen encephalitis according to Pardo *et al.* (Pardo *et al.*, 2004). **D**. Mild focal inflammation (black arrows) and gliosis (GFAP immunohistochemistry in inset) compared to patchy inflammatory foci in H (black arrow) and pronounced gliosis (GFAP immunohistochemistry in inset) with minimal to moderate neuronal loss (E&I: NeuN immunohistochemistry). Gradually increasing T-lymphocytic infiltrates (F&J: CD3 immunohistochemistry) and microglial nodules (G&K: CD68 immunohistochemistry). I-V: cortical layers. Scale bar in D and inset: 200 µm applies also for H-K.

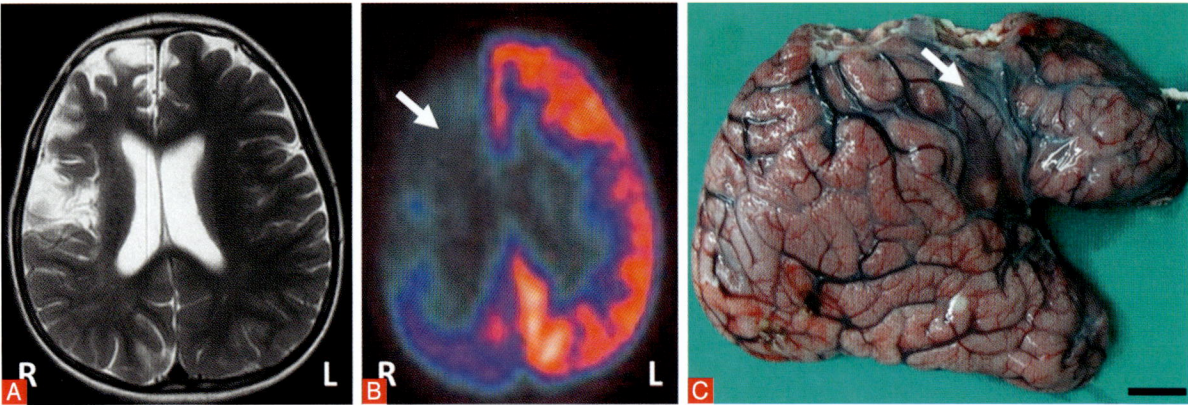

Figure 48
4-year old boy with a one year history of intractable seizures (courtesy of Dr. Dandan Wang, Beijing, China). MRI (A: T2 weighted) showed unilateral focal atrophy involving the right frontal lobe. PET (B) revealed right hemispheric hypometabolism (white arrow) also visible macroscopically in the surgical specimen (white arrow in C). Scale bar: 2 cm. Corresponding histological findings in D-K.

Figure 49
Co-occurring late (D, E-G) and end (H, I-K) stages according to Pardo et al. (Pardo et al., 2004). D. Severe cortical atrophy and gliosis (GFAP immunohistochemistry in inset) compared to total neuronal depletion in H with laminar gliosis only (above dotted line) (GFAP immunohistochemistry in inset). E & I (NeuN immunohistochemistry): severe neuronal loss (E) and complete neuronal depletion at end-stage (I). Note only few neurones (black arrow) remained in the opposed cortical ribbon. T-cell infiltration (F&J: CD3 immunohistochemistry) and microglial activation (G&K: CD68 immunohistochemistry) were variable or rare at end-stage. WM: white matter. Scale bar in D and inset: 200 μm applies also for H-K.

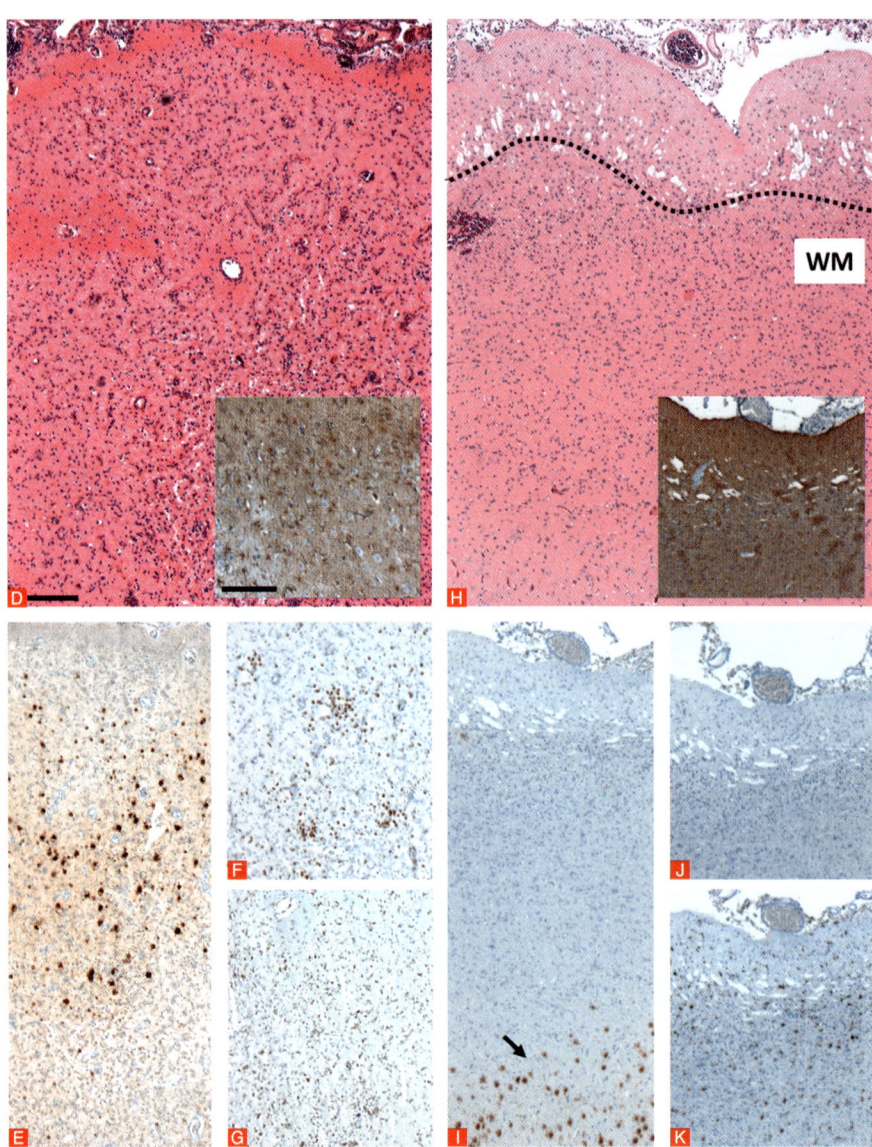

Limbic encephalitis

Clinical history

32-year old male patient with adult-onset epilepsy at age 26 years. Brain biopsy at local referring centre one year ago did not achieve conclusive diagnosis. Six months later, this patient was diagnosed with a malignant seminoma and received chemotherapy. Three months later, temporal lobe resection was performed including the hippocampus to control seizures.

Histopathology and immunohistochemistry

We received an *en bloc* resected hippocampus (3.5 × 3 × 2 cm), which microscopically showed selective parenchymal necrosis and astrogliosis (GFAP) within the dentate gyrus, as well as in CA4 and CA3 (NeuN, MAP2). No significant pyramidal cell loss within sectors CA2 and CA1 (NeuN). Microglial nodules (CD68) and T-lymphocytic infiltrates (CD3) were visible along blood vessels as well as within the brain parenchyma (*Figure 50*). Immunoreactivity directed against CD20 and p53 did not exhibit specific labelling.

Comments

The specimens revealed areas of temporal neocortex and hippocampus with severe reactive astrogliosis, microglial activation (nodules), and T-lymphocytic infiltration of the brain parenchyma, consistent with a histopathological diagnosis of limbic encephalitis (if the clinical diagnosis of temporal lobe epilepsy is conclusive). Paraneoplastic forms already were described in the 1960s, and likely are the cause in this patient. The pathogenesis of the hippocampal changes is difficult to clarify in this case, as the previous operation may have induced selective necrosis and haemorrhage. The characteristic pattern of cellular loss in CA4 also may be compatible with HS ILAE Type 3.

Microscopic findings in limbic encephalitis

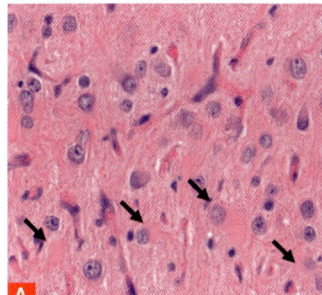 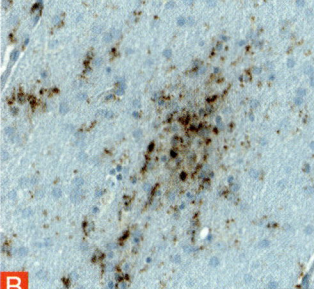 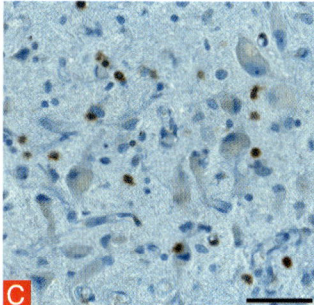

Figure 50

A. Selective parenchymal necrosis with neuronal loss and abundant reactive astrocytes (black arrows) within the dentate gyrus (H&E staining). B & C. Microglial nodules (B: CD68 immunohistochemistry) and T-lymphocytic infiltrates (C: CD3 immunohistochemistry). Scale bars in A–C: 50 μm.

Arterio-venous malformation (AVM)

Clinical history

22-year old female patient with left temporal arterio-venous malformation demonstrated by MRI and rare focal seizures.

Histopathology

We received a firm tissue specimen with convoluted vessels visible at the surface and a total size of 3 × 2 × 1.8 cm (*Figure 51*). The specimen was dissected and embedded into paraffin (2 blocs). H&E staining revealed fragments of central nervous tissue with gliosis and a large vascular malformation with vessels of irregular size and wall structure. Elastica-van-Gieson (EvG) staining was helpful to identify irregular organization of venous or arterial vessel walls, the latter often showing an incomplete internal elastic lamina (*Figure 51*). Examples in which the venous vessel directly enters a small artery (so called "shunt vessel"), are pathognomic for the diagnosis of an arterio-venous malformation. Between vessels of variable calibre were areas of central nervous tissue with varying reactive changes. Haemosiderin-laden macrophages were only visible in a very small circumscribed area (Prussian blue staining). In some instances, pre-operative embolisation may result in complete vessel occlusion.

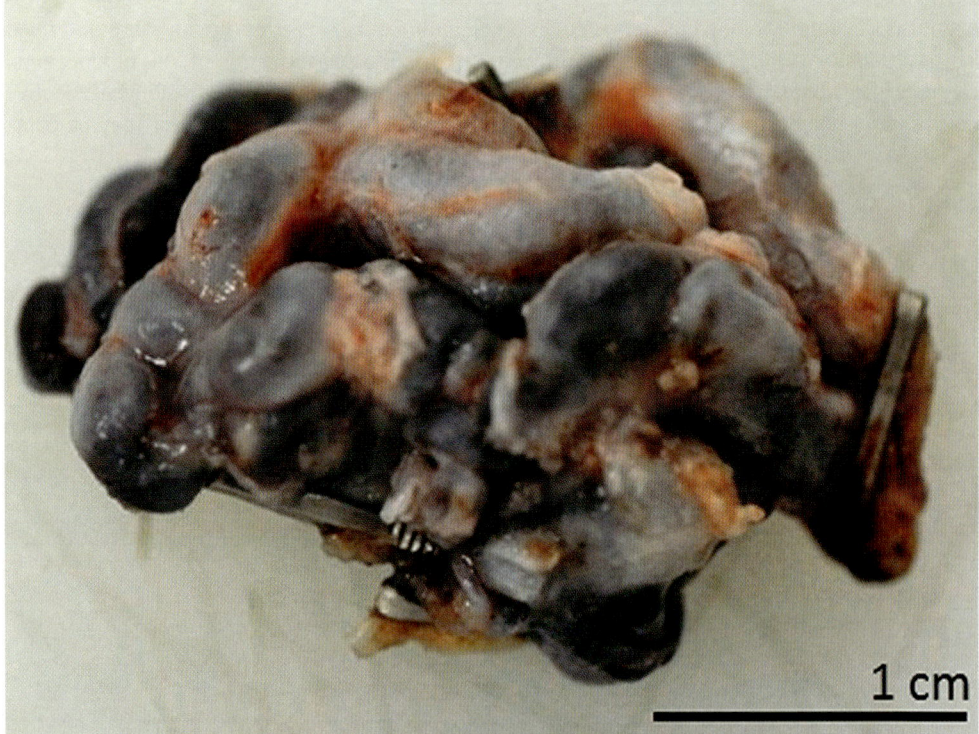

Figure 51

Comments

Microscopic inspection revealed fragments of a vascular malformation with histomorphological characteristics of an arterio-venous malformation. There were no signs of an acute inflammatory process or malignancy. The presence of an associated FCD could not be verified because the specimen did not contain sufficient cortical grey matter to enable evaluation in this regard.

Microscopic findings in AVM

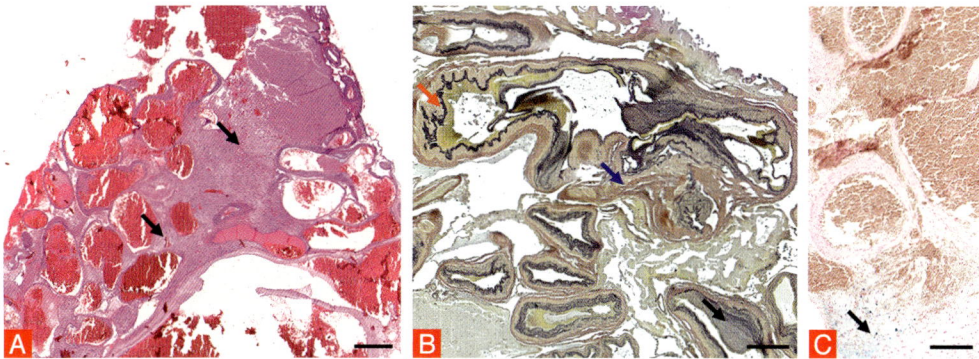

Figure 52

A. H&E staining showing a vascular malformation composed of vessels of irregular size and architecture intermingled with central nervous tissue (black arrows). **B.** EvG staining highlighting the irregular vascular architecture with arterial vessels (red arrow) containing a lamina elastica interna (visualised as black ribbon-like structure) entering a venous vessel (blue arrow). Black arrow points to pathological fragmentation of the lamina elastica interna within an arterial vessel. **C.** Haemosiderin-laden macrophages (highlighted here by Prussian blue staining) as sign for old haemorrhage were not a characteristic finding in this lesion. Such alterations were only visible in a very small, circumscribed area (black arrow), most likely due to pre-operative embolisation. Scale bar in A: 500 µm. Scale bar in B: 200 µm. Scale bar in C: 200 µm.

Cavernous haemangioma (CAV)

Clinical history

42-year old female patient suffering from auto-motor seizures with rare secondary generalized tonic-clonic seizures since age 21 years. MRI revealed a left temporo-mesial lesion suspicious for cavernoma (*Figure 53A*: T2 weighted turbo spin echo MRI; white arrow).

Histopathology and immunohistochemistry

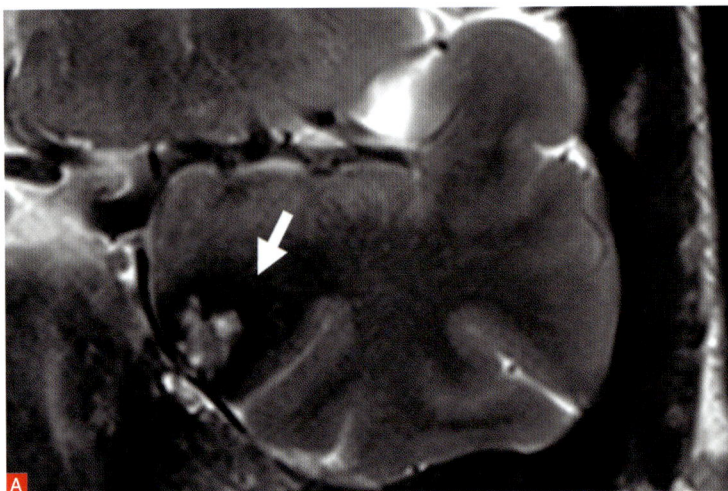

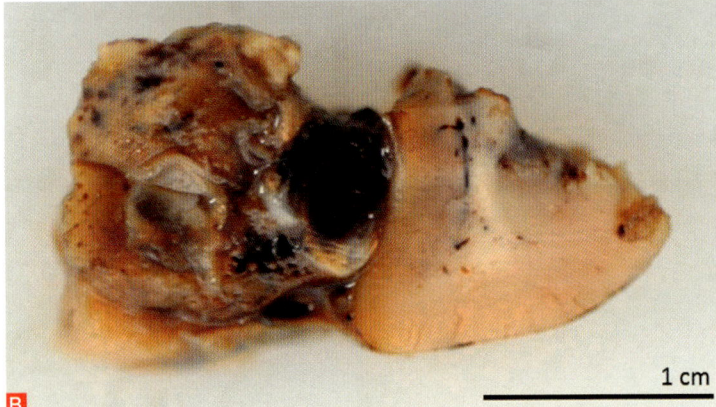

Figure 53

We received light-brownish to brownish, soft tissue fragments with a total size of 3 × 2.5 × 1.5 cm. Typical macroscopic aspect of the cortical ribbon was visible at the surface. The material has been dissected into 5 mm thin slices and completely embedded into paraffin (*Figure 53B*: left side: vascular lesion; right side: part of the medial occipito-temporal gyrus). Microscopic inspection of the H&E-stained tissue specimen revealed central nervous tissue with a vascular malformation. This vascular lesion was composed of focally thickened and hyalinised ectatic vessels, devoid of elastic lamina or smooth muscle (Elastica-van-Gieson staining, *Figure 54C*). The adjacent cortical ribbon showed a normal 6-layered architecture (NeuN and MAP2) without hypertrophic or dysmorphic neurones (SMI32), but haematoidin and haemosiderin deposits were detected as signs of previous haemorrhage (highlighted by Prussian blue staining).

Comments

Microscopic inspection revealed fragments of a vascular malformation with histomorphological characteristics of a cavernous haemangioma (syn. Cavernomas; [Rosenow *et al.*, 2013]). There were no signs of associated FCD, acute inflammatory process or malignancy.

Microscopic findings in cavernoma

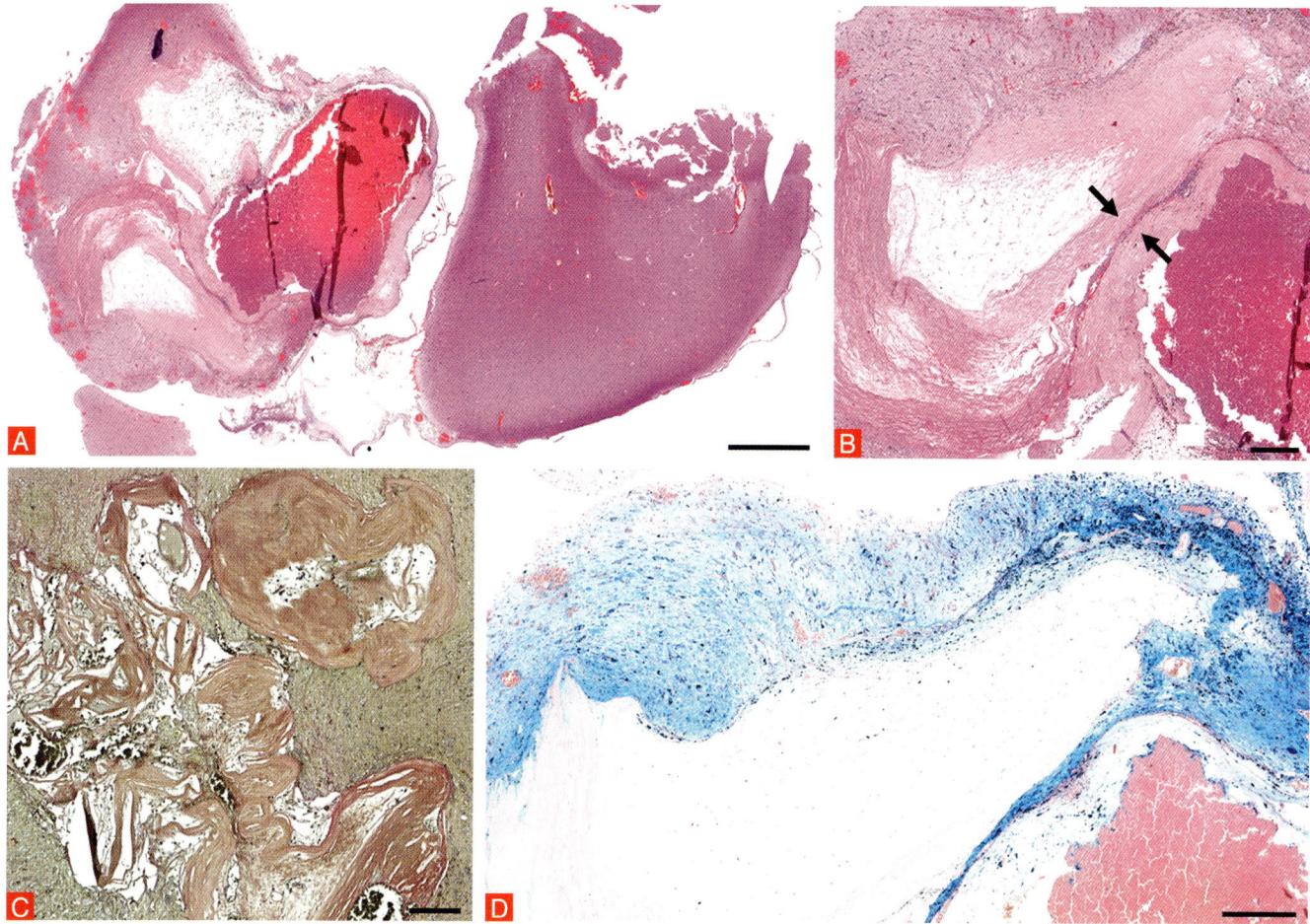

Figure 54

A. H&E staining with low magnification of vascular lesion (left side) in close association with a gyrus (right side). **B.** Higher magnification of A showing thick-walled vessels arranged back-to-back (black arrows) without intervening brain parenchyma. **C.** EvG staining at higher magnification failed to demonstrate a regular lamination of vessel walls. **D.** Typical, strong haemosiderin rim surrounding the cavernous haemangioma as sign for old haemorrhage (Prussion blue staining). Scale bar in A: 2,000 µm. Scale bar in B: 500 µm. Scale bar in C: 200 µm. Scale bar in D: 500 µm.

Sturge-Weber syndrome (SWS)

Clinical history

7-year old girl with SWS (no naevus flammeus) and epilepsy onset at the age of 13 months due to a large vascular lesion over the right hemisphere (*Figure 55A*: T2 weighted MRI with pial alterations and subjacent cortical atrophy, white arrow). Multiple drug trials with VPA, LEV, LTG, TPM and PHT failed to control seizures.

Histopathology and immunohistochemistry

We received three separate tissue samples of temporo-occipital cortex (I: 5.2 × 4 × 1.4 cm; II: 3.5 × 2.5 × 1.2 cm; III: 3.5 × 2 × 1 cm), which were dissected and completely embedded in paraffin. The sample illustrated was obtained from block I. (*Figure 55B*: occipital, pial hyperaemia suspected for angiomatosis with subjacent gyral atrophy), showing cortical grey and white matter on H&E with a leptomeningeal vascular malformation, characterized by small diameter blood vessels of irregular size. In few areas, the vascular malformation invaded the cortical ribbon, showing irregular layering in affected regions with increased micro-columnar vertical orientation of neurones in layers III and IV as well as areas of neuronal loss and hypoplastic cortical width of only 4-layers (*Figure 56*). The boundary between grey and white matter was often blurred with many heterotopic neurones in the white matter. Associated FCD IIIc became most evident by NeuN immunohistochemistry. In addition, hypertrophic neurones with neurofilament accumulation could be detected in layer III, which should not be classified as FCD Type IIa (Wang *et al.*, 2014). GFAP demarcated reactive astrogliosis throughout the cortex and white matter.

Comments

Submitted surgical specimens revealed a vascular malformation within the leptomeninges but also invading the neocortex, consistent with the diagnosis of meningeal angiomatosis in a clinically diagnosed SWS. Affected neocortical areas showed associated FCD ILAE Type IIIc with increased vertical (micro-columnar) organization, gaps of neuronal loss or a 4-layered architecture (ILAE classification 2011; (Blümcke *et al.*, 2011)). No evidence of tumour or acute inflammation was seen.

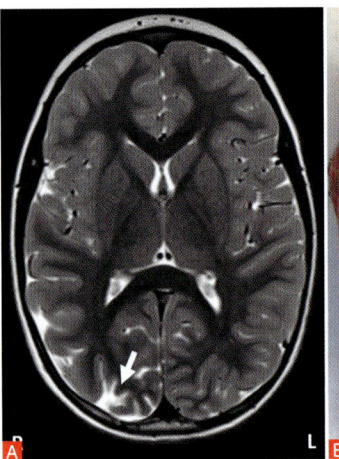
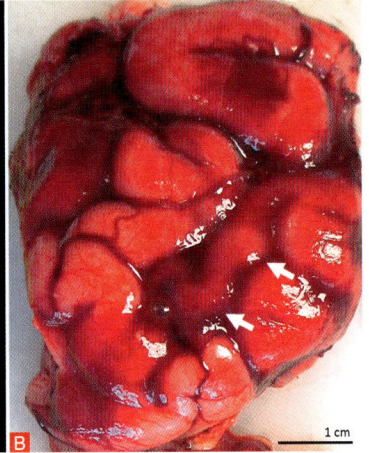

Figure 55

Microscopic findings in meningeal angiomatosis with associated FCD IIIc

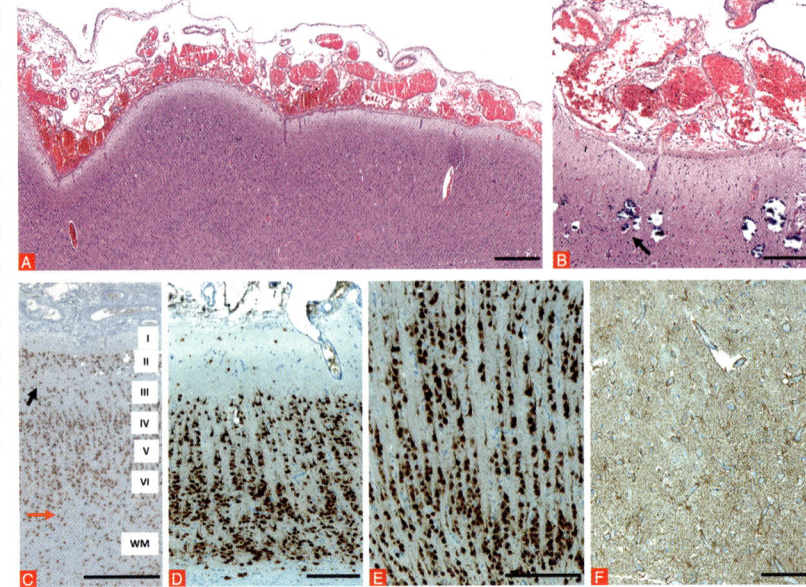

Figure 56

A & B. H&E staining showing a leptomeningeal angiomatosis with small diameter blood vessels of irregular size, some tapering into cortical layer I (white arrow in B). Note superficial calcifications (black arrow in B). C-E. NeuN immunohistochemistry demonstrated laminar neuronal loss in cortical layers II and III (black arrow) and blurred grey/white-matter boundaries (red arrow) in C, areas of hypoplastic cortical ribbon in D and focal micro-columnar arrangement in E. F. GFAP immunohistochemistry highlighting numerous reactive astrocytes within the cortex. Scale bar in A: 500 μm. Scale bar in B: 200 μm. Scale bar in C: 250 μm. Scale bar in D-F: 200 μm.

References

Bien CG, Elger CE, Wiendl H. Advances in pathogenic concepts and therapeutic agents in Rasmussen's encephalitis. *Expert Opin Investig Drugs* 2002; 11: 981-9.

Bien CG, Granata T, Antozzi C, *et al*. Pathogenesis, diagnosis and treatment of Rasmussen encephalitis: a European consensus statement. *Brain* 2005; 128(Pt 3): 454-71.

Blümcke I, Aronica E, Urbach H, Alexopoulos A, Gonzalez-Martinez JA. A neuropathology-based approach to epilepsy surgery in brain tumors and proposal for a new terminology use for long-term epilepsy-associated brain tumors. *Acta Neuropathol* 2014; 128: 39-54.

Blümcke I, Becker AJ, Normann S, *et al*. Distinct expression pattern of microtubule-associated protein-2 in human oligodendrogliomas and glial precursor cells. *J Neuropathol Exp Neurol* 2001; 60: 984-93.

Blümcke I, Giencke K, Wardelmann E, *et al*. The CD34 epitope is expressed in neoplastic and malformative lesions associated with chronic, focal epilepsies. *Acta Neuropathol* 1999; 97: 481-90.

Blümcke I, Luyken C, Urbach H, Schramm J, Wiestler OD. An isomorphic subtype of long-term epilepsy-associated astrocytomas associated with benign prognosis. *Acta Neuropathol* 2004; 107: 381-8.

Blümcke I, Thom M, Aronica E, *et al*. International consensus classification of hippocampal sclerosis in temporal lobe epilepsy: a Task Force report from the ILAE Commission on Diagnostic Methods. *Epilepsia* 2013; 54: 1315-29.

Blümcke I, Thom M, Aronica E, *et al*. The clinico-pathological spectrum of Focal Cortical Dysplasias: a consensus classification proposed by an ad hoc Task Force of the ILAE Diagnostic Methods Commission. *Epilepsia* 2011; 52: 158-74.

Blümcke I, Wiestler OD. Gangliogliomas: an intriguing tumor entity associated with focal epilepsies. *J Neuropathol Exp Neurol* 2002; 61: 575-84.

Bodi I, Curran O, Selway R, *et al*. Two cases of multinodular and vacuolating neuronal tumour. *Acta Neuropathol Comm* 2014; 2: 7.

Braak H. *Architectonics of the Human Telencephalic Cortex*. Berlin: Springer; 1980.

Fukushima S, Yoshida A, Narita Y, *et al*. Multinodular and vacuolating neuronal tumor of the cerebrum. *Brain Tum Pathol* 2014; Aug 22.

Hildebrandt M, Pieper T, Winkler P, Kolodziejczyk D, Holthausen H, Blümcke I. Neuropathological spectrum of cortical dysplasia in children with severe focal epilepsies. *Acta Neuropathol* 2005; 110: 1-11.

Huse JT, Edgar M, Halliday J, Mikolaenko I, Lavi E, Rosenblum MK. Multinodular and vacuolating neuronal tumors of the cerebrum: 10 cases of a distinctive seizure-associated lesion. *Brain Pathol* 2013; 23: 515-24.

Lellouch-Tubiana A, Boddaert N, *et al*. Angiocentric neuroepithelial tumor (ANET): a new epilepsy-related clinicopathological entity with distinctive MRI. *Brain Pathol* 2005; 15: 281-6.

Lewis FT. The significance of the term hippocampus. *J Comp Neurol* 1923; 35: 213-30.

Lorente de Nó R. Studies on the structure of the cerebral cortex. I. The area entorhinalis. *J Psychol Neurol* (Lpz) 1933; 45: 381-438.

Muhlebner A, Coras R, Kobow K, *et al*. Neuropathologic measurements in focal cortical dysplasias: validation of the ILAE 2011 classification system and diagnostic implications for MRI. *Acta Neuropathol* 2012; 123: 259-72.

Palmini A, Najm I, Avanzini G, *et al*. Terminology and classification of the cortical dysplasias. *Neurology* 2004; 62 (6 Suppl 3): S2-8.

Pardo CA, Vining EP, Guo L, Skolasky RL, Carson BS, Freeman JM. The pathology of Rasmussen syndrome: stages of cortical involvement and neuropathological studies in 45 hemispherectomies. *Epilepsia* 2004; 45: 516-26.

Reifenberger G, Kaulich K, Wiestler OD, Blümcke I. Expression of the CD34 antigen in pleomorphic xanthoastrocytomas. *Acta Neuropathol* 2003; 105: 358-64.

Rosenow F, Alonso-Vanegas MA, Baumgartner C, *et al*. Cavernoma-related epilepsy: review and recommendations for management-report of the Surgical Task Force of the ILAE Commission on Therapeutic Strategies. *Epilepsia* 2013; 54: 2025-35.

Schramm J, Luyken C, Urbach H, Fimmers R, Blümcke I. Evidence for a clinically distinct new subtype of grade II astrocytomas in patients with long-term epilepsy. *Neurosurgery* 2004; 55: 340-7; discussion 7-8.

Thom M, Blümcke I, Aronica E. Long-term epilepsy-associated tumors. *Brain Pathol* 2012; 22: 350-79.

Thom M, Toma A, An S, *et al*. One hundred and one dysembryoplastic neuroepithelial tumors: an adult epilepsy series with immunohistochemical, molecular genetic, and clinical correlations and a review of the literature. *J Neuropathol Exp Neurol* 2011; 70: 859-78.

Walther C. Hippocampal terminology: concepts, misconceptions, origins. *Endeavour* 2002; 26: 41-4.

Wang D, Blümcke I, Gui Q, *et al*. Clinico-pathological investigations of Rasmussen encephalitis suggest multifocal disease progression and associated focal cortical dysplasia. *Epileptic Disord* 2013; 15: 32-43.

Wang DD, Blümcke I, Coras R, *et al*. Sturge-Weber syndrome is associated with cortical dysplasia ILAE Type IIIC and excessive hypertrophic pyramidal neurons in brain resections for intractable epilepsy. *Brain Pathol* 2014 Jul 18.

Wang M, Tihan T, Rojiani AM, *et al*. Monomorphous angiocentric glioma: a distinctive epileptogenic neoplasm with features of infiltrating astrocytoma and ependymoma. *J Neuropathol Exp Neurol* 2005; 64: 875-81.

Wolf HK, Buslei R, Schmidt Kastner R, *et al*. NeuN: a useful neuronal marker for diagnostic histopathology. *J Histochem Cytochem* 1996; 44: 1167-71.

CHAPTER 8. Tables: Clinico-pathological findings in epilepsy surgery

Table I

Summary of all histopathological diagnosis collected at the German Neuropathology Reference Centre for Epilepsy Surgery
The 10 most frequent diagnoses explain 86.4% of the entire series (47.5% female and 52.5% male patients aged 0 to 79 years). Lesion in 49% on left and 50.6% on right hemisphere, 0.4% in other location (both sides, ventricle, callosotomy)

		All cases		Age at onset	Surgery	Duration epilepsy	Male	Main localization
1	Hippocampal sclerosis	2,082	37.2%	11.3	33.5	22.2	48.0%	T (100%)
2	Ganglioglioma	603	10.8%	12.7	24.5	11.8	52.1%	T (84.6%)
3	Focal cortical dysplasia II	444	7.9%	4.9	18.1	13.2	52.7%	Front (52.9%)
4	No lesion	357	6.4%	13.2	27.9	14.6	56.6%	T (71.7%)
5	Glial scar	351	6.3%	10.8	25.6	14.7	62.4%	T (45.0%)
6	DNT	224	4.0%	15.0	25.8	10.8	56.7%	T (71.4%)
7	Cavernoma	218	3.9%	27.2	37.8	10.7	53.7%	T (75.2%)
8	Focal cortical dysplasia I	214	3.8%	8.6	20.7	12.1	45.8%	T (49.5%)
9	mMCD	174	3.1%	9.6	22.7	13.2	58.6%	T (54.6%)
10	Focal cortical dysplasia NOS	169	3.0%	7.8	21.9	14.1	58.6%	T (49.7%)
11	Oligo (mixed)	73	1.3%	28.8	36.4	7.6	54.8%	T (43.8%)
12	Pilocytic astrocytoma	65	1.2%	14.8	26.2	11.4	53.8%	T (69.2%)
13	Encephalitis, NOS	59	1.1%	15.4	25.0	9.6	66.1%	T (62.7%)
14	Polymicrogyria	54	1.0%	2.7	8.9	6.2	53.7%	Mult (46.3%)
17	Rasmussen encephalitis	54	1.0%	7.0	11.4	4.5	57.4%	Mult (68.5%)
15	Diffuse astrocytoma	52	0.9%	26.0	31.6	5.6	51.9%	T (55.8%)
16	Cortical tuber (TSC)	49	0.9%	1.3	8.1	6.8	49.0%	Front (53.1%)
18	Hemimegalencephaly	38	0.7%	0.0	1.0	1.0	55.3%	Mult (89.5%)
19	Vascular malformation, NOS	36	0.6%	17.3	30.8	13.5	58.3%	T (58.3%)
20	Tumor, NOS	33	0.6%	17.6	28.5	10.9	57.6%	T (78.8%)
21	AVM	32	0.6%	20.7	37.3	16.6	68.8%	T (56.3%)
22	Meningoangiomatosis	31	0.6%	3	11.3	8.5	64.5%	Mult (64.5%)
23	Anaplastic astrocytoma	27	0.5%	34.1	36.6	2.4	70.4%	T (48.1%)
24	PXA	26	0.5%	18.8	30.5	11.6	46.2%	T (73.1%)
25	Epithelial cyst	26	0.5%	24.0	36.9	13.0	34.6%	T (88.5%)
26	Meningeoma	24	0.4%	39.0	48.0	9.0	33.3%	T (41.7%)
27	Nodular heterotopia	17	0.3%	7.8	20.4	12.6	52.9%	Mult (47.1%)
28	Isomorphic astrocytoma	15	0.3%	14.6	26.6	12.0	66.7%	T or Occ (66.6%)

Table I (continued)

Summary of all histopathological diagnosis collected at the German Neuropathology Reference Centre for Epilepsy Surgery
The 10 most frequent diagnoses explain 86.4% of the entire series (47.5% female and 52.5% male patients aged 0 to 79 years). Lesion in 49% on left and 50.6% on right hemisphere, 0.4% in other location (both sides, ventricle, callosotomy)

		All cases		Age at onset	Surgery	Duration epilepsy	Male	Main localization
29	GBM	12	0.2%	47.3	50.1	2.8	66.7%	T (66.7%)
30	Ependymoma	8	0.1%	9.6	25.1	15.5	62.5%	T (50.0%)
31	ANET	8	0.1%	7.0	14.6	7.6	62.5%	T (50.0%)
32	SEGA	7	0.1%	4.7	13.4	8.7	42.9%	Other (57.1%)
33	Neurocytoma	6	0.1%	12.7	23.7	11.0	50.0%	T (100%)
34	Arachnoid cyst	5	0.1%	15.2	28.2	13.0	60.0%	T (100%)
35	Callosotomy	5	0.1%	7.0	37.4	30.4	80.0%	Other (100%)
36	Hypothalamic hamartoma	3	0.1%	1.3	28.0	26.7	66.7%	Other (66.7%)
37	PGNT	2	0.0%	31	32.5	1.5	100.0%	T (100%)
	Total	5,603		12.2	27.9	15.8	52.5%	T (72.5%)

DNT: dysembryoplastic neuroepithelial tumour; mMCD: mild malformation of cortical development; NOS: not otherwise specified; oligo: oligodendrogliomas and mixed oligo-astrocytomas; TSC: tuberous sclerosis complex; AVM: arterio-venous malformation; PXA: pleomorphic xanthoastrocytoma; GBM: glioblastoma multiforme; ANET: angiocentric glioma; SEGA: subependymal giant cell astrocytoma; PGNT: papillary glio-neuronal tumour. Mean age at epilepsy onset and surgery in years. Duration of epilepsy in years. Main localization: T: temporal lobe; front: frontal lobe; occ: occipital lobe; mult: multiple lobes; other: both sides, ventricle, callosotomy.

Table II

Principle histopathological categories in adult patients undergoing epilepsy surgery
48.3% female and 51.7% male patients aged 18 to 79 years. Lesion in 48.4% on left and 51.3% on right hemisphere, 0.4% in other location (both sides, ventricle, callosotomy)

	All cases		Age at onset	Surgery	Duration epilepsy
HS	1,796	45.0%	12.5	37.1	24.6
Tumour	808	20.2%	21.4	34.5	13.1
MCD	463	11.6%	11.5	32.1	20.6
No lesion	277	6.9%	16.0	33.4	17.4
Vascular lesion	263	6.6%	26.4	38.8	12.3
Glial scar	206	5.2%	15.5	34.9	19.4
Dual pathology	140	3.5%	12.7	35.6	22.9
Encephalitis	39	1.0%	21.6	33.3	11.7
Double pathology	3	0.1%	22.0	35.7	13.7
Total	3,995	71%*	15.6	35.6	20.1

HS: hippocampal sclerosis; MCD: malformation of cortical development; dual pathology: HS and secondary lesion; double pathology: two different lesions without HS. Age at epilepsy onset and surgery in years. Duration of epilepsy in years.
* Adults comprise 71.3% of the entire series of 5,603 patients.

Table III

Principle histopathological categories in children undergoing epilepsy surgery

45.6% female and 54.4% male patients aged 0 to 17 years. Lesions in 50.6% on left and 49.1% on right hemisphere. 0.3% in other location (both sides, ventricle, callosotomy)

	All cases		Age at onset	Surgery	Duration epilepsy
MCD	604	37.5%	1.8	6.6	4.8
Tumour	353	21.9%	6.4	10.4	4.0
HS	275	17.1%	4.2	11.2	7.0
Glial scar	115	7.1%	2.8	8.5	5.7
No lesion	86	5.3%	3.9	10.6	6.7
Dual pathology	69	4.3%	3.2	8.8	5.6
Encephalitis	56	3.5%	4.1	8.1	4.0
Vascular lesion	42	2.6%	4.1	7.6	3.6
Double pathology	9	0.6%	1.7	4.0	2.6
Total	1,609	29%*	3.6	8.7	5.1

HS: hippocampal sclerosis; MCD: malformation of cortical development; dual pathology: HS and secondary lesion; double pathology: two different lesions without HS. Age at epilepsy onset and surgery in years. Duration of epilepsy in years.
* Children comprise 28.7% of the entire series of 5,603 patients.

Table IV

Topographic (lobar) distribution of principle histopathological categories

Group	Temporal	Frontal	Mult lobes	Parietal	Occipital	Other
HS	100%	~	~	~	~	~
Tumour	73.0%	12.1%	5.1%	5.0%	2.8%	2.1%
MCD	30.7%	38.1%	20.5%	5.2%	4.8%	0.7%
No lesion	70.8%	12.1%	10.7%	1.9%	1.4%	3.0%
Glial scar	42.4%	21.5%	23.7%	5.9%	6.5%	~
Vascular	65.9%	13.4%	9.8%	5.6%	3.9%	1.3%
Dual pathology	85.2%	2.4%	12.4%	~	~	~
Encephalitis	38.9%	14.7%	42.1%	3.2%	1.1%	~
Double Pathology	50.0%	8.3%	41.7%	~	~	~
#	4,063	720	492	160	122	46
TOTAL	72.5%	12.8%	8.8%	2.9%	2.2%	0.8%

HS: hippocampal sclerosis; MCD: malformation of cortical development; dual pathology: HS and secondary lesion; double pathology: two different lesions without HS.
= number of specimens in entire series of 5,603 patients.

Table V

Top 10 list of histopathological diagnosis in temporal lobe epilepsies (TLE)

49.9% on right hemisphere, 0.1% in other location (both sides, ventricle, callosotomy)

	All cases		Age at onset	Surgery	Duration epilepsy
HS	2,057	54.8%	11.3	33.5	22.3
Ganglioglioma	510	13.6%	13.1	25.2	12.0
No lesion	256	6.8%	15.9	31.3	15.4
Cavernoma	164	4.4%	28.2	39.5	11.2
DNT	160	4.3%	17.0	28.4	11.4
Glial scar	158	4.2%	15.2	34.3	19.1
Diffuse glioma	155	4.1%	23.3	32.6	9.3
FCD I	106	2.8%	12.7	27.9	15.2
mMCD	95	2.5%	13.9	29.1	15.3
FCD II	92	2.5%	6.6	20.8	14.3
Total	3,754	92%*	13.5	31.7	18.2

HS: hippocampal sclerosis; DNT: dysembryoplastic neuroepithelial tumour; FCD: focal cortical dysplasia; mMCD: mild malformation of cortical development. Age at epilepsy onset and surgery in years. Duration of epilepsy in years.
* 10 most frequent histopathological diagnosis comprise 92.4% of all TLE cases (n = 4,063).

	All cases		Age at onset	Surgery	Duration epilepsy
FCD II	235	37.0%	4.8	19.0	14.2
Glial scar	70	11.0%	12.6	25.0	12.2
Diffuse glioma	56	8.8%	28.8	34.4	5.6
mMCD	53	8.3%	4.2	16.4	12.4
No lesion	44	6.9%	7.2	20.3	13.1
FCD NOS	41	6.5%	5.2	20.8	15.6
FCD I	39	6.1%	4.9	16.1	11.2
DNT	37	5.8%	11.0	19.9	8.9
Cavernoma	32	5.0%	24.9	34.9	10.0
Ganglioglioma	28	4.4%	13.4	23.4	10.0
Total	**635**	**88%***	**9.7**	**21.9**	**12.2**

Table VI

Top 10 list of histopathological diagnosis in frontal lobe epilepsies (FLE) 40.3% female and 59.7% male patients. Lesion in 46.0% on left and 53.9% on right hemisphere, 0.1% in other location (both sides, ventricle, callosotomy)

FCD: focal cortical dysplasia; NOS: not otherwise specified; DNT: dysembryoplastic neuroepithelial tumour; mMCD: mild malformation of cortical development. Age at epilepsy onset and surgery in years. Duration of epilepsy in years.
* 10 most frequent histopathological diagnosis comprise 88.2% of all FLE cases (n = 720).

	All cases		Age at onset	Surgery	Duration epilepsy
FCD II	24	17.8%	4.5	18.5	14.0
Glial scar	19	14.1%	6.4	23.8	17.5
Diffuse glioma	18	13.3%	27.9	33.7	5.7
Ganglioglioma	17	12.6%	12.9	22.4	9.5
DNT	13	9.6%	6.8	15.3	8.5
FCD NOS	13	9.6%	3.4	15.8	12.4
Cavernoma	9	6.7%	26.2	29.6	3.3
FCD I	9	6.7%	7.1	14.9	7.8
No lesion	7	5.2%	8.3	18.4	10.1
Vascular malform., NOS	6	4.4%	16.5	31.2	14.7
Total	**135**	**84%***	**11.4**	**22.2**	**10.8**

Table VII

Top 10 list of histopathological diagnosis in parietal lobe epilepsies (PLE) 48.0% female and 52.0% male patients. Lesion in 46.6% on left and 52.8% on right hemisphere, 0.6% in other location (both sides, ventricle, callosotomy)

FCD: focal cortical dysplasia; NOS: not otherwise specified; DNT: dysembryoplastic neuroepithelial tumour. Age at epilepsy onset and surgery in years. Duration of epilepsy in years.
* 10 most frequent histopathological diagnosis comprise 84.4% of all PLE cases (n = 160).

	All cases		Age at onset	Surgery	Duration epilepsy
Diffuse glioma	25	17.6%	21.6	29.0	7.4
FCD II	22	15.5%	6.4	18.2	11.8
Glial scar	21	14.8%	7.7	21.9	14.1
Ganglioglioma	18	12.7%	9.3	21.4	12.1
FCD I	14	9.9%	3.9	12.9	8.9
FCD NOS	12	8.5%	2.3	8.9	6.6
No lesion	11	7.7%	8.4	22.0	13.6
Cavernoma	8	5.6%	23.9	28.8	4.9
DNT	6	4.2%	12.2	23.7	11.5
Callosotomy	5	3.5%	7.0	37.4	30.4
Total	**142**	**84%***	**10.4**	**21.5**	**11.1**

Table VIII

Top 10 list of histopathological diagnosis in occipital lobe or other locations (ventricle, callosotomy) 45.1% female and 54.9% male patients. Lesion in 48.6% on left and 50.4% on right hemisphere, 1.0% in other location (both sides, ventricle, callosotomy)

FCD: focal cortical dysplasia; NOS: not otherwise specified; DNT: dysembryoplastic neuroepithelial tumour. Age at epilepsy onset and surgery in years. Duration of epilepsy in years.
* 10 most frequent histopathological diagnosis comprise 84.5% of all cases with occipital lobe or other localization (n = 142).

Table IX

Histopathological diagnosis in multiple lobe epilepsies 46.6% female and 53.4% male patients. Lesion in 46.6% on left and 52.8% on right hemisphere, 0.6% in other location (both sides, ventricle, callosotomy)

	All cases		Age at onset	Surgery	Duration epilepsy
Glial scar	83	19.8%	2.8	10.8	8.0
FCD II	70	16.7%	2.5	11.1	8.6
FCD I	46	11.0%	3.7	11.5	7.8
No lesion	39	9.3%	5.1	17.2	12.2
Rasmussen	34	8.1%	6.3	10.6	4.2
Hemimegalencephaly	34	8.1%	0.0	1.0	1.0
Ganglioglioma	30	7.2%	6.8	16.7	10.0
Polymicrogyria	24	5.7%	1.8	7.1	5.3
mMCD	21	5.0%	3.6	11.5	8.0
Meningoangiomatosis	19	4.5%	0.9	6.2	5.2
FCD NOS	19	4.5%	4.3	13.8	9.6
Total	**419**	**82%***	**3.4**	**10.9**	**7.5**

FCD: focal cortical dysplasia; NOS: not otherwise specified; mMCD: mild malformation of cortical development. Age at epilepsy onset and surgery in years. Duration of epilepsy in years.

* 10 most frequent histopathological diagnosis comprise 81.9% of all cases with "multilobar" localization (n = 492).

9. Recommendations for neuropathological work-up and microscopic evaluation of epilepsy surgery specimens

Standardized operational procedure for tissue procurement in epilepsy surgery

1. Tissue procurement of en bloc resected surgical specimen(s) at operation room (OR) by local neuro-/pathologist. Neurosurgeons should clearly label the anterior-posterior axis of each sample with staples or ink. Suspected lesions or other regions of interest should be marked additionally.

2. At neuro-/path. lab: document weight (in grams) and size of tissue specimen (preferably by photo with scales).

3. Dissect each tissue specimen in 5 mm slices according to anatomical landmarks, preferably at coronal planes along anterior-posterior axis.

4. Label all slices and document order by photograph using an alphabetical or numerical system (*i.e.* I, II, III, etc., or 1, 2, 3, etc., or A, B, C,..., a, b, c). Identify lesion (if applicable; will be ideally in centre of resection) and use this tissue slice for histopathology (10% formalin fixation and paraffin embedding). From here on, we will refer to this central "lesional" slice as the "principle histopathology slice". If no lesion is present, this would be ictal onset zone as defined by intracranial EEG recordings or as determined *a priori* on the bases of the pre-surgical electro-clinical work-up by the epileptologist.

5. Adjacent tissue to principle histopathology slice should be used for tissue banking at - 80° C and/or other consented research projects (*i.e.* cell culture or formalin fixed vibratome sections). If a large specimen is available, alternate always between histopathological use and frozen storage or other procedures. Use special vials to store fresh frozen samples and label vials with ref-number (preferably lab-number), slice number and date of storage.

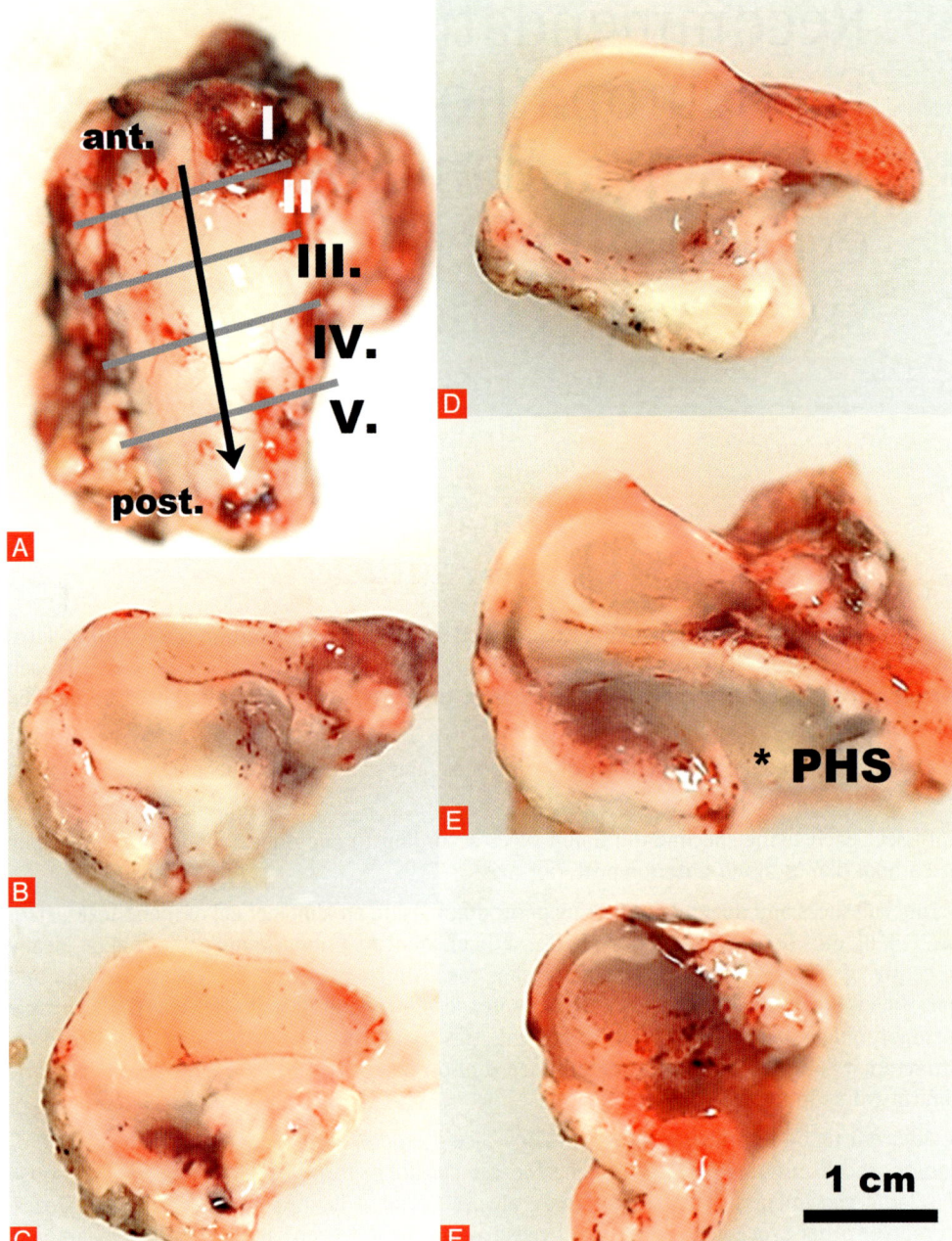

Figure 1

Tissue procurement of en bloc resected human hippocampus

Identify the anterior-posterior axis of native sample (arrow in A). Dissect tissue specimen in 5 mm slices perpendicular to ant-post axis (I. – V. indicated by grey bars). Document order and choose slice from hippocampal mid-body level for histopathology (slice 4 in E, PHS: principle histopathology slice). Fix this tissue slice in 10% formalin overnight for paraffin embedding. Adjacent tissue from PHS can be used for tissue banking at - 80° C. If available, alternate again for histopathological use, frozen storage or other approved and consented research projects.

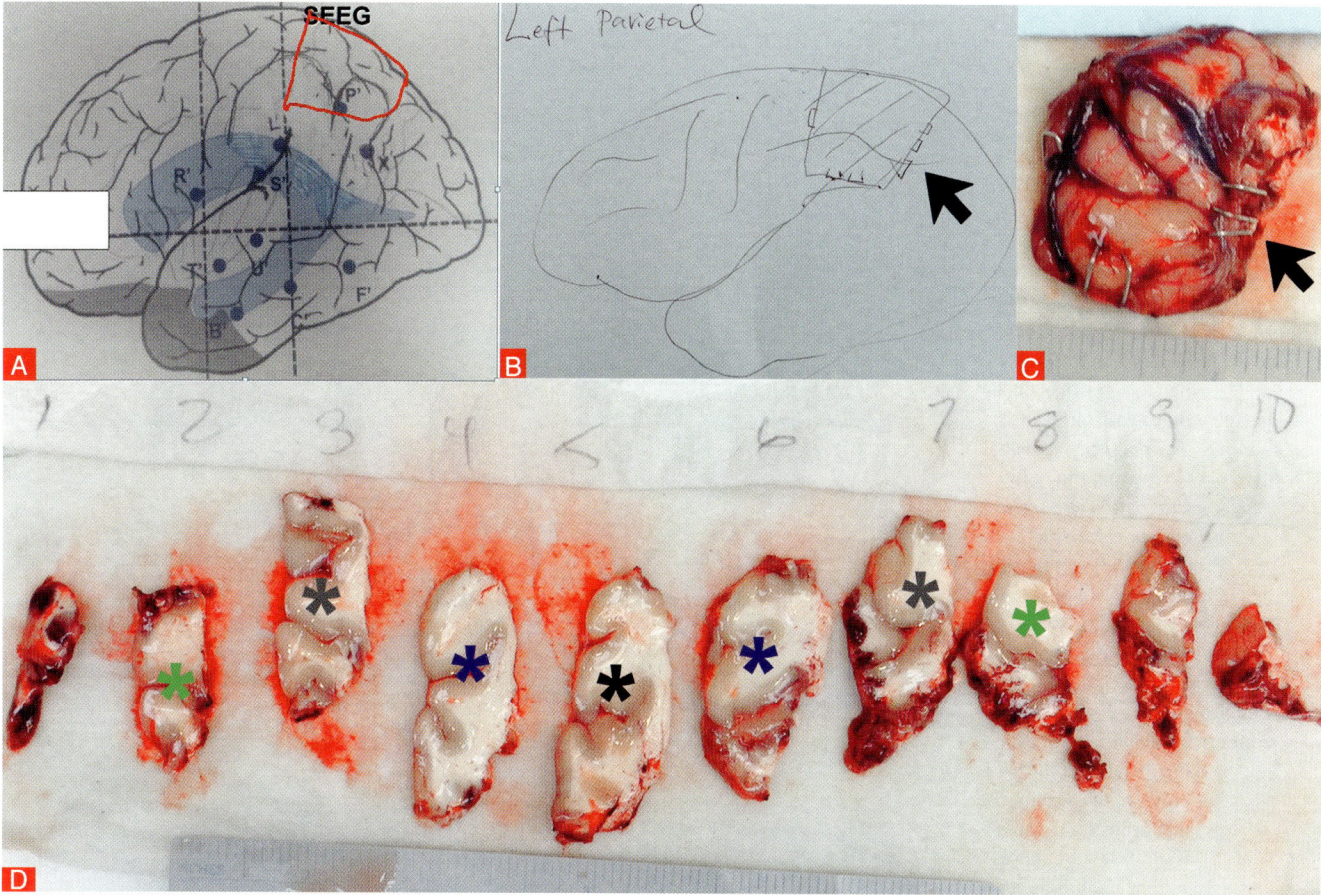

Figure 2

Tissue procurement of en bloc resected non-/lesional brain tissue

Identify the anterior-posterior axis of native sample from brain maps (A-B) and neurosurgical landmarks (B-C, staples indicating 3D orientation). Dissect tissue specimen in 5 mm slices at coronal plane in ant-post direction. Document order (slices 1 – 10) and chose principle histopathology slice (PHS) from centre of lesion for histopathology (*i.e.* 5, black asterisk). Adjacent tissue from PHS can be used for tissue banking at − 80° C (blue asterisks, slices 4 and 6). If available, alternate again for histopathological use (grey asterisk in slices 3 and 7), frozen storage or other approved and consented research projects (green asterisks in slices 2 and 8). Kindly provided by Dr. Bulacio and Dr. Gonzalez-Martinez, Cleveland Clinic, Ohio, USA.

Figure 3

Tissue procurement of en bloc resected brain tissue investigated by invasive EEG procedures

Identify the anatomo-pathological orientation of unfixed specimen and depth electrodes (preferable when left *in situ*). Label electrodes with differently coloured ink. This specimen was used only for histopathological examination and fixed, therefore, en bloc before further processing. Dissect tissue specimen in 5 mm slices. Document order and fix slices in 10% formalin overnight before paraffin embedding. If applicable, use adjacent slides for histopathology and tissue banking at − 80° C or other approved and consented research projects as stated above.
Tissue should be photographed macroscopically, both fresh and after fixation, for later correlations. Kindly provided by Dr. M. Kudernatsch and T. Pieper, Schön Kliniken Vogtareuth, Germany.

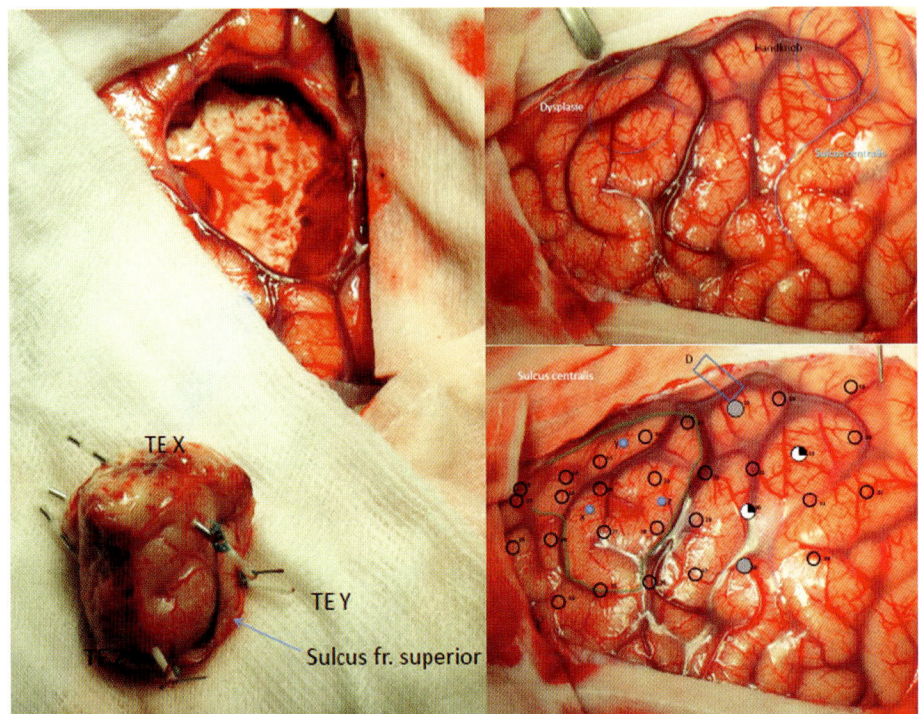
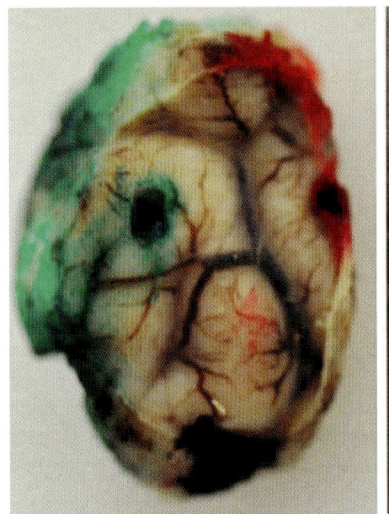
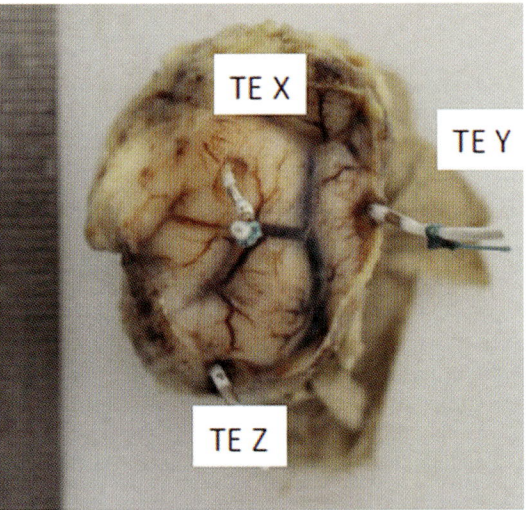
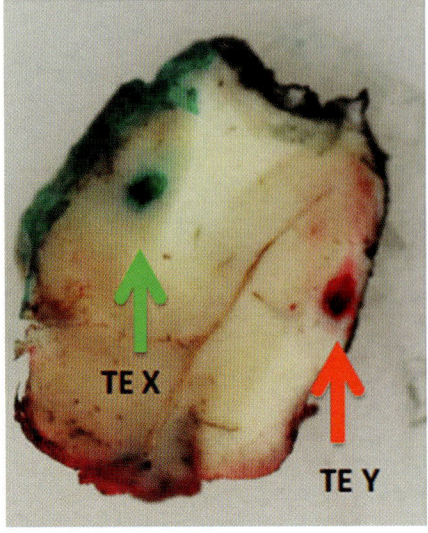
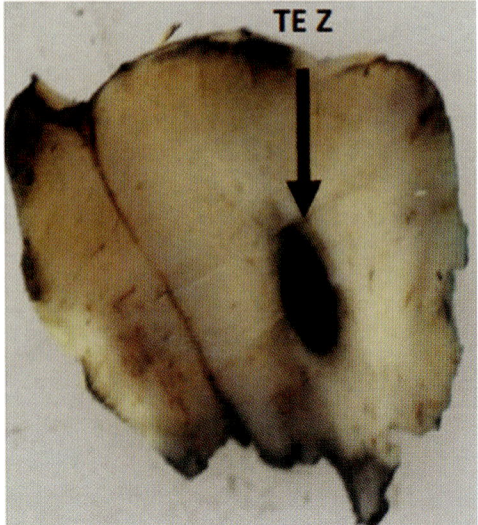

Recommendations for microscopic evaluation of epilepsy surgery specimens

• Tissue processing and storage protocols

Recommended is a standardized paraffin embedding protocol using commercially available semi- or fully automated equipment.

Paraffin-embedded tissue specimens should be cut with a rotating microtome at 4-7 μm thickness. Blocs should be cooled down to - 15° C before cutting. Sections need to be stretched in heated water bath at 40° C before mounting on coated glass slides. Allow drying for 30 min at 60° C or overnight at 36° C.

For tissue bio-banking, unfixed tissue should be snap-frozen over liquid nitrogen and stored at - 80° C in appropriate tissue container. Tissue covering in Compound Cryo Embedding Medium will prevent drying artefacts occurring during long-term storage.

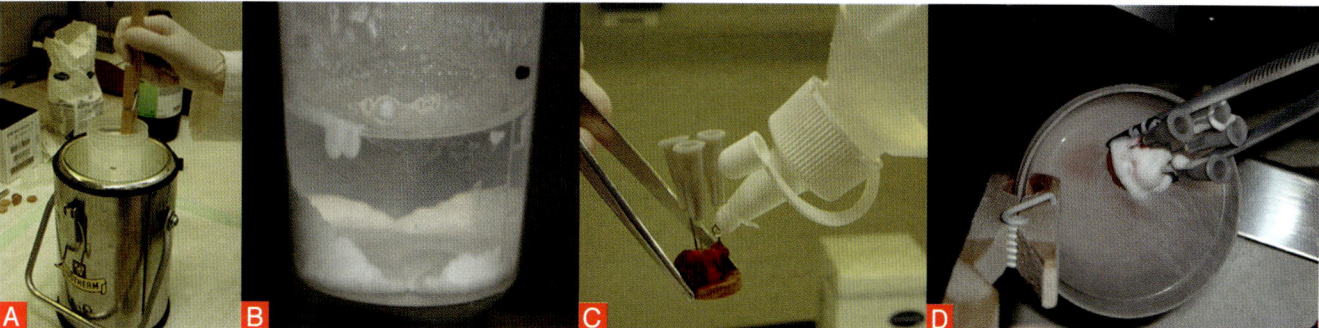

Figure 4
Frozen storage of brain tissue

Technical equipment: Liquid nitrogen with container, isopentane (2-methylbutane) in plastic bin, test glass holder and petri-dish, small and big tweezers, razor blades, cork pads and consented patient information (also check for possible infectious agents), embedding medium for frozen tissue. Fill container with liquid nitrogen and plastic bin with isopentane. Chill plastic bin containing isopentane in liquid N_2 (A-B). Patient's biopsy should be mounted on cork plate (C) and freeze sample in chilled isopentane for 1 min. Store sample in appropriately labelled cryo-vial in -80° C until further use. Always wear protection glasses and gloves when working with liquid nitrogen!

• H&E staining

De-wax glass slides and rinse in distilled water (2 min). Stain in haematoxlin for 2 min and rinse in distilled water. Differentiate in 1% HCl/alcohol. Rinse for 2 min in water (for blueing). Rinse in distilled water and stain in eosin for 40 sec. Dehydrate in ascending concentrations of alcohol into xylene and mount cover-slip using appropriate medium.

• Cresyl violet & LFB staining

1. Day: Deparaffinize in isopropanol (100%-96%). Incubate overnight at 60° C in luxol fast blue-solution.

2. Day: rinse in 96% ethanol and transfer into distilled water. Rapid incubation of each slide in 0.05% lithium-carbonate, transfer immediately into 70% ethanol. Review at microscope if background becomes clean (repeat if required). Transfer into distilled water and then stain 1 min with 0.5% cresyl violet solution. Rinse in 1% acetic acid and rinse with distilled water. Rapid dehydration through ascending concentrations of alcohol into xylene and mount cover-slip using appropriate medium.

• Immunohistochemistry protocols for paraffin-embedded sections

Day 1 (*i.e.* using Ultra Vision Large Volume Detection System; should be adapted when any other reagent is used)

1) Deparaffinize (de-wax) sections in xylene 2 x 10 min; hydrate with 100% isopropanol 5 min.; hydrate with 96% isopropanol 5 min.; hydrate with 70% isopropanol 5 min.; rinse in distilled water

2) Antigen retrieval to unmask antigenic determinants (may be required for some antibodies): Boil slides for 2 × 10 min in citrate buffer (*i.e.* microwave). Refill buffer after first round; cool for at least 10 min and rinse 2-3 times in Tris Buffered solution (TBS)

3) Block endogenous peroxidase activity: Inactivate endogenous peroxidase by covering tissue with 3% hydrogen peroxide for 15 min (45 ml methanol + 5 ml H_2O_2 [30%]) and rinse 2-3 times in TBS

4) Preventing non-specific immunoreactivity: Blocking in 3% FCS/1% goat serum/0.1% TX100 in TBS for 1 h; do not rinse! Wipe around the sections with tissue paper and apply primary antibody diluted in blocking solution; incubate overnight at 4° C

Day 2: Rinse 2-3 times in TBS; apply biotinylated secondary antibodies and incubate for 10 min; rinse 2-3 times in TBS; apply streptavidin peroxidase and incubate for 10 min; rinse 2-3 times in TBS; apply DAB chromogen to tissue section for 5-10 min (visual control of staining intensity); rinse in distilled water; counterstain in haematoxylin. (2-5 sec); rinse in water; dehydrate samples (70% isopropanol, 96% isopropanol, 100% isopropanol, xylene); mount coverslip with appropriate medium.

Epitope	Clone	Cellular pattern	Diagnostic value
GFAP	6F2	Astrocytes	Describe reactive gliosis in areas of neuronal loss and at surface boundaries (Chaslin's gliosis)
NeuN	A60	Neuronal nuclei	Subfield analysis of neuronal cell loss (ILAE classification of HS)
CNPase	11-5B	Myelin sheets	Myelin architecture in the hippocampus
CD45	LCA	Lymphocytes	To exclude limbic encephalitis
CD34	QBend10	Oncofoetal marker	To exclude ganglioglioma
MAP2	HM2	Neurones and glial tumour cells	To exclude diffuse glioma

GFAP: glial fibrillary acidic protein; NeuN: Neuronal nuclei; CNPase: cyclic nucleotide phosphodiesterase; CD: cluster of differentiation; MAP2: microtubule associated protein 2; HS: hippocampal sclerosis; ILAE: International League against Epilepsy.

Table I

Recommended antibodies for the diagnosis of hippocampal sclerosis and glial scars

Epitope	Clone	Cellular pattern	Diagnostic value
Neurofilaments	SMI32	Dysmorphic neurones	FCD ILAE Type II, but present also in aged pyramidal cells of cortical layers III and V
pS6	Ser 235/236	Dysmorphic neurones and balloon cells	Activated mTOR in FCD Type II, TSC and HME
Vimentin	V9	Balloon cells	FCD Type II, but also expressed in reactive astrocytes
NeuN	A 60	Neuronal nuclei	Architectural abnormalities of cortical layering in FCD I, II and III, PMG
MAP2	HM2	Neurones	Heterotopic neurones in white matter and nodular heterotopia
Synaptophysin	pc	Axosomatic and axodendritic synapses, non-specific for type or neurotransmitter, site or function	Late maturational marker; radial orientation of synaptic layers in FCD; synapses in white matter heterotopia and grey matter dysmorphic neurones and some balloon cells
Calretinin	pc 7696	Cytoplasmic marker in specific populations of interneurones	Identifies GABAergic inhibitory interneurones arriving in cerebral cortex by tangential migration; distribution may be reduced or altered in some FCD

pS6: phosphor-S6 ribosomal protein; NeuN: neuronal nuclei; MAP2: microtubule associated protein 2; pc: polyclonal; FCD: focal cortical dysplasia; ILAE: International League against Epilepsy; PMG: polymicrogyria.

Table II

Recommended antibodies for the diagnosis of cortical malformations

Epitope	Clone	Cellular pattern	Diagnostic value
CD34	QBend10	Gross tumour, diffuse tumour infiltration or satellite tumour cells	Majority of ganglioglioma and diffuse glio-neuronal tumours, typically not expressed in diffuse gliomas
MAP2	HM2	Neurones and neoplastically transformed glia	Majority of glial cells in diffuse glioma; only neuronal expression in glio-neuronal tumours
IDH1	H09	Neoplastically transformed glia	Reacts specifically with the R132H point mutation not present in glio-neuronal tumours
Ki-67	Mib1	Proliferation active nuclei	Low proliferative index (< 5%) in glio-neuronal tumours
CD68	KP-1	Macrophages and microglia	Helpful to explain regions with increased proliferation due to reactive macrophages or activated microglial infiltration

CD34: class II epitope; MAP2: microtubule associated protein 2; IDH1: mutation-specific antibody against isocitrate dehydrogenase 1.

Table III

Recommended antibodies for the diagnosis of long-term epilepsy associated tumours

IMPRIM'VERT®

Achevé d'imprimer par 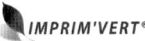 Corlet, Imprimeur, S.A.
14110 Condé-sur-Noireau
N° d'Imprimeur : 173827 - Dépôt légal : août 2015
Imprimé en France